W9-BAL-482

Social Discord
and Bodily Disorders

Carolina Academic Press
Medical Anthropology Series

Pamela J. Stewart *and* Andrew Strathern
Series Editors

❧

Curing and Healing
Medical Anthropology in Global Perspective
Andrew Strathern *and* Pamela Stewart

Physicians at Work, Patients in Pain, 2nd Edition
Biomedical Practice and Patient Response in Mexico
Kaja Finkler

Healing the Modern in a Central Javanese City
Steve Ferzacca

Elusive Fragments
Making Power, Propriety and Health in Samoa
Douglass D. Drozdow-St. Christian

Endangered Species
Health, Illness, and Death Among Madagascar's People of the Forest
Janice Harper

The Practice of Concern
Ritual, Well-Being, and Aging in Rural Japan
John W. Traphagan

The Gene and the Genie
Tradition, Medicalization and Genetic Counseling
in a Bedouin Community in Israel
Aviad E. Raz

Social Discord and Bodily Disorders
Healing Among the Yupno of Papua New Guinea
Verena Keck

❧

Social Discord and Bodily Disorders

Healing among the Yupno of Papua New Guinea

Verena Keck

Carolina Academic Press
Durham, North Carolina

Copyright © 2005
Verena Keck
All Rights Reserved

Library of Congress Cataloging-in-Publication Data

Keck, Verena.
   Social discord and bodily disorders : healing among the Yupno of Papua New Guinea
/ by Verena Keck.
      p. cm.
Based on author's thesis (doctoral)—Universitaet Basel, 1991.
Includes bibliographical references and index.
   ISBN 0-89089-404-3
   1. Yupno (Papua New Guinea people)—Diseases. 2. Yupno (Papua New Guinea people)—Medicine. 3. Yupno (Papua New Guinea people)—Psychology. 4. Traditional
medicine—Papua New Guinea—Finisterre Range. 5. Medical anthropology—Papua New
Guinea—Finisterre Range. 6. Ethnopsychology—Papua New Guinea—Finisterre Range.
7. Finisterre Range (Papua New Guinea)—Social conditions. I. Title.

DU740.42.K435 2004
615.8'8'0899912--dc22

                                                             2003026872

Carolina Academic Press
700 Kent Street
Durham, North Carolina 27701
Telephone (919) 489-7486
Fax (919) 493-5668
E-mail: cap@cap-press.com
www.cap-press.com

Printed in the United States of America

Contents

v

List of Charts, Documents, Figures, Illustrations, Maps, Surveys and Tables

Series Editors' Preface

Medical Anthropology Series

Social Discord and Bodily Disorders:
Healing among the Yupno of Papua New Guinea

—Pamela J. Stewart and Andrew Strathern

This a unique ethnographic study, one of a very few detailed monographs covering the experience of sickness and its treatment in Papua New Guinea. This study is built on two strategic axes: the first is a descriptive analysis of the social organization of the Yupno people, especially with regard to debts arising from marriage prestations (gifts made between the groom's and the bride's side at the time of a marriage), and how these give rise to "social discord." The second axis is the experience of illness, with an extended discussion of the sickness and eventual death of a baby boy, Nstasiñge, and how his condition was differentially diagnosed in the village where he lived by comparison with the biomedical health care center to which his mother took him when his "bodily disorders" worsened. The link between these two axes of discussion is the concept of *njigi*, "oppressing problems". Bridewealth payments in particular (comprising gifts made to the bride's kin by the kin of the groom) may give rise to long-standing and sometimes intractable disputes between people, and the negative feelings these disputes generate are held to produce sickness in children born of the marriages concerned. If the disputes are not settled, it is held that the children may die.

The attribution of sickness to social causes, connected with issues of morality, balance, and harmony in the world, is common throughout Papua New Guinea and in many other social contexts where kinship relations are prominent in the social order. Kinship is a crucial site where the moralities and expectations of nurture, reciprocity, obligation, and emotions of dependency and personal constraint and rebellion, all play confusingly together. It is from the emotional nexus of conflict, defined by anger, desires, frustrations, and resentment that the genesis of diagnostic notions regarding the causes of illness emerges. In turn, remedial action has to begin with attempts to settle the perceived wrongdoings or omissions that are in play. Kinship is an important source of morality; it is also a chronic source of conflict between people in Papua New Guinea (for example, see Strathern and Stewart 2000a) as elsewhere.

In Papua New Guinea morality is also frequently bound up with proper performance in exchanges of wealth between people. In the Yupno case bridewealth is the crucial nexus around which such notions of proper performance center. While there is a generalized expectation between groups that if a woman marries into an outside group, that group will reciprocate at some later date by sending a female member back in marriage, there is a more specific expectation that the bridewealth, or brideprice, for the daughter will repay that for the mother: that is, that those within the kin network who helped the father to pay for the mother's brideprice can later reclaim their debts from the brideprice for the daughter. This interesting stipulation is paralleled from materials among the Duna people of the Southern Highlands Province in Papua New Guinea (see Strathern and Stewart 2004), and may perhaps constitute one of the older rules by which brideprice debts were settled in a number of ethnographic cases. It is evident that the claimants to such debts have to wait a long time before they can receive repayment through their claims. In the meantime many things can go wrong. What, for example, if there is no daughter? Or the mother remarries and takes her daughter with her to a hostile group? Or memories become hazy and conflicted or some claimants die without clearly passing on their knowledge of debts/claims to their successors? Moreover, as Verena Keck also points out, brideprices are in general high, yet some people on the bride's side may be left out because of ill-will or inadvertence, and as a result their anger may subsequently cause illness in the children of the marriage. Such claimants, of course, derive their claim in turn from the earlier marriage of the bride's mother. This rule of debt thus continuously implicates cross-generational sets of kin on both sides of any given marriage.

In the Duna area (see Stewart and Strathern 2002) many of the marriage customs share features with the Yupno ones, e.g. special gifts to the bride's mother and presentation of netted bags (that can be used to carry a newborn child as well as other items) to the new bride by her in-laws. But differences exist also: in the Yupno case the problems arising from debt or unmet claims have resulted in a greater elaboration of ideas about sickness than seems to be found in the Duna case, even though among the Yupno, there is a return payment, *pelok*, made for the initial brideprice, which liquidates a part of the debt incurred by the groom with respect to his helpers. This is because *pelok* gifts repay these helpers' contributions; while in the Duna case no such return gift is made. In this particular feature, Yupno custom resembles Hagen (Melpa) practices, from the Western Highlands of Papua New Guinea (Strathern and Stewart 2000b), rather than Duna ones. Similarly to Hagen expectations also, recipients of the brideprice may claim they were tricked into receiving a sickly pig that died later, or because of subsequent disagreements they may make more demands for further payments over time. If these payments are not met, trouble is thought to emerge and this can lead to sickness; as in the Yupno case where disputes can arise out of "inadequate" *pelok* gifts.

The matrix of marriage payments themselves, then, can generate sickness as a result of anger that brings about "oppressing problems." Both suspicions of highly individual manipulation and a sense of overwhelming, even malevolent, relationships are clearly shown in this set of ideas. From this foundation, Keck builds her skillful account of how sickness is handled, beginning with essential ideas about the components of the person, organized around notions of energy *(tevantok)*, humors of the body, and the breath and shadow spirits of the person, all of which may be implicated in processes of illness and its treatment. The shadow spirit is said to share experience with other such spirits through dreaming, as happens with the Melpa *min* (see Stewart and Strathern 2003), and if the separation from the body is too long, illness or death may result (a classic set of notions in New Guinea). Health lies in the human being remaining "cool" (*yawuro* in the Yupno language), as opposed to "hot" or "cold," which are both undesirable states and are marks of illness. Magical aggression may make a person too cold; the bush spirit *sindok* may make them too hot. Remedies for illness involve the use of "hot" objects to counteract a "cold" state and vice-versa, always with the aim of producing a balanced, "cool" condition. A menstruating woman's energy and breath spirit are thought of as too hot, and so she must wash and cool down before she cooks for her husband again after menstruation is over. Male or female specialists known as "soothers" or "heat extinguishers" use a wide variety of plants and barks seen as "cool" to bring a patient suffering from a "hot" disorder such as a fever back into the cool state. Hot disorders in turn may be induced by the actions of specialists in *mawom* or *sit* sorcery (*sit* means to burn, heat, or cook). These ideas parallel ones found in Pangia in the Southern Highlands Province (see Strathern and Stewart 1999). In extended detail, Keck demonstrates the salience of humoral ideas of the body/person and their central significance for treating illness conditions. This again is likely to be a widespread feature of New Guinea societies which until recently was insufficiently explored or acknowledged in the literature (see A. Strathern 1996, Stewart and Strathern 2001).

Humoral ideas come into play in the context of practical treatment, but recovery from sickness depends, for the Yupno, on further diagnosis of oppressing problems, triggered by anger among the living and transformed into sickness by the agency of ghosts, whose intentions may be deduced from the evidence of dreams. So it was in the case of the small boy, Nstasiñge. People may be confused and search for various causes in past disagreements as an illness proceeds and is resistant to treatment. Gossip about sexual misdemeanors may cause anger and lead to violence and oppressing problems. Gossip appears here in its guise of negative social action rather than as a mechanism for solidarity. Generally, in New Guinea, this is how gossip is perceived (see Stewart and Strathern 2004 for an extended discussion of this theme in the context of witchcraft and sorcery accusations). Competing and conflicting accounts of wrong-doing add to the confusion of diagnosis. In a fascinating vignette, Keck describes how the relatives of Nstasiñge attempted to achieve reconciliation and harmony (and so relief from oppressing problems) by touching a one-Kina coin (the introduced state money of Papua New Guinea) and hanging it on the sick baby's neck, and also by giving the baby some water to drink from a bowl consecrated by a Christian prayer. The intrusion of new ideas derived from state and church organizations and their incorporation into the humoral ideas of the body are shown clearly here, since both the coin and the water were said to be "cool"; and the coin, as the equivalent of a traditional valuable, was thought to be able to entice the baby's shadow soul to return to his body.

One of the many interesting features of Keck's analysis is that she gives equally detailed accounts of attempts made in Nstasinge's home village to treat his illness and to the treatment given at the Teptep Health Centre by biomedically trained personnel. In both contexts a major problem was difficulty of diagnosis and a concomitant "failure of treatment" (see Lewis 2000 for this phrase). At the Health Centre, translation problems compounded the difficulties. Older people tend not to speak the lingua franca Tok Pisin, still less English, and the health personnel are largely from outside the local area and do not understand the Yupno language. Patients are sometimes afraid of these medical personnel. The situation is reminiscent of the account we ourselves received in the Duna area in 1999 of an unsuccessful visit to the Lake Kopiago Health Centre by a couple with a sick child who subsequently died; although in this case the child's father could speak Tok Pisin fluently, the parents of the sick child found it hard to gain the attention of the health personnel (Strathern and Stewart 1999: 88). More efficient and well-stocked local health centers for patient care, staffed by trained native-language speakers, would help in solving some of these problems. Keck does note the interesting point that a female Papua New Guinean nurse at Teptep incorporated the idea of a 'hevi' (or oppressing problem) into her own diagnosis of why Nstasiñge's illness did not improve with treatment. Medical pluralism may be at work in the biomedical context, just as the use of the Kina coin in treatment indicates the incorporation of new items by the Yupno into their own cultural scheme of thought.

Throughout her account, Keck gives us the kind of detailed ethnography that not only elucidates customs but also poignantly reveals individual and collective experience. Her analyses are comparable to those given by Stephen Frankel on the Huli people of the Southern Highlands of Papua New Guinea (Frankel 1986) and by various authors in the volume edited by Frankel and Lewis (1989); and her careful, detailed descriptions parallel those given by Lewis in his ethnography of the Gnau people of the West Sepik in Papua New Guinea (Lewis 1975, 1980, and especially 2000, which also centers on the extended illness and death of a single person, Dauwaras). These are classic studies in medical anthropology generally as well as in Papua New Guinea ethnography. Verena Keck's study belongs to this same genre, and will take its place alongside the work of Frankel, Lewis, and others dedicated to comprehensive ethnography and careful, insightful analysis.

We are delighted to include Verena Keck's book in the Ethnographic Studies in Medical Anthropology Series. The other titles in this Series include:

"Curing and Healing: Medical Anthropology in Global Perspective," 1999 (by Andrew Strathern and Pamela J. Stewart)

"Healing the Modern in a Central Javanese City," 2001 (by Steve Ferzacca)

"Physicians at Work, Patients in Pain," 2nd edition, 2001 (by Kaja Finkler)

"Endangered Species: Health, Illness and Death among Madagascar's People of the Forest," 2002 (by Janice Harper)

"Elusive Fragments: Making Power, Propriety, and Health in Samoa," 2002 (by Douglass Drozdow-St.Christian)

"The Gene and the Genie: Tradition, Medicalization, and Genetic Counseling in a Bedouin Community in Israel," 2005 (by Aviad Raz)

"The Practice of Concern: Ritual, Well-Being and Aging in Rural Japan," 2004 (by John Traphagan)

References

Frankel, Stephen (1986) *The Huli Response to Illness*. Cambridge: Cambridge University Press.

Frankel, Stephen and Gilbert Lewis (1989) *A Continuing Trial of Treatment: Medical Pluralism in Papua New Guinea.* Boston: Kluwer Academic Publishers.

Lewis, Gilbert (1975) *Knowledge of Illness in a Sepik Society.* London: Athlone Publishing.

Lewis, Gilbert (1980) *Day of Shining Red: An Essay on Understanding Ritual.* Cambridge: Cambridge University Press.

Lewis, Gilbert (2000) *A Failure of Treament.* Oxford: Oxford University Press.

Stewart, Pamela J. and A. Strathern (2001) *Humors and Substances: Ideas of the Body in New Guinea.* Westport, Conn. and London: Bergin and Garvey, Greenwood Publishing Group.

Stewart, Pamela J. and Andrew Strathern (2002) *Remaking the World: Myth, Mining and Ritual Change among the Duna of Papua New Guinea.* Washington, D.C.: Smithsonian Institution Press.

Stewart, Pamela J. and Andrew Strathern (2003) Dreaming and Ghosts among the Hagen and Duna of the Southern Highlands, Papua New Guinea. In *Dream Travelers: Sleep Experiences and Culture in the Western Pacific,* Roger Ivar Lohmann (ed.), pp. 42–59. New York: Palgrave Macmillan.

Stewart, Pamela J. and Andrew Strathern (2004) *Witchcraft, Sorcery, Rumors, and Gossip.* New Departures in Anthropology Series, No. 1, Cambridge: Cambridge University Press.

Strathern, Andrew (1996) *Body Thoughts.* Ann Arbor: University of Michigan Press.

Strathern, A. and Pamela J. Stewart (1999) *Curing and Healing: Medical Anthropology in Global Perspective.* Durham N.C. : Carolina Academic Press.

Strathern, A.J. and Pamela J. Stewart (2000a) Kinship and Commoditization: Historical Transformations. Special Issue of *L'Homme* on kinship, Nos 154/155, April/September, pp. 373–90.

Strathern, A. and Pamela J. Stewart (2000b) *Arrow Talk: Transaction, Transition, and Contradiction in New Guinea Highlands History.* Kent, Ohio and London: Kent State University Press.

Strathern, A. and Pamela J. Stewart (2004) *Empowering the Past, Confronting the Future: The Duna People of Papua New Guinea.* New York and London: Palgrave Macmillan.

January 2004
Department of Anthropology
University of Pittsburgh
Pittsburgh, PA 15260 USA

Author's Preface

This study is based on my experiences and perceptions gained during 22 months of fieldwork among the Yupno people in the Finisterre Range of Papua New Guinea between 1986 and 1988, and in two shorter visits in 1992 and 2000. The research formed part of a larger interdisciplinary project, in which two other anthropologists, a psychologist, a botanist, an ethnomusicologist and two physicians participated; the research topics of the other anthropologists were ethnobotany (Christin Kocher Schmid) and concepts of space, the Yupno counting system, and environmental classification based on a hot-cool-cold continuum (Juerg Wassmann). My own subject was the medical system from the Yupno point of view. A central element of the whole project was co-operation with scientists from other disciplines: zoologists, botanists and a developmental psychologist, Pierre Dasen, from Geneva, Switzerland. I worked with two medical doctors, Sandra Staub and Andreas Allemann, both from Basel, Switzerland, who, apart from working on their own Ph.D. theses, carried out a series of examinations amongst the population of Gua village. Their adviser was Prof.Dr.med. Niklaus Gyr from the Kantonsspital Basel. Robert Kiapranis, botanist at the Wau Ecological Institute, supervised the botanical classification of the various plants. Ethnomusicologist Don Niles, of the Institute of Papua New Guinea Studies in Boroko, worked on the melodies and instruments of the Yupno.

My fieldwork was financially supported by a doctoral grant from the Studienstifung des Deutschen Volkes. My sincere gratitude goes to this institution. I wish to thank all those who helped me during fieldwork, with the analysis of the data and later in discussions (of the German version of my thesis): Meinhard Schuster, at that time Head of Department at the Basel Institute of Anthropology, my teacher and Ph.D. supervisor; Niklaus Gyr, medical director at the Kantonsspital Basel, for his help with the medical components of my subject, including assistance with the biomedical evidence and terms; Andrew Strathern, for his helpful comments on issues of theory and on Melpa-Yupno concepts of "souls;" Sandra Staub, who, with her intensive involvement and sense of humor, made it possible to cooperate especially well in the village and who contributed substantially to the analysis of the medical data in the post-fieldwork period. Many thanks also to Ingrid Bell, who translated the text from the original German into English, and especially to Bob Tonkinson, who edited the English version. I also cordially thank Don Gardner, ANU, Canberra, who during his time in Heidelberg suggested the title of this book, and Dan Jorgensen, who helped with the very last changes. My greatest thanks are to my partner and colleague, Juerg Wassmann, for his intellectual and emotional support, in the field and since then. Above all, I owe an enormous debt of gratitude to the villagers of Gua for their cooperation, warmth and generosity in allowing me to share their daily life.

Conversations with the older male and almost all the female informants were translated by interpreters from the Yupno language into Tok Pisin, the Neo-Melanesian Pidgin-English and lingua franca of Papua New Guinea, and vice versa. Only the younger men were fluent enough in Tok Pisin to converse. The Yupno language is Papuan in type and has so far not been fully recorded; the only document is a preliminary grammar, in manuscript form, by Wes Reed of the Summer Institute of Linguistics (SIL), but even that was compiled in a different dialect-group at Kewieñ. Despite my intensive attempts to learn Yupno, I did not achieve fluency in this language; however, I was able to converse in a broken version and get the gist of most conversations.

It was extremely important for me to grasp Yupno notions and concepts in the vernacular, so, with considerable effort and a lot of patience on the part of my informants, we managed to overcome the language barrier and dissect central terms, i.e. split them into their basic components and essential meanings in order to render them understandable. However, in order not to overload the text with Yupno terms and thereby make it unreadable, most such terms have been replaced by English glosses, which render the meaning and are not always literal. Especially relevant terms are dissected into their components and translated; they can be found in the glossary. Two exceptions to this are the central terms *moñan* and *aminwop*, both referring to essential parts of the human being. The many shades of meaning implied in these Yupno terms cannot be captured by an English translation, but the two English terms in brackets have been added as auxiliary labels.

This monograph comprises seven chapters. In the first part, I introduce the topic and situate this study among existing medical-anthropological studies in Papua New Guinea. The second chapter centers on Gua, the village of little Nstasiñge, who is the protagonist of this book, and introduces the inhabitants and their social and kinship relations. Chapter 3 concerns the concept of person from the Yupno point of view and is essential for the understanding of illness. The fourth chapter, which is the core of the book, outlines the history of the sickness of the little boy, Nstasiñge, from both the Yupno point of view and the biomedical perspective. These contrasting perspectives demonstrate how very differently the same sickness episode can be interpreted. In the first section of this chapter, the child's mother and the relatives are heard, their stories being interrupted by explanatory excursi. The second section of the fourth chapter contains the biomedical data, based on the report of Madang Hospital, compiled by the physician Sandra Staub and formulated by me in cooperation with her. In Chapter 5, I present an attempt on to systematize the Yupno medical system, placing the concepts mentioned during the child Nstasiñge's illness into a broader frame; in addition, further aspects not mentioned in this particular case are described. Chapter 6 contains my concluding comments, and Chapter 7 briefly sketch the situation years later (1992 and 2000) during subsequent fieldwork visits.

This book is based on a longer and more detailed German Ph.D. thesis (Keck 1992). Some materials in this book are adapted from the article "Two Ways of Explaining Reality", published in Oceania 1993 (63): 293–314, with the permission of the Editor.

Notes on the Text

The special symbols used are:

- (*i*) is a volatile upper vowel. It is best reproduced by attempting not to pronounce it at all. E.g. *amin* (man) is best pronounced as if the i was not present: *amn*.

- (ñ) is a velar sound pronounced like in "to sing"

- Yupno terms are rendered in the text in italics, Tok Pisin words are put into simple quotation marks. Proper names, names of clans and topographical designations are written with capitals.

Social Discord
and Bodily Disorders

Chapter 1

Introduction

1. Orientation

Medical anthropology, "internationally, the most rapidly burgeoning subfield of the discipline" (Keesing 1989: 58), is a special field recognized by some as a discipline in its own right, and by others as a subdiscipline of anthropology. Whatever its classification, it has been experiencing a marked increase in prominence since the 1970s, manifested in specific journals, a profusion of publications, conferences and newly established societies, and a rapid growth in the number of practitioners who label themselves medical anthropologists. Linked to this burgeoning of the field of study are rapidly changing theories and numerous articles replete with discussions about models as well as methodological and theoretical approaches.[1]

According to Foster and Anderson (1978: 4–8), the beginnings of "medical anthropology" are to be found in four different disciplines: first, physical anthropology, whose representatives, who are for the most part physicians or natural scientists, deal with genetic and serological questions or the influence of nutrition on bodily structure as well as the occurrence of diseases such as arthritis, diabetes, anemia and so on. Secondly, the "culture and personality" movement, which for a period from the 1930s was a prominent component of American "cultural anthropology." Its best known representatives included Margaret Mead, Ruth Benedict, Cora DuBois, Ralph Linton and psychoanalysts such as Abraham Kardiner and Erik Erikson. A major concern of this school of thought was personality structure, whereby, given the notion of culture as learned, the personality structure of its carriers was thus a characteristic expression of the culture under investigation. Increasing interest in culture-specific forms of social transgression and psychological disorders later led to the establishment of "ethnopsychiatry." The third discipline is "international public health," research in which originated in the 1940s. In 1942, the gov-

1

ernment of the United States initiated health programs in several Latin American countries as part of extended technical aid; and after the end of World War II, this support was expanded to African and Asian countries. In 1948, the World Health Organization (WHO) was founded as a special organization of the United Nations. The development planners employed in these programs soon realized that the simple transfer of the health service of industrialized nations did not meet the needs of the so-called developing countries. Only for some of the health-programs were anthropologists taken on as advisers because of their regional expertise. In 1978, WHO, in its Alma Ata declaration, proclaimed a new strategy in health politics for "Third World" countries by way of a Primary Health-Care Program (PHC), wherein it was proposed (Article 82) to train and involve "traditional medical practitioners and birth attendants" in the PHC (WHO 1978).

Ethnomedicine, a field of research within cognitive anthropology (formerly also called ethnoscience), which deals with non-Western concepts of sicknesses and curing practices, was the fourth disciplinary point of departure for "medical anthropology." By comparing an earlier definition of ethnomedicine (Hughes 1968: 88) and a more recent one (Nichter 1991: 138), some indication can be gained of the rapid change that has occurred in this field of research. For Hughes (1968: 88), "The term 'ethnomedicine' will be used to refer to those beliefs and practices relating to disease which are the products of indigenous cultural development and are not explicitly derived from the conceptual framework of modern medicine." Nichter (1991: 138), in contrast, outlines the field as follows:

> All too often, ethnomedicine is simplistically compartmentalized as a subfield of 'medical anthropology' and delimited as the study of folk illnesses, traditional medical systems, herbal remedies, and healing rituals. While these subjects are central to ethnomedicine, they are points of departure, not the focus of a fixed gaze. Ethnomedicine is... grounded in the study of everyday life, perceptions of the normal and natural, the desirable and feared, and that form of embodied knowledge known as common sense as it emerges in efforts to establish or reestablish health as one aspect of well-being. Ethnomedical inquiry entails the study of how well-being and suffering are experienced bodily as well as socially... (Nichter 1991: 138).

Nichter's 1991 definition contains key terms that have become guidelines for contemporary approaches and stances adopted by practitioners in medical anthropology, including my own research: an emphasis on everyday life; a focus less concerned with predominantly static concepts (as, for instance, classifications of illness) than with the agency of the patient and his or her therapy managing group, understood as being embedded in their social space of experience ("Erfahrungsraum," as Mannheim 1982 calls it), and involved with strategies and actions aimed at maintaining or restoring well-being within the affected group. As a clear rejection of the strongly biomedically marked perceptions of a physical ailment (reminiscent of Descartes' body-mind distinction, so important for biomedicine), the majority of medical anthropologists today endeavor to provide a holistic view of this well-being, which, while it may definitely have physical aspects, is also characterized by social and spiritual components that are frequently of the greatest significance. Furthermore, biological and biomedical data are no longer accepted as "an assemblage of incontestable natural facts" (Lindenbaum and Lock 1993: X).

Now often regarded as the classic study in "ethnomedicine" (which, however, did not call itself by that name until thirty years later), *Medicine, Magic and Religion* (1924) was written by the eminent physician, psychologist and anthropologist, W. H. R. Rivers. He was a member of the first significant interdisciplinary field-study, the Cambridge Anthropological Expedition (1898/99), led by the zoologist (and later anthropologist) A. C. Haddon, in the islands of the Torres Strait, which lie between Papua New Guinea and Cape York in Australia and are predominantly Melanesian in cultural character. (Further participants were the British physician and anthropologist C. G. Seligman and the psychologists, Myers and McDougall.) Rivers has become closely identified with the ethnomedical perspective because he systematically linked traditional medicine with other aspects of culture and social organization. He defines medicine as

> a term for a set of social practices by which man seeks to direct and control a specific group of natural phenomena...phenomena which lower his vitality and tend towards death....society has come to classify these phenomena together, and has distinguished them from other groups of natural phenomena under the name of disease [Rivers 1924: 4–5].... when we speak of the concept of disease...we mean no exactly formulated definition, but a more or less vague system of ideas, which, though not distinctly formulated by a people, yet directs their behaviour—their reactions towards those features of the environment which we have classified together under the category of disease (Rivers 1924: 7)

and

> ...the practices of these people in relation to disease [are]...not a medley of disconnected and meaningless customs, but are inspired by definite ideas concerning the causation of disease. Their modes of treatment follow directly from their ideas concerning etiology and

pathology....the important point is that...their practices are the logical consequence of those beliefs [...] We may say even that these peoples practice an art of medicine which is in some respects more rational that our own, in that its modes of diagnosis and treatment follow more directly their ideas concerning the causation of disease (Rivers 1924: 51–52).

For Rivers, traditional medical practices are therefore rational acts. However, his approach has been criticized by Wellin (1977: 50):

Despite his training as a physician, Rivers is indifferent to biological factors and allows no place in his model for them...By focusing on world view, and its linkages with belief and behavior, Rivers can find no way to accommodate magico-religious and naturalistic-scientific world views within the same domain of inquiry. As a result, Rivers' model precludes consideration of Western medicine and is limited to medicine among primitive groups (Wellin 1977: 50).

This criticism draws attention to an alleged shortcoming that, in my view, is a virtue. Despite his training as a physician, Rivers became deeply involved in the study of traditional medical concepts, and attempted to understand them emically, as we would say today; that is, in terms of the worldview of the carriers of the culture in question, and he avoided mixing these indigenous concepts and understandings with his own biomedical system of reference.

Another important scholar, Erwin H. Ackerknecht, held by some scholars to be the father of "medical anthropology" (Foster and Anderson 1978: 52), is another pioneer whose theoretical approach includes elements that we may regard as meaningful for "ethnomedicine." Like Rivers, Ackerknecht was initially trained in medicine and only later began to work in anthropology. His publications, most of which first appeared in the 1940s, are for the most part based on literary studies and museum collections. For Ackerknecht, who was to a great extent influenced by Ruth Benedict, the most important unit of investigation is the total "cultural configuration" and the space which the "medical pattern" occupies within this totality. True to cultural relativism, for him there is not one indigenous medicine but possibly as many as there are indigenous cultures (Ackerknecht 1971: 53), and these indigenous medicines were best understood in relation to cultural concepts, that is, without regard to biology, epidemiology, or environmental factors, though perhaps with the aid of material culture. As a special characteristic of indigenous medicine, he stresses its social function:

In many primitive societies, disease becomes the most important social sanction. [...] The social concept of disease in primitive society is also reflected in the belief that the disease sanction may affect every member of the family as well as the sinner himself (Ackerknecht 1971: 20).

"Ethnomedicine" proper, in its stricter definition, originated as a thematic domain within cognitive anthropology, a field established by W. Goodenough and F. Loundsbury in 1956 as a new theoretical orientation in anthropology. Its aim was to first discover the cognitive principles according to which members of other cultures classify the world around them, their "world order" so to speak, and then to describe it using the own categories of the culture in question.

While, in the opinion of the cognitive anthropologists, this "order of the world" in other cultures had been formerly described using pre-formulated principles and categories originating from our own culture, hence etically, cognitive anthropology attempts to render this "order" emically, "in their (the members of the culture) own concepts," culture-specific or culture-immanent. A well-known claim of this approach is that it would no longer look for "words for things" but for "things for words" (Frake 1962: 72).[2]

In the 1960s, cognitive anthropology climaxed in a series of famous field studies that investigated the cognitive orders in singular, conceptually precisely structured cultural domains, such as color terms, botany, zoology, kinship terms and categories of disease. The methods used (establishing a taxonomy, componential analysis and representation in a paradigm, etc.) were borrowed from structural (pre-transformational) linguistics.

Frake's study *The Diagnosis of Disease among the Subanun of Mindanao* (1961) stands as a typical and highly successful example of this period of cognitive anthropology.[3] Rigorous in his methodology, Frake presents a taxonomy of the terms for skin diseases on several contrasting levels as well as their ever-changing names during the course of the sickness. He regards the diagnosis of a disease as a cognitive process.

While in the 1960s and even at the beginning of the 1970s cognitive anthropology was represented by a series of individual studies, it reached a turning point around the mid-1970s. Its practitioners realized that it was not possible with this method to examine domains that in linguistic terms were structured either weakly or barely at all. (Gatewood, in 1985, aptly expressed the dilemma by invoking the adage, "actions speak louder than words"). Nor was it possible to investigate values, decision making and more complex correlations such as causality. The relatively static models anthropologists had hitherto been able to construct ideally with an "omniscient informant" (Boster 1985) did not explain any cultural deviations, such as differing models within one culture; thus variations in cultural knowledge within a culture, on the bases of age, sex, specialization and other factors, could not be comprehended. Criticism of nearly all the studies from this period of cognitive anthropology consists of the question whether these categories so clearly represented in taxonomies and paradigmata were really those that people in a specific culture applied when thinking, or were only rendered in accordance with the way the researcher was structuring them. The severest critics look upon all of these models as nothing but constructs by the anthropologist and deny them any relevance for the culture in question.

Realizing these shortcomings, cognitive anthropology turned towards the subject of the acquisition and application of this knowledge in everyday life— towards what actually happens (and is not elicited) in observable everyday life; with few exceptions, however, this remained for the anthropologists Western everyday life. New methods such as the establishment of "prototypes" (Rosch and Mervis 1975: 574) or of "cultural models" (Holland and Quinn 1987: 4) have been initially tested in the Western world (predominantly in the USA[4] and in various subgroups). However, because of the highly complicated methodological procedure and heavy dependency on language entailed, their application in a culture foreign to the researcher seems hardly feasible.

2. Concepts

To help understand the terms and concepts used in this book, first some definitions are necessary: the concepts "biomedicine," "traditional medicine," "medical system," "disease," "illness" and "sickness."

Modern medicine, biomedicine, Western medicine, scientific medicine, allopathic medicine and cosmopolitan medicine are terms for the medical system which historically had its origin in Europe, building on a paradigm from natural science (Cartesian), which in now ubiquitous and is no doubt taught at universities worldwide. Amongst its characteristics are a high degree of technology, the attempt to control and fight disease by surgical interventions, drugs and measures of public health care, and the positioning of its highly specialized representatives in status hierarchies (McElroy and Townsend 1979: 107). Like any other medical system, biomedicine is not a static discipline independent of other influences but a dynamic field, confronted with new insights and selectively incorporating new influences. Nor is it by any means totally homogeneous worldwide: biomedicine as practiced for instance in Europe may be a far cry from its manifestations in a "borrowed" form in Third World countries.

As a demarcation from the above-mentioned biomedicine, the terms "traditional medicine," "non-Western medicine" or "indigenous medicine" are used. This opposition recalls the old, out-dated dichotomy "we/the others" and, accordingly, no anthropologist today would adopt such a crude methodology; rather, the term "traditional medicine" would be used to designate the medical system found in an ethnic group, in order to differentiate it from imported biomedicine. In addition, the dualism represented in an idealizing typifying way, based on an ahistoric, static comprehension, to oppose traditional medicine in its many forms and imported biomedicine, does not exist, because either both systems have influenced each other or else traditional medicine has incorporated parts of other traditional medical systems.

The term, "medical system," which has become widespread in medical anthropology,

> properly embraces the totality of health knowledge, beliefs, skills, and practices of the members of every group. It should be used in a comprehensive sense to include all of the clinical and nonclinical activities, the formal and informal institutions, and any other activities that, however tangentially, bear on the health levels of the group and promote optimum functioning of society (Foster and Anderson 1978: 36).

There are opposing opinions on what a medical system is and what it includes. According to numerous authors, a culture has by no means only one medical system but several. Leslie (1976) demonstrates this in his contribution to his famous book *Asian Medical Systems* where he points out nine parallel medical systems for India; in our society also, we can find next to the medical system "biomedicine" other medical systems, such as homeopathy, and a series of medical systems of a psychotherapeutic or religious persuasion. These diverse co-existing medical systems are studied under the concept of medical pluralism. One view of "medical traditions," however, is that they "are distinctive combinations of ideas, practices, skills, apparatuses and materia medica....a given medical tradition can be practiced in more than one medical system. A pluralistic medical system is one which incorporates more than a single medical tradition" (A. Young 1983: 1206–7).

For the Yupno and their medical system, then, either their traditional medicine is regarded as one medical system and the biomedicine they are offered as another, in which case we can either talk of medical pluralism or of two parallel medical systems—a point of view which I adopt. Or, if one were to adopt A. Young's perspective, then traditional medicine and biomedicine are no more than different medical traditions within a pluralistic total Yupno medical system, which historically is not the case.

Two further central concepts of medical anthropology are disease and illness. That there is a clear distinction[5] between them is today a taken for granted in medical anthropology and discussed in most textbooks (Strathern and Stewart 1999). Nevertheless, both terms have undergone a change of meaning between the 1970s and the 1990s.

For example, Fabrega (1971: 213) writes:

> Disease: Designates altered bodily states or processes that deviate from norms as established by Western biomedical science. This state is presumed to have temporal extension. This state may or may not coincide with an illness state.

In the literature of the 1970s, diseases are for the most part formulated as belonging to the biomedical model, according to which they are classified by only one taxonomy of (presumed) universally valid and culture-independent categories.[6] In the 1980s, it is linked with the professional sector and its practitioners, who, in the Western world, are part of the biomedical establishment (Kleinman 1980: 73, Chrisman and Johnson 1990: 110). Connected with the term disease is "curing," referring to "practices which are efficacious, from the point of view of biomedical science, in either [sic] reversing, limiting, or preventing disease" (A. Young 1983: 1208). A. Young then provides the following contrast:

> Illness refers to people's perceptions and experiences of disease and other socially disvalued states which they lump together with disease. These 'people' can be sick people, their relatives, practitioners or other people immediately affected by the course of the sickness. Healing refers to practices which are efficacious, from the point of view of these people in affecting illness or illness behavior in a desirable way (A. Young 1983: 1208).

The term "illness" refers also to the culturally defined perceptions and experiences of the patient and his/her social group. Kleinman introduces "sickness" as a generic term and subdivides this into the two aspects, "disease" and "illness":

> Disease refers to a malfunctioning of biological and/or psychological processes, while the term illness refers to the psychosocial experience and meaning of perceived disease. Illness includes secondary personal and social responses to a primary malfunctioning (disease) in the individual's physiological or psychological status (or both). Illness involves processes of attention, perception, affective responses, cognition, and valuation directed at the disease and its manifestations (i.e., symptoms, role impairment, etc.). But also included in the idea of illness are communication and interpersonal interaction, particularly

within the context of the family and social network (Kleinman 1980: 72).

As Leslie (1980: 193) clearly states, illness and disease may, but do not necessarily have to, coincide: "People have diseases without being ill or assuming sick roles, and they experience illness and take sick roles when they do not have diseases." Also apposite here is the comment by Kleinman (1978: 88) that: "Neither disease nor illness is a thing, an entity, instead they are different ways of explaining sickness, different social constructions of reality."

Most medical anthropologists find the distinction between disease and illness useful,[7] a means "to create a single language and discourse for both clinicians and social scientists" (Scheper-Hughes and Lock 1987: 10). As the same authors note, though, "one unanticipated effect has been that physicians are claiming *both* aspects of the sickness experience for the medical domain. As a result, the 'illness' dimension of human distress (i.e. the social relations of sickness) are [sic] being medicalized and individualized, rather than politicized and collectivized" (Scheper-Hughes and Lock 1987: 10).[8]

In addition, as Brown and Inhorn (1990: 189) indicate, "[the distinction between disease and illness] is based on a questionable assumption that the biomedical definition of disease is objective and culture free." For most medical anthropologists today, it is understood that biomedicine is not a culture-independent discipline either; being heavily influenced by the values of the Western world, it is "international, cosmopolitan, dominant, and hegemonic" (Brown 1998: 109) and is only one (our) "emic" system among others.[9] As Nichter (1991: 139) aptly points out: "Biomedical research is not the 'objective other' which it is often made out to be. 'Scientific reasoning' is motivated and as much a product of culture and practical reason as are traditional systems of ethnomedicine." For Singer (1989: 1194, citing Taussig 1980), "disease, seen only as a malfunctioning in biological or psychological processes, possesses a phantom-objectivity." Rubel and Hass (1990: 118) define biomedicine succinctly as "the ethnomedicine in which physicians are trained," and, for Wright and Treacher, it is certainly not "clearly and distinctly independent of social forces by virtue of its special scientific status" (1982: 5), but a "social construction" (1982: 9).

3. Two Ways of Explaining Reality: An Example of Interdisciplinary Cooperation

My medical-anthropological topic was chosen out of the conviction that concepts of and practices for disease and illness form a central complex of ideas for every ethnic group, because disease, illness and health are essentially linked with the origin, quality, maintenance and loss of life. The judgement of what it means to be ill or healthy and people's opinions and attitudes towards "illness" are closely linked with their particular culture's worldview, hence with the ways they perceive their environment, the characteristics of their social and religious system, and their system of social values. There is also a connection to the concept of the person, such as the dimensions that define the body-mind and the self, and therefore these themes belong to the anthropology of the body and the anthropology of the self; in short, ethnomedicine in this sense presents itself as "multidimensional and metamedical" (Nichter 1991: 137).

During the preparation for fieldwork, when I became engaged in "ethnomedicine" and worked through the existing medical-anthropological studies on cultures in Papua New Guinea,[10] I became increasingly uncomfortable about the methodology of some of these works, and began looking for alternative ways of tackling the problem. The focus of these studies often lay in the biomedical domain, and the research was based on a global approach. The indigenous medical system of the community or group in question, its social, moral and religious context (for example, its concepts of the person and defining aspects thereof, ideas about body-mind, the hereafter, and so on), received little attention. In other words, I looked in vain for a detailed and well-rounded account of the emic point of view. In the majority of cases, these investigations were conducted by physicians or—less often—by scientists who had been trained medically as well as anthropologically (as in the case of Stephen Frankel or Gilbert Lewis). Anthropologists, in turn, hardly dared touch upon this subject since they were often accused by medical and anthropological colleagues alike of being professionally incompetent to investigate such a complex topic without a degree of medical training. The point of view of biomedicine was therefore dominant, so the local perspective, the traditional concepts of illness, did not receive the attention it warranted.

Even the one discipline that could have been expected less to order and classify cultural phenomena according to Western criteria, namely anthropology itself, found it difficult to contextualize culturally the concepts it labeled "sorcery," "witchcraft," "magic" and so on in connection with sickness, illness, and people's behavior during illness and curing. In the volume edited by Stephen in 1987, *Sorcerer and Witch in Melanesia*, various articles identify "sorcerers" as traditional causers of sickness and, at the same time, occasionally as healers, but what is emphasized is the position of these practitioners in the traditional religion system, their functions during warfare, their role in community social control, and so on. Their central importance for the medical system of the group in question is dealt with only in passing.

Stephen Frankel's study, *The Huli Response to Illness* (1986), is one of the best-known ethnomedical investigations of a Papua New Guinea people. Like Gilbert Lewis (see below), Frankel was trained as a physician as well as an anthropologist and, with this dual education, seemed predestined to carry out ethnomedical research. In the introduction, he describes his approach as follows:

> I am therefore handling two distinct analytical frames: on the one hand the Huli's particular culturally determined set of ideas through which they interpret instances of illness, and which guides their responses to it; and on the other the disease pattern which can be described in medical terms (Frankel 1986: 5)....A key methodological issue in a study of this sort concerns the problem of translating between the terms of scientific medicine and those of a folk taxonomy of illness (1986: 61–62).

Gilbert Lewis was the author of another well-known ethnomedical study from Papua New Guinea, *Knowledge of Illness in a Sepik Society: a Study of the Gnau, New Guinea* (1975). In an anthropological mode, he attempts emically to grasp Gnau concepts of illness, but then he transfers these concepts of illness onto those of biomedicine, making it his system of reference for much of the study. Statements such as "One question lying behind my account of the Gnau view of illness is to know how it corresponds to ours..." (Lewis 1975: 129) confirm his point of departure, and he does not seem strictly to follow his own recommendation: "the anthropologist who intends to study illness in another society from his own...should also in my opinion try to keep in mind a distinction between disease defined by external modern medical criteria and illness as it happens to be recognized in the society he studies" (Lewis 1975: 129).

However, in his monograph *A Failure of Treatment* (2000), he describes a case study of the prolonged illness of a Gnau man, and here clearly employs a culturally-grounded, local perspective.

> To follow the course of his illness was to see in practice how social ties were woven and how strong they were; how people interpreted an illness and reasoned about its causes, what credence they gave to dreams, spirit revelations, and divinations for understanding it; as to treatment, I followed their hopes of success, the pacing of interventions, how they timed them and judged their efficacy (Lewis 2000: 2).

In their medical-anthropological landmark studies on Papua New Guinea societies, Lewis (1975) and Frankel (1986) both introduced biomedical terms as components of an analytical concept into the investigation of traditional medical systems. However, in the more recent reader about medical pluralism in Papua New Guinea they jointly edited (Frankel and Lewis 1989a), they use a much broader, less biomedically-determined approach, as the following statement shows: "Illness may be seen as a sanction for misconduct, a mystery, a sign of revenge, or a sign of the power of spirits, a natural risk, and so on" (Frankel and Lewis 1989b: 4).

Another classic ethnomedical contribution is that of Glick (1963, 1967), whose approach had a strong influence on my research. He was the first anthropologist (1960–1962) to choose as his research topic the medical system of a people, the Gimi in the Eastern Highlands of Papua New Guinea. In earlier studies of this region, ethnographic data concerning concepts of illness could be found here and there but were far from the primary interest of a study. Glick (1967: 35) proposed that "ailments," physical states without socially significant cause and treated with simple "remedies," should be excluded from an anthropological analysis of illness. Critics, such as Welsch (1987: 208) and Panoff (1970: 68) claimed that Glick had thus to a great extent omitted the whole realm of home remedies or family-based therapies. Despite this, though, his division into positively and negatively directed treatments was regarded by other scholars as a heuristically acceptable complex of categories (Johannes 1980: 51, Welsch 1982: 333–35, Welsch 1983: 48–49).

According to Glick, one must first clarify what constitutes an illness in a culture, what kinds of illness are recognized and upon which criteria a diagnosis is based. Every diagnostic statement about an illness contains three dimensions: the evidence (namely the symptoms), the process (the pathological aspect) and the cause, which is the most important dimension in most cultures. This causality concept (formulated by other authors as "the why question") is highly important in personalized systems (in medical systems where the concept of illness as caused by an agent predominates) since "illnesses are caused by agents who in some way bring their powers to bear against their victims.... they are conceived as willful beings, who act not indifferently but in response to consciously perceived personal motives" (Glick 1967: 36).

To summarize my point of view and departure: with its emphasis on the emic approach, my study stands indeed in the tradition of cognitive anthropology or "ethnomedicine" respectively. These early methods of cognitive anthropology, including the construction of models as a taxonomy or a paradigm, however, were not feasible among the Yupno, just as among the Gnau (Lewis 1975: 141) and the Huli (Frankel 1986: 8), since the Yupno do not have a complex taxonomic hierarchy of concepts of illness.

To do justice to a representation of the Yupno medical system from the Yupno point of view and avoid the unfortunate blending of two different models of explanations while also considering the biomedical point of view, I chose a different method, which favored interdisciplinary cooperation with physicians and thus allowed an efficient division of labor. The physicians, Sandra Staub and Andreas Allemann, examined the physical condition of the Yupno from the biomedical point of view, which meant dealing with the concept of disease, while I was able to concentrate on the concept of illness by endeavoring to understand as fully as possible the Yupno point of view. I was, and still am, convinced that my lack of professional medical knowledge made it easier for me to understand Yupno concepts of illness, their practices, reactions and therapies; right from the beginning of the study, I had neither the urge nor the knowledge to put a biomedically defined label on any incident of illness. During the initial stages of fieldwork, however, this open approach, while free of reliance on the existing Western system of reference, was confusing and it was some time before I began to understand the logic of the Yupno system.

In the center of the study stands the case example of the little boy Nstasiñge, which permits a syntheses of the aims of this investigation, namely, the presentation of concepts of illness from the point of view of the Yupno themselves plus interpretations of data specific to this case that was collected on an interdisciplinary (anthropological-biomedical) basis. It thus becomes possible to consider the two points of view of a single illness/disease incidence, which demonstrate two contrasting modes of interpretation. The detailed case study contains an additional aim, which approaches the goal of medical anthropology and contemporary cognitive anthropology: to include the processes and dynamics of mundane Yupno life. Cultural concepts of illness are present as knowledge "in the heads of the members of a society," but it is far more important to understand how they are used in everyday life to make decisions in an actual case. They are not monocausal but change over the course of an illness, being influenced by the cultural knowledge of the participants, which varies within an ethnic group, and they may change according to the social constellation of the people in question; in other words: they are pluralistic.

Chapter 2

Gua, the Village of Little Nstasiñge

1. The Surroundings and the Village

I

The Yupno inhabit a wildly rugged, isolated highland region in the Eastern Finisterre Range of the Huon Peninsula in the northeastern part of Papua New Guinea. A mighty massif with high, treeless summits between 3500 and 4000 meters, the Finisterre Range traverses the northern part of the Huon Peninsula, running northwest to southeast. Towards the northeast, it declines steeply to a hilly countryside, covered with grass and crossed by wide rivers, which flattens into a coastal strip bordering the Bismarck Sea. To the southeast lies the high Saruwaged Range, the southwestern side of which adjoins the wide Markham Valley.

The name Yupno[1] (literally, "it deposited [flotsam] on its banks") refers to the action of the river that flows down the main valley. According to Yupno mythology,[2] the first people originated from the bamboo, *teet*, that was washed up by the river and deposited on its banks. In fact, almost all culturally important things, from special kinds of banana to objects used for rituals (such as the special stones, *sulek*), were deposited by the river in this fashion.

The Yupno River eroded its bed so deeply that—especially around its middle and upper course—this created a narrow, steep-sided valley. From its source on the eastern side of a high mountain, it flows together with the Kewieñ River though an impassable ravine, below which it is joined by two more important tributaries, the Daldal and the Kael. The Yupno then rushes down through a deep gorge, an especially impressive part of the river where, on both sides, big waterfalls cascade down several hundred meters over huge

Map 1: The Finisterre Range

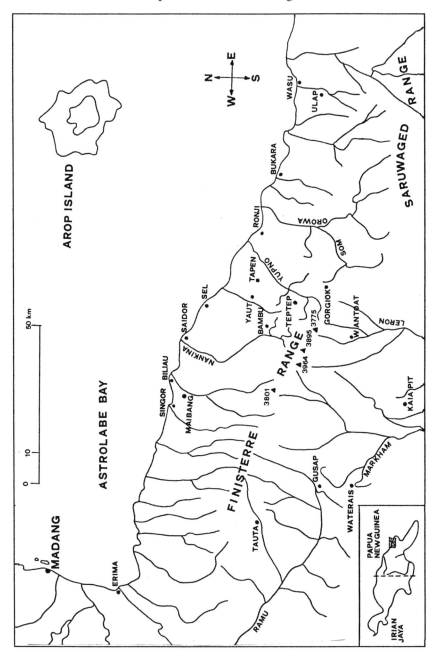

Illustration 1: View of the upper Yupno and Kewieñ Valleys
(towards the southwest)

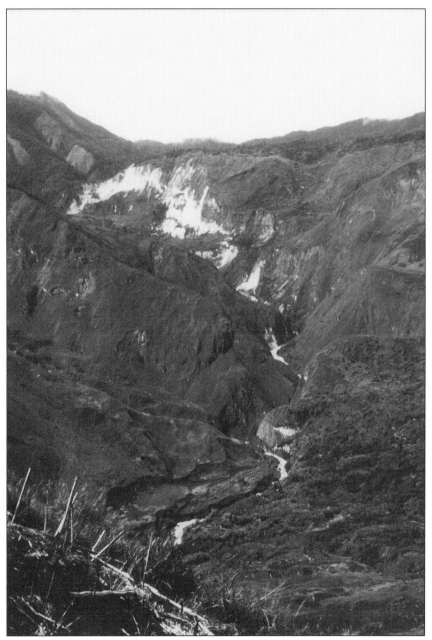

sandstone cliffs. The river then slows and begins to meander, presses through a narrow gap and down into the coastal region before it empties into the sea a few kilometers north of the village of Ronji.

With all its twists and turns between source and estuary, the Yupno is about 50 kms long. Flatter stretches of countryside, such as small plateaus suitable for settlements and garden lands, are found only in the valleys of the smaller tributaries around the upper reaches of the river.

II

The Yupno Valley contains two types of landscape:[3]

- the lower Yupno region is almost completely covered with rainforest. The climate is humid and warm. The villages of Kwembun, Windiluk, Wandaboñ, Bonkiman, Kwaup and Tapen[4] are situated at altitudes of between 700 and 1200 m and, according to the census book of 1985, have approximately 1200 inhabitants,[5] one fifth of the Yupno population, who cultivate mainly taro, yams, to a smaller extent also sweet potatoes, bananas, sugar cane and fruit (pineapple, papaya). These people of the lower area are called by the upper Yupno *molit*, "the people from down there." They live in rectangular, relatively airy gabled houses with built-in bamboo platforms.
- The upper Yupno region, to which little Nstasiñge's village, Gua, belongs, is clearly bleaker. The villages are situated in the side valleys on both sides of the Yupno, which flows some hundred meters below. The vegetation in the inhabited parts of the upper course region (1600–2200 m) consists of grassland and rainforest, and on the higher mountains (up to almost 4000 m) the ground is covered with sparse grass and stones. The climate is severe, with temperatures in the higher villages dropping to 8° C. at night, while during the day, even in sunny weather, it rarely gets warmer than 22° C., and during rainfall may reach only 18° C. In the dry season (May to November), the day generally starts with a cloudless, bright morning, then towards the mid-afternoon heavy clouds slowly creep up the valley, and by dusk, about 6 p.m., envelop the village in a dense fog. During the rainy season, a clear morning is followed by the almost daily heavy afternoon downpour. Dull days, during which it is constantly cloudy or raining, are very rare.

The upper Yupno live in fourteen villages[6] and form the largest part of the population, totalling 5279 people in 1985. They are called *oskoron*, "people from the upper bush," by those living in the lower course of the river.

Map 2: Yupno Valley

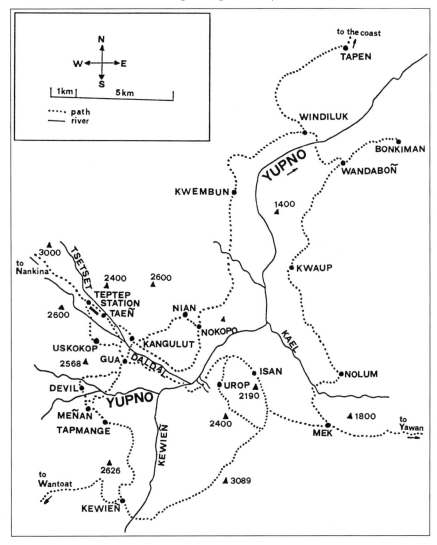

The Yupno form an autonomous group, despite cultural differences that become particularly manifest in the distinctions they draw between inhabitants of the lower and the upper valley, and despite linguistic and cultural similarities with some neighboring groups. Traditionally, however, they had no proper name for themselves. Younger people—especially if they dwell in towns—today call themselves Yupno to distinguish themselves from other ethnic groups (which they experience as firmly established entities in towns). Wurm and Hattori (1981) classify their language as Papuan, the "Yupna family," belonging to the "Finisterre-Huon Stock"; and subdivide this language family into nine dialects. Structurally, there are always two villages where the same dialect is spoken. The dialectal differences between these pairs of villages are very large and increase along with spatial distance. Many Yupno are multilingual, or at least can understand the people from the culturally-related Wantoat and Nankina region without being themselves able to speak their language.

In each case separated by a high pass, the neighboring groups of the upper Yupno, with whom they have trade relations (and partly also kinship links), are the Nankina to the northwest, the Wantoat to the southwest and the Orowa to the east. Owing a very high level of linguistic and social fragmentation, however, not all the Yupno villages are embedded in these relationships, which tend to be restricted to the respective neighboring settlements.

Until the early 1990s, the Yupno were to a large extent an undocumented ethnic group. An article by C. A. Schmitz (1958) was the only anthropological publication.[7] Other information on the Yupno, recorded in Patrol Reports and in annual reports from Tapen Mission station, is unpublished.

III

Gua, the village of little Nstasiñge, is situated on the left side of the Yupno River in a fertile side valley, about 6 kms long, on a northeastern slope. This valley is formed by the two rivers Tsetset, "the one split on both sides," and Daldal "the one which swirls [things in the water] around," which join below Gua and from there, as the River Daldal, flow into the Yupno further down. The other settlements in this side valley, whose inhabitants are closely connected to the Gua people, are Kangulut on the other side of the Daldal, Taeñ with Teptep station, and Uskokop, "upper place," which is on the same slope as Gua but higher and towards the northwest, and forms a single dialect group with Gua. All these places are between 20 and 45 minutes walking distance from Gua.

The name Gua[8] derives etymologically from *guam*, "centipede," an animal with special importance for the village. Today's Gua village, the "place of the centipede," is not a traditional settlement but, like all the other Yupno villages, a construction forced into being by the Lutheran Mission and the administration. In former times, the inhabitants lived at Gua-*mbema*, the "place next to the *mbe* tree," a fenced-in settlement which (in the ideal case) was divided into two parts: one half for the women, where women, children and unmarried youths lived, and the part of the men: where the men's house (also called *mbema*) and a house for religious objects were to be found. Within this

Illustration 2: The "official" part of Gua village (Gua 1)

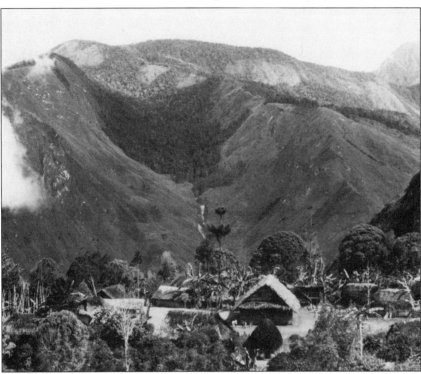

mbema, every kinship group lived in its own fenced-in section. The former Gua-*mbema* stood a bit below the actual village of Uskokop in the midst of a bamboo grove. Apart from this *mbema* (the central settlement around the men's house), each kinship group owned one or several houses in the garden- or bush-land, which they often inhabited over a long period of time. To the Neuendettelsau Lutheran Mission, this dispersed settlement pattern seemed to be an impediment to the realization of Christian communities, while the administration (or its representative, the Patrol Officer) took it to be a hindrance to economic and infrastructural development, including schools and health care, and to the development of political consciousness; and so the people were compelled—in the case of Gua, by armed force—to leave their traditional settlements (*mbema* and the bush- or garden-shed hamlets) and move into larger villages to facilitate missionary and administrative control.

The history of Gua village can be reconstructed with the help of Patrol Reports and Mission Reports as follows: the first visit to the Yupno Valley by an Australian government officer, L.G.Vial, took place in 1936. Starting out from

Wantoat, he marched through the valley, visiting Kewieñ and Isan[9] (Vial 1938). He did not meet the people who were later to move together into Gua village and who then lived in Gua-*mbema,* and nor did many of his successors, since this place lay somewhat away from the usual patrol route. There were no patrols during World War II. Biographies of older people in Gua show that the former inhabitants of Gua-*mbema* had moved down to the Yupno out of fear of the Japanese, who, during their short time in the Yupno Valley, shot at people and looted their gardens. Down by the river, the Yupno hid under cave-like cliffs for a long time. After the Japanese retreated, part of the population returned to Gua-*mbema,* which was slowly disintegrating, while a large kinship group split off and settled at Wamɨnoka, the "place of many tree-beetles."

In 1945, Patrol Officer M.W.S. Rylands first mentioned Gua, probably referring to the settlement of several houses at Wamɨnoka, which he spotted from Kewieñ, on the ridge of the mountain above present-day Gua: "9th [September]. Checked census. The deserted villages of GUA and NOKOPO can be seen across the valley on the MADANG side of the YUPNA. Natives are living in the bush and there is said to be dysentery" (Rylands 1945: 3).

In 1952, the inhabitants of Gua, to whom an evangelist from Finschhafen and from Kewieñ had been assigned, were pressured to found a village. The missionary K. Munsel, working at the Tapen mission station, writes about it:

> Two bigger villages [Gua and Teptep] are being built at present in the Gua plain and another one [Nian] above Nokopo on the suggestion of the government patrol officer, to gather the hundreds of scattered people who are living along the hill slopes. Prior to that our evangelists were successful in gathering the people of the village of Teptep. These, together with their fellowmen, who are still living in the forest, have recently also abandoned the things they had formerly used when employing magic and sorcery. They also have started with baptismal instruction (Munsel 1952: 4).

In June of the same year, A.D. Steven, the first Patrol Officer, visited the settlement of Gua (probably meaning: the enlarged settlement Wamɨnoka above present-day Gua) and took the first census (Steven 1952/53a). In November of the same year, he visited the settlement again, noting that, in addition to the construction of a settlement in Wamɨnoka, the inhabitants had also begun to build a new village, today's Gua, further down the hillside (Steven 1952/53b). During his next patrol in 1953, Steven noted:

> The three newly established villages NIAN, TEP TEP and GUA all showed large increases in population as a result of new names being

recorded. At GUA alone there were 82 new names. It is certain that all will not settle permanently in the village but given time most of them may be enticed in. GUA is now divided into two groups. Half the village has built on a new site nearer the floor of the valley. The other half is still living on a ridge 20 minutes above the new site.... Two recruiters were recently operating on the MOROBE District side of the YUPNA and eight men from GUA offered themselves for work in RABAUL (Stephen 1953/54: 5).

In 1953, therefore, a part of the population was living in Wamɨnoka ("on a ridge") and the other in present-day Gua ("nearer the floor of the valley"). Missionary work was showing results, as missionary H. D. Klemm, who substituted for missionary Munsel in Tapen, documented:

> A remarkable and joyful event was the first baptism in the Tetep [sic] Plain at the village Gua. It is hoped that the other four big catechumen classes in the Tetep Plain, which have shown very unsatisfactory results in their examinations every year, being encouraged by the example of the Gua people, will learn the Biblical stories with greater zeal and probably get ready for baptism in 1958 or in the beginning of 1959 (Klemm 1957: n.p.).

The construction of Gua village was finished toward the end of the 1950s. Two men were designated by the administrators to the function as official village representatives, a 'luluai' and a 'tultul'. Since 1976, they have been replaced by the 'komiti'.[10] For a time, Gua seemed to be accepted as a village by the people and also remained inhabited, as the following two excerpts indicate. "Gwar. Village found to be in good order..." (Nixon 1965/66: 2); "Thursday 27th February...1100 [sic] hours to Gua, a twenty minutes walk S.E. from Wasikokop [Uskokop] along valley side. Gua lined and censused 1130 hours and completed at 1300 hours" (Somers 1968/69: 3).

One year later, however, Patrol Officer F. X. Alcorta found the village deserted:

> Sunday 30th November.... Afternoon — Conducted census for TEPTEP, WASIKOKOP [Uskokop] and GUA. GUA was found completely deserted and overgrown with secondary growth. Const.1/c HOVIA was sent to surrounding bush with instructions to fetch people to TEPTEP. Read the riot act to Luluai and Tultul. No appearant reasons for preference of bush life over village life as there is plenty of fertile land available nearby. Conducted census and held talks. Very apathetic and surly hearing...Slept night TEPTEP. Monday 1st December. 0600 people from GUA returned to their village. It was re-

quested that they clear up their place and make it habitable again. A couple of small disputes settled arbitrarily (Alcorta 1969/70: 3).

With this entry, the available reports of missionaries and administrators on Gua end.

IV

Today, the settlement is divided into three village sections, sometimes called by the young people simply Gua 1, Gua 2 and Gua 3, which are situated a few minutes walk apart from one another, at between 1850 and 1970 m altitude. The village numbered 392 inhabitants in 1987. The settlement is almost completely surrounded by gardens, except that, to the southwest, a steep rock towers over the village, and below it the houses of Gua 3 crouch close to the rock face. The small hamlets consist of relatively compact groups of houses linked by little paths. Some of the dwelling houses that do not belong to these hamlets are surrounded with a fence, and stand quite isolated around the village.

Approaching the settlement from the direction of Teptep, across (the plain) Mbɨvɨka (1) "place of the broken-up ground" and Gomevɨlka (2) (no translation, where the garden land of little Nstasiñge's parents lies), directly before Gua 1 there is a "by-pass path" to the right via Gowañowa (3), "above below," and Gualbok (4) (no translation) up the hill to Kewieñ village and to the left between Gowañon (5), "below," Kokndekmon (6), the "toilet mountain," and Makumbaga (7), the "hill of the *makum* tree," down to the place Kangulut, as well as to the Yupno River. Straight ahead, one first enters the "official" section of the village, a leveled, plateau-shaped space where the church (A), a small trade store (C) and the houses of the teacher, the evangelists and some villagers stand. This area is known by the name Teetmevilgowañ (8), area "below the *teet* bamboo grove." Directly adjacent towards the mountain is Bapiayutyoma (9), the "school-fence," where the small 'tokples skul', the village school, stands (B). This official section of the village is very well cared for; unlike all the other sections, there are flower-beds in front of the houses and, on the otherwise totally uncovered ground (which turns to mud during the rainy season) there are a few lawns that are regularly cut. The empty space between the church and the trade store serves as a gathering ground for official events like church proclamations or the weekly meetings for the organization of the 'komyuniti de'.[11] Behind it, in Lepmonkwagɨlɨn (10), the "garden of a bare ass," the houses of the Gua people stand closely together; towards the mountain in Kaparɨkandom (11, where little Nstasiñge's house (D) is also situated), the "hill of the *kaparɨ* sweet potatoes," and Ngopmbaka (12), the

Chart 1: Gua Village

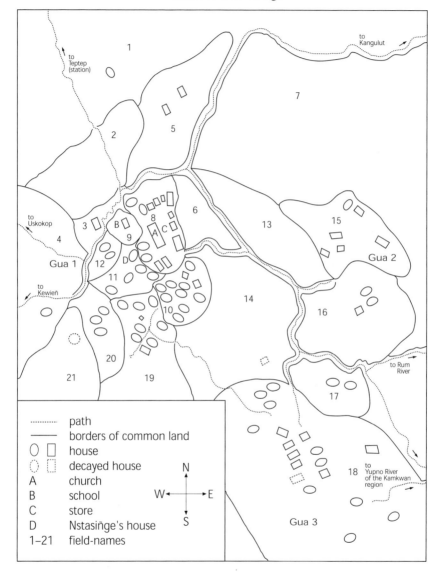

"place of many shelters," they are mostly fenced-in, as was formerly the custom. The footpaths in this area partly lead to the individual entrances, like sunken roads between high fences plaited from reed-like grass.

From this main place, namely Gua 1, a narrow, steep paths leads across a grassy plain, Lepmonkwagilin, the "garden of a bare ass" and through fields of

sweet potatoes, to Mpagmbekagowañ (14), the location "below the many
sources," to the hamlet Mpagmbewoñok (15), the "place of the emerging lake,"
a fenced-in group of houses where single dwellings are in turn surrounded by a
second fence. The houses of this hamlet, Gua 2, do not stand as closely together
as those in Gua 1; there are trees between them, barren ground or smallish gardens. Just before Mpagmebwoñok, the path leads further down and forks off:
the left path leads past Jogakluk (16), the "place of the *jogak* tree crowns," and
the little hill Sindalin (17), the "place with a view," past the water hole of Gua at
the River Rum and on to the warmest and lowest area, Kamkwam, the "place
where everything grows fast," that is, the large garden area of Gua, then further
on down to the Yupno river and up towards Isan village; the other path leads
through a bamboo grove to the village sector Mundogon (Gua 3) (18), the region of the "falling rocks," a settlement with two rows of houses surrounded by
other relatively scattered houses. Mundogon lies in a gully directly below the steep
mountain cliff towering over Gua. From Mundogon, in turn, a steep path leads
through a bamboo grove to the eastern part of the main place Gua 1, to Mundagalgowañ (19) (no translation) and Njapnjapilin (20), the "slope of the many *njapnjap* plants," a small group of houses that are counted in with the main village,
Gua 1. Behind this group of houses, higher up the steep mountain, is the cemetery of Gua, Siñgoronbaga (20), the "cemetery hill." From here one can return to
the main place within five minutes. The round trip takes about 25 minutes.

V

Many foreign visitors have been attracted by the traditional Yupno houses,
the *tedetedetyut*, "houses in circles," which they have labelled variously: from
the dull unimaginative "bee-hive hut with an oval ground-plan" (Schmitz
1958: 346) to a more vivid "igloo type houses" (Hanrahan 1955/56: 7) or "like
a small haystack" (Dyer 1955/56: 6). These houses are constructed by sticking
thin poles into the ground in an oval, then linking them with vines in circles
(*tedet*) that become narrower towards the top; the ridge pole is added and all
of it is covered with a thick layer of dried 'tiktik' grass, which forms the outer
skin. This method offers several advantages:

- the Yupno live in an environment with little wood; for the construction
  of a house of this sort, no thick trunks are necessary, thus obviating their
  cutting and transport over a long distance, which would be an extremely
  tedious endeavor and would further decimate the scarce supply.
- The houses are highly windproof and warm and therefore optimally
  adapted to the cold and often humid highland climate.

- Because of their self-supporting construction, they are relatively earth-quake-proof in a region where earth tremors or earthquakes occur repeatedly.
- Finally, the construction time for such a house is short.

However, one disadvantage is that these houses catch fire easily and thereby can become a trap for their inhabitants. Through a low, narrow entrance, traditionally closed with pandanus leaves as well as some sticks (and today often with a door and a padlock),[12] one reaches a small ante-room at ground level. Separated by a bamboo-plaited dividing wall from the main room, this is where gardening tools, household utensils and sometimes firewood are kept. From here, people climb via a tree-fork or ladder into the dome-shaped main room. Its floor consists of a plaited bamboo platform elevated about one meter above the floor, and in its middle an elongated fireplace is suspended. Above this fireplace, along the whole length, hangs a wooden rack on which different things are dried: firewood, but mainly plant seeds, split bamboo pipes and *bumbum*-bundles made out of reed grass, which serve as torches and lighters. Along the walls to the right and left of the fireplace, the smoked nuts of the pandanus palm are kept in large sausage-shaped plaited *bumum*-baskets (up to four meters long). These houses differ in length and height, but the largest of them will easily accommodate 60 people.

The other type of house found in Gua, called *mbumbumayut*, "wrapper house," is a rectangular gabled house. The Yupno consider these houses to be more modern, but they are smaller, colder and much more difficult to construct than the traditional dwellings. Of the 72 houses in Gua, 46 have been built in the traditional oval style and 26 as rectangular gabled houses.

As a rule, a house is inhabited today by a nuclear family, meaning that parents and their children form a household to which adopted children may also belong. Depending on the family situation, unmarried female siblings and widowed parents or those needing care also live in this household. Added to them are single women whose husbands work in town. They have no permanent residence but spend months at a time with one or another related family.

VI

Apart from this village-house, every family, especially the ones whose garden-land lies far from the village, owns a fenced-in garden- or bush-house, built in traditional or modern style, where its members spend the night dur-

Illustration 3: A traditional Yupno house

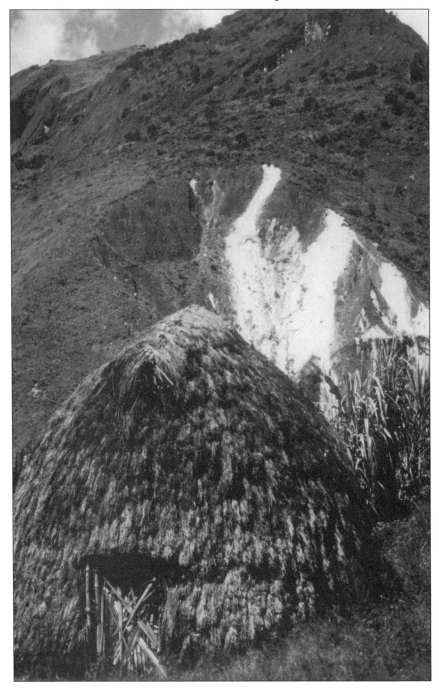

Illustration 4: Evening in a dwelling-house

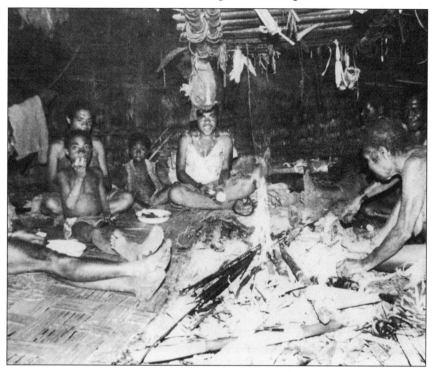

ing planting time or when doing other work in the gardens. It also serves as a possible refuge if someone temporarily or permanently wishes to avoid contact with the village community, a tendency noticeable mainly in older people in order to avoid pressure by the mission or other modern influences. Most of these garden-houses are situated in Kamkwam, the "place where everything grows fast," i.e. the large slope that stretches south of Gua to the Yupno River, a flat plain of big gardens, in which many mythologically important locations are to be found: certain small rivulets, which originated from the Yupno, as well as bamboo groves with special kinds of bamboo which the river washed ashore at the time of creation. Since the region lies somewhat lower than Gua and is therefore warmer climatically, small quantities of plants like yams and papaya can be cultivated there. On "normal" days (with no market in Teptep or other obligations), two thirds of the Gua population are certain to spend the day in Kamkwam. The smaller region north of Gua, in contrast, is less intensively used by the Gua people; here, a few gardens are owned by inhabitants of Uskokop.

The Gua people mainly subsist on the cultivation of sweet potatoes, potatoes (to a smaller extent also taro and, less frequently, yams), bananas, sugar cane and different native and European vegetables ('pitpit', *kwawɨl*, pumpkin, cabbage, onions, beans).[13] This food is supplemented by the gathering of certain wild plants. Also, large amounts of pandanus nuts are collected at harvest time and their kernels are later smoked on racks that hang above fireplaces. As part of an agricultural Lutheran development project, some people, mainly younger ones, also grow cash crops: coffee, European vegetables such as spring onions, cucumbers, carrots, radishes, cauliflower, silver beet and garlic, which are marketed in Teptep, the nearest station and the only airfield. The cash-crop produce is hardly ever eaten by the producers, since it is "foreign" and therefore can only be incorporated into the traditional concept of nutrition[14] with difficulty. People certainly know how these plants have to be cultivated but not whether they are eaten raw or cooked or roasted.

Hunting plays only a minor role in Gua, since the village is situated several hours on foot from the actual hunting grounds in the dense highland forest. When men, with their hunting dogs, set out to hunt, their main quarry is typically marsupials and birds. Every family owns pigs, but these are killed only on special occasions: for a brideprice, at a death, or as payment of compensation. They are kept in pens outside the village and fed once or twice a day. Smaller piglets often sleep with the family in the house, then in the mornings are tied to a rope by the women and dragged along to the gardens, where they are tethered on an uncultivated plot. Since there are frequent fights because of escaping pigs despoiling other peoples' gardens, Gua village is surrounded by a bamboo fence as well as by planted *umban* (Cordyline) on the sides facing Kamkwam, the "place where everything grows fast" and Gualbok, where many pigs are also kept. The fence intersects the footpath, and must be crossed via forked branch.

Almost all garden work (making a new plot, digging, planting, loosening the ground and harvesting) is done by the women. The men help to cut down trees (when new gardens are made) and assist with the clearing; and today they are also responsible for the construction of houses and fences and for the cutting of firewood. Looking after the pigs is wholly women's work, besides household tasks and cooking, as is the cutting of *bumbum* (the reed-like grass already mentioned) which is used in bundles as lighters, torches and often the only source of light in the house, as well as the fetching of water, which is poured into large bamboo pipes at the sources of the Rum or other small streams in the neighborhood, and is often carried to the houses over long distances.

2. Social Organization

I

The Yupno are divided into *jalap*, a term that has two major connotations. It can mean "entry" or "entrance in a fence" and refers to the traditional settlement pattern *mbema*, the "fenced-in place," where the different kinship groups lived in fenced-in small hamlets and every group had its own entrance, or *jalap*, to the area. These hamlets in turn consisted of separately fenced-in family farmsteads, *yɨmakon*. The term *jalap* can also mean the community living inside this fence, the people who can be reached through this common entrance. This group of males and females is residential, and its membership is regulated through patrilineal descent, exogamy and common land ownership.

Not all *jalap* (kin groups) are able to name their mythical founder (which, in many definitions of "clan" is a postulated criterion), but they, nonetheless, have a notion (often vague) of their common mythological descent, and of their place of origin, which almost always lies in a bamboo grove, and they have a definite feeling of solidarity, so such groups can be fairly labeled 'clans'. Each *jalap* comprises one or several lineages, which can prove their descent from a known but not always named ancestor but seldom comprise more than four generations and have no proper name. To put it differently: some *jalap* consist of several lineages on the same level, whereas others are only represented in one lineage. The concepts "clan" and "lineage," which are on different categorical levels, and are formed by using different criteria, thus coincide in these *jalap*. If a *jalap* is only represented by a very small lineage, for example by only two men and their families, it often cannot act out its social duties any longer, and so it attaches itself to another clan. Following this same principle, smaller lineages immigrating into Yupno territory were absorbed into already resident clans. However, the opposite case is also possible: lineages that are too large split up, either within a *jalap* into new lineages, or else the *jalap* itself is subdivided into several clans.

Today there are ten clans in Gua:

- the largest clan Talon, represented in many lineages, is the group that lives at the "slope of the *ta* tree"; two lineages of this Talon-*jalap* live in the neighboring village of Uskokop. The Talon originally came from Arop Island (Long Island, cf. Map 1). The ancestor Sopm left Arop, stayed briefly on the coast at the river, Panjewik, and then wandered up the Yupno via Kwembun to Kangulut where he founded a settlement on the piece of land called Pɨragon. Later this group, his descendants, moved across the river Daldal to the already resident Mam-

bap people (see below) who offered land to the group, called Mambapbaga, the "hill near the big ginger," in order to found Gua-*mbema*
together (situated below today's village of Uskokop).

- The clearly smaller *jalap* Tuwal I, Tuwal II and Tuwal III, represented
  by one to three lineages, are an example for the above-mentioned fis-
  sion of a larger clan into several smaller clans. The name Tuwal means
  "keel, spit of land," and as their place of origin the Tuwal people name
  the piece of land Salimbaga, the "hill where the *sal* tree grows." Little
  Nstasiñge belongs to the Tuwal I clan.
- The following clans are represented by only one or two lineages:
- the clan Umban, "Cordyline-plant," gives as place of origin Gualbok,
  the region above Gua.
- The clan Ngandum, the people from the "hill of the pandanus trees,"
  claims as its place of origin Guagowañ, "below Gua-*mbema*," a piece of
  land below Uskokop village.
- The clan Komin, the people of the "*komin* tree," originates from the
  area Eka, "landslide," situated below Gua-*mbema*.
- The clan Kapbaga, the people with the "head-covering," gives as its
  place of origin Ekatuwal, "sliding spit of land."
- The clan Mambap, the people from the "big ginger plant," today a
  minor clan, is held to be the first and oldest *jalap* in Gua, originating
  from Mambapgowañ, "below the big ginger plant."
- The clan Ngangalbuk, "those who come from far away," originally from
  the Nankina region to the Northwest, from the village of Sap. Some
  generations ago, it settled first at Devil and found permanent residence
  there by a marriage into the Gua-*mbema*.

While the Talon and Ngangalbuk clans are clearly immigrant groups, the origin of the other clans remains a mystery. Some of them have definitely immigrated within the past five to eight generations.[15] It is therefore conceivable, as
Schmitz (1960b: 51) writes of the neighboring Wantoat, that the Yupno immi-
grants, too, either took possession of an already existing bamboo grove or else
planted a new bamboo grove and thereby created a new place of origin, and that
this taking possession or new planting, then, was lost to memory over generations, perhaps for ideological reasons, and that the descendants think of themselves with reference to this bamboo grove as "always having been here." Thus
the clans of today's Gua are not kinship groups that have been resident for cen-
turies and possess a long continuous tradition, but are relatively recent groups.

Before the arrival of the mission, all these clans lived in the Gua-*mbema*,
even though at times they also inhabited their scattered garden houses.

Today, garden land can be loaned, since not all the clans either originally had rights to land or else small and declining clans disposed of land to growing, land-poor clans. With population increase and intensified horticulture for cash crops, land for cultivation is slowly becoming scarce in Gua, a trend of which the younger men, especially, are aware. If land is "loaned" over several generations and if the descendants of the "borrower" come to think of themselves as the owners, this often leads to bitter land disputes, which may be taken as far as the 'kiap'.

II

There is a special relationship between two clans that form a unit. This paired relationship is called *ngapma ngapma* (from *ngampa*, "deep hole") and means the indissolubility of this especially close relationship as well as the stability of the arrangement, just like a deep hole from which one cannot escape and where everything thrown down into it stays forever. Each clan has its *ngapma*, "partner clan," and combined they face each other as *ngapma ngapma*. This special relationship of paired clans was established by the common mythological origin of its founders: a bamboo pipe washed up by the Yupno River burst and set free the two first clan members. As a rule, this pair of clans was exogamous. Just as by birth and the principle of patrilinearity one is born into a clan, simultaneously with clan membership one also receives a *ngapma*-connection. In former times, in the Gua-*mbema*, the clan settled directly adjacent to its partner clan, its *ngapma*. Today, this settlement pattern has been abandoned, but every *jalap* tries at least to live together with its relatives of the same lineage and the members of the other lineages in its clan. This principle of a *jalap* as a cohabiting unit living on its own land has not been followed through in Gua either, but when new houses are constructed today there is discussion about where depending on the owner's clan-membership this house "actually" should be standing, and there is a detectable tendency to adhere to this principle more strictly. This could mean a slow dissolution for Gua 1, where most of the clans have settled on land not belonging to them.

Before missionization, the *ngapma ngapma*-relationship was of major importance during male initiation and in fights against other hamlets. Today, it still plays a role in relation to brideprice, the distribution of land, and in cases of sickness and death. The special characteristic of this relationship is the reciprocity that is entailed; thus, in former times in the men's house *yut bap*, ("big house"), the *ngapma ngapma* exchanged food and betel nuts in differently shaped special bowls, with one partner clan owning longish bowls, and the other round bowls.

On the one hand, the *ngapma ngapma* stand opposite each other as two *jalap*, two groups; on the other hand, this relationship is not only kept up by the clan as a group towards the other partner clan, the *ngapma*, but also between the individuals of these clans. This relationship, however, is far more important to men, because of domains like initiation and brideprice (and sickness-inducing activities linked with it) than to women. Each man from a clan looks upon the individual male members of his partner clan as *ngapma*. In former times, the *ngapma ngapma*-connection was primarily a collective relationship; today, in contrast, this relationship (since initiation and fighting have been given up) stands on a much more individual basis. Every individual is continuously conscious that this partner relationship cannot be dissolved, but it becomes outwardly manifest only in activities which can solely be undertaken in common.

The clans forming a *ngapma ngapma*-relationship in Gua are:

- Tuwal I and Umban
- Tuwal II and Ngandum (including Komin and Kapbaga)
- Tuwal III and Ngangalbuk
- Talon and Mambap.

The two clans, Komin and Kapbaga, were formerly connected as a *ngapma ngapma*, but have joined the Ngandum. Their membership had sunk so low that they were no longer able to conduct the *ngapma ngapma*-activities on their own. Together with the Ngandum people, they now have as a common *ngapma* the Tuwal II clan. Since the small Tuwal I clan, little Nstasiñge's clan, has as a *ngapma* the Umban clan, which is also not very numerous, it tends to join the Tuwal II clan for brideprices, and together they look upon the Umban, Ngandum, Komin and Kapbaga as *ngapma*. Depending upon the context, there are thus three or four pairs of clans in Gua.

In conclusion, Yupno social organization is based on clans (*jalap*), "openings in the fence," groups of people who used to live within one fence because of their kinship origin. Within this fence, the individual families lived in single homesteads, which are also fenced. Two clans at a time are linked by a *ngapma ngapma*-connection, which is founded on a common mythical origin and which today, in contrast to the formerly more collective emphasis, stands on a predominantly individual level. The existence of surprisingly large villages, going back to the politics of mission and administration, is deceptive in that the basic unit of social organization above the level of the family is the clan, whose members typically lived, and still live, in scattered garden houses.

3. The Kinship System and Brideprice

I

The Yupno kinship system is centered on the principle of patrilineal descent. A (male) Ego calls all the members of his clan (*jalap*), *nut* (I),[16] a term encompassing the largest group, regardless of whether this clan is represented in one or several lineages. *Nut* or *nutno*, "my *nut*," is also frequently used outside of this kinship context for 'wantok'.[17] The male members of one's own patriline (FaBr, FaFaBrSo) and patrilateral kin (FaFaSiSo) in the first ascending generation are lumped together as *waunyi;* if a single person is referred to, it is *wauno*, my *wau. Wau* also means a name-sharing relationship between two people, "the one with the same name" or a "namesake," an (older) person who has to fulfill certain duties towards his *wau*, the (younger) "namesake," who is always in the generation below. A *wau* should from time to time present gifts to his younger *wau*, today help him raise his school fees, substantially collaborate in the first wearing of the *nsaguo*-wheel of feathers (the large dance-decoration, cf. Chapter 3.3.), organize and finance the feast connected with it, and give special brideprice gifts to the mother of the future wife of his younger *wau*. In short, the *wau* accompanies the growth of his younger *wau* with permanent attentiveness and by discharging special responsibilities. On these terms, *waunyi*, owing to the system of name-giving (cf. Chapter 3.3.), means potential *wau*. Since these persons are all male relatives of Ego's father, *nan*, they are also called *nanjok*, "little fathers." The wives of these "little fathers" (FaBrWi, FaFaBrSoWi, FaFaSiSoWi) are called *meñ*, like one's own mother. Father's sister (FaSi) and also FaFaSiDa and FaFaBrDa are called *mami*, the "nameless." The husbands of these "nameless" are the *murum*, "the cool ones." The "nameless," the "cool ones" and their descendants as a group are called *maminyi*, the "group of the *mami*" (II).

Ego's matrilateral kin are called *pek* (III). The mother and mother's sister are called *meñ*, their husbands (Fa and MoSiHu) *nan*. Mother's brother is *a* or *ano*, "my *a*." All of a male Ego's patri- and matrilineal relatives of the second ascending generation, his grandparents on the father's and the mother's side, are called—as men—*mbawo* (no translation) and—as women—*owa* (no translation). All the grandchildren of either sex in the patriline, i.e., persons in the second descending generation, are also called *mbawo*. Ego calls his brothers and parallel cousins in the patrilineage (Br, FaBrSo) *pe*, but the elder brother is more specifically called *patogo* (both terms without translation). Their wives are *waunomi*, "mother of my (potential) *wau*" (see above). *Sami n* (no translation) is used for the sisters (Si) and parallel-cousins (FaBrDa) in the patriline. Patri- and matrilineal cross-cousins (FaSiSo, FaSiDa, MoBrSo,

Figure 1: The Kinship System

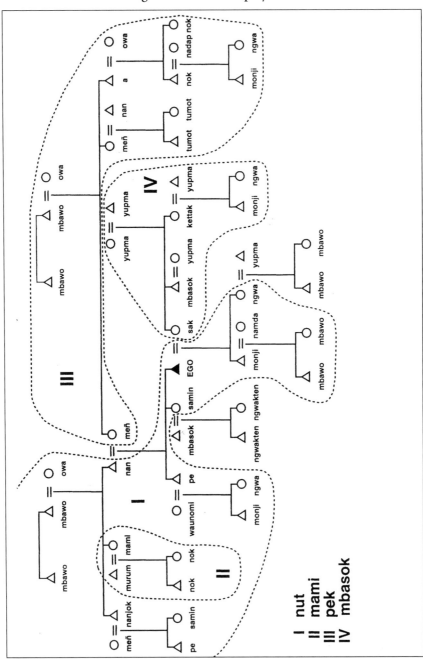

MoBrDa), plus persons in Ego's generation related to him via the patrilateral grandparents and his matrilateral parallel-cousins (MoSiSo, MoSiDa) are the *nok*. The matrilateral parallel-cousins (MoSiSo, MoSiDa) can also be called *tumot*. Ego calls the marriage partners of a male *nok*, i.e., their wives, *nadap* (no translation), and the marriage partners of a female *nok*, i.e., their husbands and the husbands of his sisters, *mbasok* (no translation).

One's own sons as well as the brothers' sons and the *nok*'s are *monji*, "the small ones"; one's own daughters, brothers' daughters and *nok*'s, in contrast, are *ngwa* (no translation). If they are children of a *waunomi*, a "mother of my *wau*" (BrWi), they are correspondingly also called *wau* since they are potential *wau*, "namesake-children," for Ego. The wives of the "small ones" are *namda* (no translation), and the husbands of the women are called *ngwa* are *yupma* (no translation).

Ego's sister's children, since they do not belong to Ego's clan, are called *ngwakten* (no translation), their male marriage partner is *kamɨt* (no translation), and the female marriage partner *namda* (no translation).

At Ego's wedding, his patriline *wau* and his maternal kin group *pek* are joined by a third group, the relatives of his wife *sak* whom he calls, as a group, by the term *mbasok* (no translation) (IV). Ego's patrilineal relatives and especially his parents *meññan*, "mother-father," in contrast, call this kin group newly joined by marriage *kasok* (see below), the term used for the money transferred as a brideprice, which this group receives. The parents of his wife as well as her brother's wife Ego calls *yupma* (no translation), his wife's sisters (WiSi) are *kettak* (no translation), their husbands (WiSiHu) and her brother (WiBr) *mbasok*. The children of his wife's sisters (WiSiCh) are *monji* (the sons) and *ngwa* (the daughters).[18]

II

Regarding the formerly existing system of marriage rules, I could ascertain only that women normally came from other *mbema*, "fenced-in areas," the traditional settlement units, and that a clan and its partner clan (i.e. the two *ngapma ngapma*) formed an exogamous unit. Looking at the kinship terminology, it is surprising that mother's sisters' husbands (MoSiHu) are called *nan*, father, even though they are from different clans (today at least), and that the children of mother's sister's son (MoSiSoSo, MoSiSoDa) are called *wau*, a term reserved for members of Ego's patriline. This can be explained upon consideration[19] that, formerly, there had been marriage rules according to which the men of one clan could take their wives only from one specific other clan. The children and grandchildren of these anomalous *nan* would thereby belong to the same clan as Ego, as to be expected. Of course, according to this logic the wife's sisters (WiSi) would have to be called by the same name as the brothers' wives (BrWi), which, however, is not the case.

From the kinship system, yet another marriage preference becomes clear: the exchange of sisters. It is striking that, disregarding this preference, the terms for totally different persons are the same: sister's husband (SiHu) and wife's brother (WiBr) are both called *mbasok* by a male Ego, husband's sister (HuSi) and brother's wife (BrWi) are called *maniok* by a female Ego. In the case of an exchange of sisters (or an exchange of brothers respectively), these persons are identical. Owing to the lack of present-day information, both considerations concerning a system of prescriptive marriage rules have to remain hypothetical.

III

The kinship system has been presented in detail for a very important reason: every illness is closely connected with the kinship relations and the family situation of the patient in question, and can only be understood against this background. Avoidance rules also form a part of the domain of concepts of illness. Thus there is still a quite strictly observed avoidance taboo (concerning a male Ego) in connection with three kinship positions: *nadap* (the wives of the cross-cousin *nok*, FaSiSoWi, MoBrSoWi), *kettak* (WiSi) and *yupma* (WiFa, WiMo, WiBrWi, DaHu, BrDaHu). In no case may people in such a relationship have close contact; they may not sit next to each other in the house, or touch or offer anything to each other (e.g. betel nuts). If by accident physical contact should occur between them; for example, if somebody enters a dark house and sits down without first making sure who is sitting next to him, the offender will feel *miyaga*, "shame," and will recompense the "victim" of this thoughtless act with a pig, money and betel nuts, and the victim, some time later, will reciprocate in like manner to the offender. By this exchange, the deed is at least mitigated and there are no lasting consequences. Also, no one else may touch both these people at the same time and thereby indirectly create contact between them.

The consequence of a breach of this avoidance taboo is socially expressed as an illness: both will get swollen knees and, in the worst case, lose the ability to walk. There is no cure against this illness. This is why, in a strange house and before sitting down or passing something to somebody, one asks as a precaution: "*yupma bo nadap yikndak bo ndɨma?*" "sits [in this house] a *yupma* or a *nadap* or not?" Any such person present would answer "I am here," and then both can keep their distance accordingly.

All of the three kinship terms *kettak*, *yupma* and *nadap* indicate affinal relatives, people incorporated into a kinship group through marriage. This extension of kinship through marriage is extremely important for the Yupno, because of resulting pathogenic conflicts over the presentations of brideprice, and therefore the brideprice will now be described in detail.

IV

For the Yupno, the most important event in which the whole village generally participates is the transfer of the brideprice, *aññok*, "to prepare food [and give it away]." The brideprice goes to the relatives (clan and partner clan) of the wife, who at a later date will return part of the gifts received. This restitution is called *pelok*, "can you [give back]?." Should the transfer of a brideprice not be correctly executed and should somebody feel left out (at the brideprice transfer, *aññok*, a member of the wife's group; at the restitution, *pelok*, a member of the husband's group), this frequently causes bitter conflict involving all the participants, which can manifest itself in sickness, often years after the actual brideprice event.

How important the brideprice is to the Yupno is documented in numerous biographies and illness narratives, where this topic is mentioned as a constant, be it a wedding, i.e., one's own experience of brideprice, or a brideprice where one assisted or should have received something. For the Yupno, brideprice transfers also serve as a measure of time: "at the time when we bought a wife for X, the Japanese (or the missionary Y, etc.) came," are common ways of speaking.

Brideprices, even if transferred years before, are the subject of many heated debates, and their exact amount as well as the names of the participants (both donors and recipients) are remembered for generations. Because of the high importance the Yupno attach to the brideprices, which are often the cardinal points in the search for causes of illness, a detailed description of *aññok* is now given. The main participants of a brideprice transfer are the groom's clan and his partner clan as the donating group and the bride's clan plus her partner clan as the receiving group. Both groups call each other, although at different times, *kasok*, after the name of the money, which is attached to bamboo-sticks;[20] the first *kasok*-group is the recipient of the brideprice *aññok*, the subsequent *kasok*-group is the recipient of the retribution, the *pelok*. The protagonists (from the Western viewpoint, the future marriage-partners) step into the background as individuals at the brideprice transfer, and play a role only as representatives of two clans. Their wedding is arranged and organized by their paternal relatives, who do not consult with them, and they themselves "officially" do not know of the planned event for a very long time. I participated in brideprice transfers where the groom was either staying in town and was to be surprised with his completed wedding after his return or else where the groom, out of horror, fear or shame, had fled into the bush for a few days.

People are married between the ages of sixteen to twenty years, often before the young develop an interest in the opposite sex and start having relationships. Thus marriage also serves as a kind of prophylaxis against forbidden sexual relations and, above all, its result, a pregnancy, which often causes
pathogenic conflicts. This only solves the problem of forbidden sexual relations officially, "on the outside," since many young men who have been married to a partner against their will, whom they do not really like, are carrying
on love affairs with unmarried girls. As long as affairs among young unmarried people are discreet and without consequences such as pregnancies, they
are tolerated, though in the couple's peer group they may be the subject of
many gibes.

It is the responsibility of the father's brother of the future groom to look for
a suitable young woman. His choice depends on several interconnected criteria.

- The woman should be qualified, i.e., industrious, able to cultivate a
  garden properly, to look after the pigs well and also be young, healthy
  and sociable; the husband's clan expects a capable new member who
  moreover will help guarantee its continuity by bearing children.
- Even though there are no definite marriage relations[21] between the villages, and marriages also take place within a village, a bride's place of
  origin is nevertheless important: if, for example, one or several elder
  sisters of a groom from Gua were married into a clan of the neighboring village of Uskokop, it is customary that a woman from there marries, "as an exchange," a man in Gua, a relative of the sisters. The
  chances of the father's brother agreeing to such a wedding are therefore good. Should the groom's mother already come from Uskokop and
  if, in the meantime, no women of the groom's clan have been married
  to Uskokop, the chances are poor. The Uskokop will not want to continue such a one-sided relationship in which their gift of daughters to
  Gua men is not reciprocated with Gua women.
- If the bride's mother's brideprice was very high, her own brideprice is
  also put very high since now the people who assisted in "paying" for
  her mother have a claim to the brideprice of the mother; the father's
  brother of the groom thus must consider whether such a high brideprice can be raised by his clan and his partner clan after all.
- The amount of the brideprice is also partly determined by the size of
  the woman's clan and her partner clan (the rightful recipients, the *mbasok*) as well as by the size of her husband's clan and his partner clan
  (the donors, the *kasok*), and a high brideprice *aññok* also means a correspondingly high restitution *pelok*.

Brideprices carry a lot of prestige. Even though they are "calculated," they are not given close-fistedly and are reminiscent of the potlatch of the North American Indians of the northwest coast with respect to self-presentation and power of the groom's clan and partner clan. Meagre brideprices ruin not only the reputation of the clan but that of the whole village as well. The brideprice transfer is also not looked upon as a "payment" or "sale of the woman," but as the gift of a valuable, esteemed member of a kinship group with whom one only reluctantly parts (and who one does not want to get rid of at a profit) to another kinship group, with the aim of helping insure its continuity. Accordingly, it is expected that, in compensation at a later date, this kinship group will help one's own clan in the same way through a reciprocal wedding. Thus the woman is not primarily thought of as a "new labourer" but as the mother of future children, who are then looked upon by the husband's clan as the "products" of this brideprice—and to a certain extent as property.[22] Once the choice is made, the father's brother of the groom contacts the father's brother of the bride or a man of his partner clan (*ngapma*). He in turn discusses with his male relatives how high the required brideprice should be. This price (as mentioned above) depends on how high the bride's mother's brideprice was, i.e. how many people formerly assisted the father of the bride to buy his wife and therefore now have a claim to the brideprice of the "product" of this purchase, the bride.

How important the brideprice is to the Yupno can also be judged from its size. An observation by the administrator Neal in the 1950s shows that it has not inflationarily increased in recent times because of the introduction of Western money but had been very substantial traditionally:

> Bride price throughout the area is extremely high, varying according to the choice of bride and also to the wealth of the bridegroom's family. It is not uncommon, however, for the exchange of gifts to exceed the value of fifty pounds. At one such wedding in the Yupna valley recently the following articles were exchanged, eight pigs, varying from one to three years in age, twenty five new earthenware saucepans, eight long strings of Siassi beads, highly valued in the area, over thirty net bags, each filled with leaf tobacco and betel nut, a dozen new bark loin cloths, dogs', oppossums' and flying foxes' teeth and black cockatoo feathers, highly valued in the local traditional singsing. Finally ten new bows and between ten and fifteen arrows with each. On top of all this a large quantity of food was distributed at the same time as the wedding took place (Neal 1954/55: 6–7).

On average,[23] the brideprices recorded by me between 1986 and 1988 consisted of at least 20 (and at the most 30) fully-grown butchered pigs, some live piglets and, apart from other gifts, of at least 200–300 Kina in cash.

To every potential brideprice recipient a little stick (*njul*, no translation) is ascribed. This means that a man from the woman's kin group will receive a butchered pig (including money and several store-bought goods) at her brideprice. Should a claimant to the brideprice with whom there are also perhaps bad connections be "forgotten" or left out on purpose, he may be angered enough to later cause illness, which most often affects the newlyweds' child. These little sticks, *njul*, are counted, bundled together and given to the father's brother of the bridegroom. Together with his relatives, he in turn now counts the sticks, and in this way learns how many pigs the other party expects and can then calculate how many pigs he and his group must procure for this brideprice. He discusses it with his relatives and together they ponder over which man (even from another clan) still has debts because he in turn was helped with the brideprice for his wife or for a son, or who at the time owns a suitable pig and would contribute it—to be compensated later. This group of pig suppliers is called *tinyikabɨ*, "some good [people]." All the clans of a village are woven into this net of interdependencies through a brideprice, and the more a man is enmeshed, that is, the more people owe him something or vice versa, the more far-reaching are his social relations and the more strongly is he socially integrated and actively participating in village events. This is a desired state, which is prolonged by new debts or credits given again and again. The amount of the reciprocal debts and credits is recorded in people's memories over generations. Everyone who wants to assist in this brideprice (or is pressured to do so) breaks such a *njul* stick in two: thereby he is bound to give a pig. When all the sticks are broken, the brideprice is theoretically held to be guaranteed. A special role falls to the older "namesake" (*wau*) of the bridegroom: helped by assistants, he prepares a special gift, *meñi kong*, "for the eyes of the mother," to the bride's mother, who should be especially compensated for her efforts and pains taken while raising her daughter.

During this preparatory phase, a member of the partner clan or the father's brother of the bride himself will repeatedly come to the bridegroom's village "completely by chance" and inquire about the state of affairs, the number of broken sticks. Once it becomes obvious that the brideprice can be raised, the trial period for the bride begins. Suddenly, one night, male relatives from the bridegroom's clan and his partner clan enter the bride's house and take her, often against her and her mother's[24] fierce resistance, to the house of her future father-in-law. Earlier, the bridegroom had been induced, on often vague pretexts, to go and sleep in another house[25] for the time being.

The next morning, the bride publicly receives a large number of grass skirts, net bags, blouses, pieces of cloth, soap, biscuits and some money from the female relatives (from the clan and the partner clan) of the groom. During this presentation, the bride stands in front of her future father-in-law's house, encircled by the women, who bring their gifts. Men watch as spectators from a distance. One woman, most often the wife of the father's brother, receives the gifts, calls out the name of the donor and puts everything on a big heap, counting exactly how many grass skirts, net bags and so on each woman contributed and how much the total is. Once everything is heaped up, the bride has to wear as many grass skirts as possible (up to ten) on top of one another, as well as several pieces of cloth; then the grass skirts are fitted, that is, cut knee-high. Finally, all the heaped up gifts are hastily stuffed into net bags by the bride and her future sisters-in-law and carried into the father-in-law's house. This concludes the first part of the brideprice transfer, *añgumgumañ*, "to soothe." The bride is meant to be "soothed" or calmed down and "made welcome," as she has in most cases been taken by surprise (and, depending upon the circumstances, is also saddened or furious) when put into this new situation. Women from other kinship groups may also make contributions to these "arrival gift"; as with the actual brideprice, there is a network of dependencies, gifts and countergifts that includes all the women in the village. From this perspective, the prelude to the brideprice can be interpreted as a system of exchange reserved for the women alone—a female counterpart to the more male-dominated formal brideprice transfer. Details of these transactions are also stored in the people's memories for generations.

A share of the many grass skirts, net bags and so on will be kept by the bride for herself. She gives a further share to the relatives of her paternal clan, and yet another share is kept for the next brideprice of her "new" clan (her husband's), when she will then give net bags and grass skirts to the "new wife" as a gift of welcome. Many such gifts, therefore, are not personally worn or used but are redistributed again and again in a constant cycle.

During the next period, which can last between two weeks and three months, the bride stays in the household of her parents-in-law. From my talks with various women, it became obvious that this time was, for many (especially those from other villages), the worst of their lives because they felt totally isolated, and for the first time torn from their familiar surroundings, facing the prospect of a wedding to a virtual stranger, or to a man known but not liked. During this time, conversation between the future marriage partners is taboo and they must avoid each other (if the bridegroom is present at all). Many women abscond during this interval and return to their parents, who almost always take their daughter back to the house of her future parents-in-law.

After the trial period has been successfully completed, the actual brideprice transfer takes place. The father's brother fixes the date, and the killing of the pigs begins. For this purpose, they are tethered close to the garden houses and killed with an arrow shot through their heart. The woman who raised the pig in question mourns it vehemently and keeps its tail as a memento. Then the bristles are scorched and the pig is completely disemboweled. Its body is cut lengthwise into four to six portions, which are tightly bound with vines. At the same time, a big earth oven is prepared in a dug-out hollow. First, stones are heated in a big fire and a portion of them carefully lifted out. Banana leaves are laid on the hot stones in the hollow, then the bundled pieces of meat are put on the top of them, then the pig's head, a thick layer of leaves, the remaining stones and more banana leaves. After a few hours, the cooked meat is carried into the houses. During the killing of the pigs (which lasts two to three days), a relative of the bride's partner clan or her father's brother comes and watches the preparations.

On the set date, a rack of bamboo pipes is erected in front or near to of the bridegroom's father's house, with a number of vertical sticks corresponding to the pigs to which the money sticks will be attached (e.g. 22 pigs = 22 vertical sticks). At the same time, the pigs and the other gifts are stored in the houses around the neighborhood. Special gifts are piled up in a house for the mother of the bride.

Now everybody awaits the arrival of the bride's relatives,[26] that is, the bride's clan and partner clan as well as all the other claimants to the brideprice. They arrive at the village together and very formally, in a long row, and are then invited into the houses of the father of the bridegroom and his relatives, where they are first given a feast (today, it consists mainly of rice, fish, vegetables, sweet potatoes and potatoes) as well as betel nuts. In the meantime, the brideprice donors, following strict rules, arrange their gifts like show-pieces above and below the rack. Banana leaves are put underneath first, as a foundation, then cooking bananas, betel nuts, taro and yams as well as 'pitpit' (a kind of wild sugar-cane, the shoots of which are a favorite food) are heaped on them. On top of these foodstuffs are placed the pigs, and the pieces of meat are arranged to form an opened-up whole pig. At the very top, the pigs' heads and the trotters are set, protruding from bamboo pipes.

On the rack itself, grass skirts, pieces of cloth, tree bark cloths and painted back blankets, packets of bought food (rice, tins of fish, salt, biscuits, oil, sugar), cooking pots, soap, net bags and blouses are laid and hung, and onto the vertical poles are attached the *kasok* gifts of money towering above it all, with two-Kina bills artfully fixed on top of each other between two bamboo sticks. The live piglets are not displayed but are directly handed on their leads to the recipients once the latter have packed up their gifts.

Once everything is prepared, the bride's mother is the first to receive her gifts, in a small group consisting of the family of the bridegroom and his relatives. As a rule, a part of it is called *añnok* (meaning that she must later give some of it back), and the rest is given to her as her *manimi*, "without name," that is, without expectation of reciprocity. After this, the recipients of the brideprice position themselves next to the rack. A member of the bridegroom's partner clan makes the rounds of the displayed pigs and pauses at each one to call out the name of the donor. Then the bride makes the rounds of the pigs and dribbles onto each of them milk from a coconut she has cracked.[27] She is followed by a member of her father's partner clan who calls out the name of the recipient at each pig. This distribution is observed with the greatest attention. As soon as the proclamation is over, the recipients hurry nearer, and with lightning speed stuff all the gifts into the net bags they have brought along, take the *kasok* money sticks apart and carry everything off to their village or village section, heavily burdened and dragging the piglets behind them. This concludes the brideprice transfer, which to an outsider seems to be quite an abrupt ending.

In former times, the father's brother or a member of the partner clan concluded the wedding in the evening when, in the bridegroom's house, he handed two bowls of food to the couple, who now for the first time sat officially with all the relatives. Facing each other across the fire, the married couple exchanged the bowls,[28] thus sealing the marriage.

V

The compensation for the brideprice, *pelok*, "can you [give back]?," follows between one month to one year after the *añnok*. The bride's relatives now have to give back part of the brideprice they received to the contributors to the brideprice, those individual men from whom they had received pigs and money. Thus the bride's group becomes the *kasok* or "donor"-group. Pigs are returned at the same amount (1: 1), and money, grass skirts and everything else at half the amount. The brideprice compensation proceeds in the same way as the brideprice transfer, *añnok*, but now takes place in front of the house of the bride's parents. The former brideprice donors now come to collect the gifts prepared for them as *pelok* recipients. In the bridegroom's village, the pork is later eaten communally. With the return of the brideprice, the whole brideprice procedure is said to be finished.

Very frequently, however, the bride's clan and its partner clan feel themselves inadequately paid, though this resentful feeling of having been "short-changed" is not expressed until some time after the brideprice transfer and its return. It may be that a piglet received at the brideprice has died, and therefore the re-

Illustration 5: The transfer of the brideprice: the gifts (tied up pieces of pork, netbags, grass skirts, money, and so on) are being arranged.

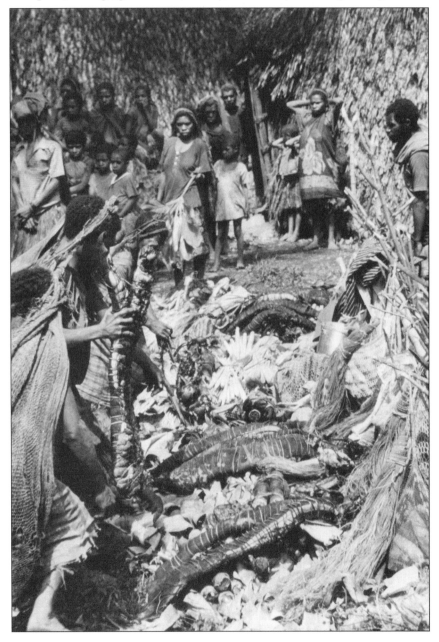

cipient complains of being "fobbed off with a bad pig," or a new dispute may arise between the two parties, which subsequently increases people's dissatisfaction. Since this unhappiness, too, may develop into an "oppressing problem" that can sometimes manifest itself in the wife's failure to become pregnant, the husband now has to make additional payments (pig and/or money) to his wife's kinship group. This support or transaction is called *ngopmo*,[29] "my covering." Should he not be able to make such payments, a relative or fellow-villager will help him out (against a guarantee of compensation).

If the two marriage partners in the course of time do not settle down, that is, if they do not like each other at all and are incompatible, one of the still-unmarried brothers of the husband "takes over" the wife so that she stays since she is a "paid for" member in her husband's clan. If no suitable man is available, or if the woman, even after strong coaxing, does not want to live with the other man either, she returns to her parents, who, together with their relatives, must give back the brideprice.

4. Changes

I

Like all the other groups in Papua New Guinea, the Yupno have increasingly been confronted with Western impacts that are changing their traditional culture in many ways. Missionization began in the 1930s (cf. Wassmann 1992), but Gua itself was not affected until the early 1950s, when its inhabitants were forced to move to the present location and had to destroy all their religious objects and burn down the men's houses. In Waminoka, which is above modern Gua, a deep hollow was dug, all the religious objects were thrown into it and a big tree was planted on top. Today, more than thirty years after this decisive experience of the destruction of major symbols of the traditional religion, this hollow and its surroundings are still deemed "dangerous"—a sign that these objects have lost little of their significance.

Since that time of upheaval, no more initiations or other religious ceremonies involving the joint participation of all the initiated men have been held, so information about them is scarce and contradictory. With the loss of the men's houses, the men's collective rituals were also given up. In other words, an important component of the religious system, partly esoteric and partly exoteric, and one that concerned all the Yupno, along with its cosmogonical and anthropogonical contents, was destroyed. Morap, "the one who lives in abundance," the Yupno creator god, was replaced by Anutu (the

Kâte name[30] for the Christian god); the bush-spirit *sindok* was interpreted by the mission as the figure of satan; and *moñan*, "breath," the personal substance proper to every human being (cf. Chapter 3.1.) became the "Holy Spirit." The world beyond was dissociated from its traditional place, the sea, and placed in heaven. Christian services replaced the traditional religious meetings. The new religion, with its rituals emphasizing "Christian" communal institutions (services of which everybody should partake) included the women, which partly put the men out of work. There were also new religious functionaries such as mission helpers, evangelists and pastors, who were to be kept by the village, and this led to a new kind of hierarchy.

At such collective events, the church divided, and still divides, the population into the "good," "Christian" ones living "in the light," and the "bad" or "heathen," those "dwelling in darkness." Such statements, which certainly do not further the integration of the village community (a declared aim of the mission), mostly derive from sermons preached in Kâte, however. Since few Yupno understand this language, such pronouncements do not affect village life and everyday social relations.

What opened the way to disintegration was the forced abandonment of male initiation, the institution that traditionally strengthened communality by consciously and explicitly integrating young, growing men into the community and teaching them the knowledge and skills required for social adulthood. The work of the mission prohibited this transition, which had been so decisive for social cohesion, and failed to introduce a replacement. Larger villages were established, prompted by mission politics, but were losing their cohesion because of an enduring and ever-increasing tendency towards individualization among the Yupno. Few men remain competent in the total traditional religious system, and the younger and middle generations know only fraction of it.

The "new" Christian religion, though, is likewise understood poorly and in a fragmentary manner, so its supplanting of the traditional religion has been incomplete and rather superficial. The "exterior" is Christian, but behind it as always has remained the individual (and clan-specific) esoteric knowledge that expresses itself in certain rituals for gardening, and for successful hunt, as well as in acts that cause or cure illness. These practices have never been executed in groups; traditionally, they were done very discreetly and today remain an intrinsic element of everyday Yupno life. Even though this knowledge, too, is slowly being lost, exacerbated by Western schooling and the phenomenon of generational conflict (new to the Yupno), there are still young bachelors who learn this knowledge from their fathers, along with with a Western-style education.

> If one does not go to school and learn all this [Western knowledge],
> one will live in the village with nothing to do, have no work and live
> like in a 'kanaka' place....But it is bad to be like a woman [without
> traditional esoteric knowledge]. Women do not know anything about
> it. If you want to live like a man you have to know this, you must have
> the traditional knowledge. That is good.

This sentence by a young, 18 year old man who had attended school but
was also instructed by his father in the traditional knowledge of "sorcery," expresses the attitude and the wish of many young men who are endeavoring to
find their way in both systems, the traditional and the Western.

However, the majority of the younger men are in fact disoriented and without occupation, standing between the two systems rather than inside both of
them, while not really belonging to either. In former times, men predominantly worked under contract[31] on the plantations on Buka, and after completion of their contract in most cases came back[32] to the village, whereas
young people today are mainly attracted to the cities of Lae and Madang.
Above all, the out-of-work school leavers (in Gua, an adolescent who finished
"grade 10" level and several youths at "grade 6"), whose parents went to great
financial pains and held highly hopes for their education, feel like "mis-in-
vestments" and superfluous when they come back to the village. Some of these
Yupno youths founded a 'raskal gang' in Lae, which later dissolved after an
unsuccessful raid on a trade store, yet for some of them it had been an excit-
ing time full of positive memories.

The traditional knowledge of women, encompassing the rearing of pigs, tending gardens, the classification of plants and food (Wassmann 1993a, 1993c), the
wellbeing of infants and children seems to have been altered less by christianization and influences from outside worlds. Women still perform their gendered
traditional roles and tasks with more self-assurance than men; this might be due
to the fact that girls are significantly less likely to be sent to school or have an opportunity to spend time away from the village. In any case, they seem to be more
at home in the village and show little desire to venture into the world beyond it.

With the opening of the airstrip at Teptep in 1972 and the construction of
a government station, a nationally run "community school" was opened up
(at first to "Grade 3," but later to "Grade 6"), though it was mainly the boys
who were sent to school. Some of them later underwent further schooling at
distant places and there became acquainted with a modern, urban lifestyle.
Back in the village, their new knowledge was not helpful; mundane traditional
skills, such as how to plant a garden or hunt successfully or detect the causes
of illness, had barely been passed on to them. They were called by the older

Illustration 6: The Teptep airstrip

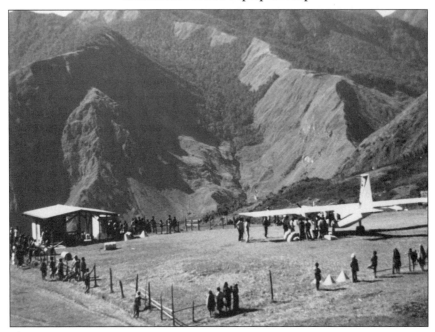

men 'man nating', totally insignificant men, and they in turn showed little re-spect for their male elders anymore. Often married off against their will, they were bored, and longed for the modern life and its Western consumer goods that they had experienced away from home. Their dissatisfaction grew, and some tried to oppose the old structures of authority in the village, which led to social tensions and a conflict of generations. Others have withdrawn from this situation by increasingly frequent and longer stays in town. Yupno women, in contrast, have experienced far less disruptions in their lives.

II

The construction and enlargement of the station at Teptep also set in train an economic change. At the beginning of the 1980s, the Lutheran church ini-tiated a vegetable project, motivating the population to cultivate European vegetables. This cash crop gives the people the opportunity to make money, which in turn is meant to make life in the villages more attractive and thus decrease migration to the cities. The vegetables are marketed at Teptep and flown out into the cities of Madang (daily) and Lae (one or twice a week). A market that is held three times a week for the station employees enables women from the less distant upper Yupno villages to sell their garden produce. The younger women make much use of this opportunity to earn money. Trade stores offering Western goods have also been opened: the traditional dress (for women the grass skirt, for men a bark-cloth belt) is more and more replaced by Western clothing, available at low prices in second-hand shops in Teptep. New kinds of food (rice, tinned fish and so on) supplement meals. New household articles and utensils (plastic buckets, aluminum pots, spades, knives, etc.) replace traditional vessels and utensils, such as bamboo pipes, wooden bowls, digging stick and bamboo knives.

Since 1963, with the opening of an Aid Post and its later extension into a small Health Centre, the medical facilities available to the Yupno have also increased. Along with their traditional medicine, they can now also make use of the Western medical system with its pharmaceutical products.

Teptep, because of its airstrip and resident foreigners a window to the outside world, is a favorite destination for excursions among the younger people. They stroll about on market days, visit different stores and observe and comment on the often eventful landings and take-offs of the airplanes. Here they meet people of the same age from other villages and from Nankina, and here news is heard and exchanged.

III

Despite these changes, in comparison with many ethnic groups in Papua New Guinea the Yupno were still living in a traditional way in 1987. Information about events outside the valley hardly reached the village, not even via Teptep. A remark by Patrol Officer Morrison almost 20 years ago to a large extent still applies: "…there is virtually no constant source of outside information for the area. I did not see one radio throughout the whole patrol and of course no literature.…at present communications between this area and the outside is virtually non-existent" (Morrison 1969/70: 3), and Patrol Officer Sailoia commented with some resignation some years later on his attempts to teach the Yupno "political consciousness": "Interest is…shown in newspapers, but this is mainly used for rolling tobacco" (Sailoia 1976/77: 3).

The population was thus barely affected by the debate waged for decades by the Madang and Morobe government about the Provincial affiliation of the Yupno valley, which lies right on a border line. Even though Gua, like Teptep and other villages, officially belongs to Madang Province, the best educated young man from Gua, the first representative of all the Yupno, decided to join the opposition side in the Morobe Provincial Government.

In 1987, at the election for the National Government, there was an intensive campaign by several parties in the Yupno region, but the people from Gua could not cast their votes. From a report in the Wantok newspaper (No. 679, 2–9 July 1987, cf. Niles 1987):

> In the villages of Goa (Gua) and Kangulut at the border between Madang and Morobe Province, the people did not vote. When the first date for voting, the one for Morobe Province, had arrived and the people went to the voting place, the administrators told them their names were on the list for Madang. Alright. When the date for the election of Madang Province arrived, the population of both places was told their name stood on the Morobe list. The people did not vote because the government agents had done their job wrong and in a contradictory sense [translated from the original, in Tok Pisin].

This event, which probably for the first time put Gua village in the headlines, confirmed the younger people's view that no Provincial Government represented their interests. After this incident, the people very soon turned back to their private and village affairs, and life in the village continued as before.

Chapter 3

The Background: The Concept of Person

1. The Complete Human Being

I

As with all human societies, no adequate investigation of health and illness among the Yupno would be possible without an understanding of the concept of the person. To put it simply, illness always means being in a state that is "exceptional," "different," situated "above," or "hot." The question then is: which spiritual or emotional or body parts of a human being are in this exceptional condition, and which "human-being parts" can change their state or can themselves be changed?

The external, visible component of a human being is its body, *ngodɨm*. To be more precise as to what kind of body is meant, the term is preceded by the respective noun, as, for example, with *amɨn ngodɨm* (*amɨn*: human being, man) "human body," *sak ngodɨm* (*sak*: woman, grass skirt) "female body," or *minam ngodɨm* (*minam*: bird), "body of a bird." The task of holding this body upright, to give it a frame, is done by the bones, *kɨrat*. As becomes evident from the following terms, two "qualities" are connected with this word: the *kɨrat* prevent the collapse of something (a human being, a house) and thereby provide (for the human being, the house, the world) stability. *Kɨrat* is used in the following compounds: *yut kɨrat*, "house post," *kɨnam kɨrat* (*kɨnam*: bamboo), namely "bamboo pipe" (in which vegetables or other foods have been cooked). Thus, *amɨn kɨrat* (*amɨn*: man) means "the human skeleton," and *mbisoñ kɨrat* (*mbisoñ*: head) the "skull."

The body is surrounded by a wrapping, *ngop* or *ngopm*; *ngop* means skin when talking about human beings, specifically *amɨn ngop*, "skin of man." In other compounds it means "peel" (*nalok ngop*, from *nalok*: banana, *ondeñ ngop* from *ondeñ*: sweet potato), "bark" (*kandap ngop* from *kandap*: tree, wood), "pod" (*mbɨrap ngop*, from *mbɨrap*: bean), something also that envelops, surrounds, protects against the outside. This wrapping is vulnerable, since all "pests" coming from the outside settle on it first: like dirt or lumps of earth sticking to the peel of a sweet potato, a bean pod can be nibbled at by a caterpillar, thus the invisible, pathogenic "oppressing problems" in human beings settle on the skin. Between the bones and the wrapping is *tsabom*, flesh, muscles, a word also used for the meat of birds, pigs and so on.

II

Far more important than the biological concept of the body and its organs is *tevantok*, which is inherent in every human being and can be translated as "vital energy," or "inner strength." *Tevantok* is impersonal, not individually imprinted; every human being possesses it in about the same amount (although men generally have a bit more *tevantok* than women), and it resides at an unspecified location in a person's body. It is also immanent in certain objects with religious meaning, like the *kokop kɨrat*, a term deriving from *kokop*, "settlement," "place," and *kɨrat*, "bone," which means "strength-holder of the settlement," or is more loosely translated as "center of energy" of the village. It is thus an object where the "vital energy" inherent in every individual (as a member of the village) is also present, but in an especially concentrated and condensed form. A *kokop kɨrat*, or local "strength-holder of the settlement," can be a certain animal, or its imitation, a bird, a lizard (or, in the case of Gua, a centipede, *guam*), a snake, a stone, a bullroarer, or a human skull—such that, as a rule, today every village[1] owns one such object in common. These objects had either been brought into the Yupno region by the mythological founders when they "immigrated" or followed them, flew after them or were dreamt by the ancestors. The forms of the *kokop kɨrat* are as diverse as their respective origins or creation. Formerly, they used to be carefully stored in a special house, the small men's house *tɨlagɨ yut*, the "exceptional house."

Tevantok, "vital energy," is subject to change by certain circumstances or acts, and can temporarily be increased and then bring a person or an object to a state called *tɨlagɨ*, "to be different." Someone with increased *tevantok*, "charged" by certain acts, is *tɨlagɨ*, "different," "exceptional." *Tɨlagɨ* is also used for the description of states of qualities of different phenomena (like social relations, objects like *kokop kɨrat*, "strength-holders of the settlement," and also certain parts of the landscape) which are "different"; the term may signify "to be forbidden," "inflicted with a taboo," "to be hot," "to be sacred"; and at the same time and very significantly, it can also mean "to destroy." To put it differently: "normal" *tevantok*, "vital energy," which is immanent in every human being, may lead, if increased or strengthened, to a *tilagi* state to "being different." This "being different" is at the same time an exceptional, "hot" state, which carries with it an element of destruction. This, above all, becomes meaningful in the traditional religious context, and for intentional acts aimed at causing someone to be ill, i.e. "hot," "different." For this purpose, the *kokop kirat* (objects that are especially charged because of the particularly concentrated *tevantok*) may be used as to reinforce the power of the ritual.

III

Apart from the impersonal "vital energy" (*tevantok*), two souls or spiritual aspects, *moñan* and *wopm*, are part of a human being. *Moñan* means wind, breath, steam (when it has rained and the sun shines on the wet ground) and breeze. It causes a human being to see, hear, smell, walk around and possess his or her own personality, and is contained in every particle of the body— in the hair, saliva, and excrement, but as well in all things that have been touched by someone, such as a betel nut or a cigarette stub. Since *moñan* is especially concentrated in a human being's breath, I will refer to it as "breath spirit"; it dissolves at death. *Tevantok*, the above-mentioned impersonal "vital energy" of each human being, is connected to *moñan*.

The other spiritual dimension that forms part of a complete human being is *wopm*, "image, shadow," also often called *aminwop*, "shadow of man"; I will refer to it as "soul" or "shadow soul." It is not precisely localized but is hidden in the body, from which it can escape during sleep (when somebody is dreaming), or in the case of illness; at death, however, it leaves the person for good and becomes a *koñwop* (*koñ*: "ghost"), a "soul of a dead person." In time, the *koñwop*, the "soul of a dead person," loses the personal attributes of the deceased and becomes an always anonymously conceived *koñ*, a "ghost." All the animals (pigs, dogs, chicken) kept by human beings also have a *wopm*.

Moñan, "breath spirit" and *wopm*, "shadow soul," are both personal, individual dimensions of a human being, and together form his or her personality. *Moñan* has a substantial quality, since part of it remains on everything with which it comes into contact, regardless of spatial and temporal distance. Although part of it constantly leaves its owner (as, for example, via the breath), its amount or intensity does thereby not decrease. It perhaps could be compared to a small cloud that leaves little veils on everything it brushes against (tree, house, protruding rock) without itself dissolving. In contrast, *wopm*, frequently called more precisely *aminwop*, "shadow of man," is without substance. It is a sealed, indissoluble unit held to be easily frightened and "sensitive," which can leave a person in a dream, or in case of illness or death, as a whole and without "leftovers." Temporary separations from it, as in a dream where it meets the "shadows" of other people and shares "dream experiences" with them, do not harm a person, yet the Yupno never abruptly wake up somebody who is sleeping, lest his or her *aminwop* be away and not have time to slip back into its owner. Longer separations between a person and his or her *aminwop*, however, may cause illness and death, as will be shown.

This dualistic concept of a "breath spirit" and a "shadow soul" is widespread in Papua New Guinea cultures. Among the Rawa people, for example, who distinguish between "breath" (*yuka*) and "spirit double" (*kapokapoyi*) (Dalton 2002: 125), their concept is similar to Yupno ideas. Other well-known examples are the Ngaing, for whom, according to Lawrence (1967: 207), breath (*kitang*) and shadow (*ananuang*) are manifestations of a living person. The Kabana-speaking people in New Britain assert that, besides the physical body, the *tautau* (spirit, soul, vital essence, principle) and *anunu* (reflection, shadow, mirror image, persona) are necessary conditions for a human being. Their ideas, as depicted by Scaletta (1985: 225–26), come very close to the Yupno concepts of *moñan* and *wopm*. Other well known concepts in Melanesian anthropology, for example, the Melpa terms *min* (life, force, spirit, soul) and *noman* (mind, will, intention), are complex and central for indigenous understandings of a person.[2]

IV

To the complete human being also belong his or her social relations. Their frame or social space is for the most part defined by the social structure (clan, partner clan) as well as by the kinship system (one's own patrilineage and matrilateral and affinal relatives). If these relationships do not "click"—either on a dyadic level or between two kin groups, and are thus burdened with conflict or are "tense," which is almost always the result of wrong behavior (e.g., the breaking of norms) and ensuing "hot" emotional states—a person can become ill because of such "oppressing problems." This illness may not only befall the actual instigator of the conflict-laden relationship but also any member of his or her kinship group. Thus it becomes evident that individuals are not only responsible for their acts and the consequences thereof but that their individual behavior is embedded in the social structure and therefore affects relatives as well: each individual therefore also carries the responsibility for his or her relatives, since a person is a socially-tied being. These close social or kinship ties are constantly confirmed in everyday life. All activities, whether garden work, erecting fences, cutting trees, hunting, killing a pig, eating the evening meals or just resting in the house, are undertaken in company, frequently in novel combinations of personnel drawn from the partner clans (*ngapma ngapma*). Only very rarely does one meet a Yupno on his or her own.

V

A component of the personality of every human being is his or her own *koñgap* melody,[3] the "voice of the ghost." Like a name (which is less relevant, see Chapter 3.3), it belongs to every human being. Shortly after birth, the mother is the first to invent a *koñgap* melody for her child, which it later exchanges for another, its "own." There are various possibilities for finding one's own *koñgap* melody: some people dream their melody, others playfully try out different melodies until one of them seems suitable. Children and adolescents often sing their own melody in a relatively "unregulated" way, for example, while working in a garden or walking on a path. Other people repeatedly hear a melody and relate it to the appropriate person, and this *koñgap* melody is then considered to be that person's *koñgap*.

The *koñgap* has several characteristic aspects: it comprises an extremely short succession of notes, seldom more than five, and serves as a "recognition call" across the mountainous countryside. At the same time, it is the only traditional melody that men have for a dancing feast. It is more important to the men and more often sung by them than by women, and its use by men is also more strictly regulated than among women.

Every adult Yupno stores in his memory several hundred[4] different *koñgap* that he can readily ascribe to the respective owner, and even dead people's *koñgap* are memorized over a long period of time. Three possible interpretations, none of them definitive, come to mind for this cultural element: the *koñgap* might be the "melody of the ghost," the voice of one's own "ghost" (of the owner of the melody); it may serve to communicate with the "world beyond," with one or all of the "ghosts"; or else it wards off these "ghosts." As the following "rules" for the everyday use of the melody show, it expresses social position (to rise above somebody and thereby make that person "small," or to declare oneself as a friend), relations between the sexes, feelings (mourning someone who is absent) or else aspects of communication, and all are phenomena that concern the "here and now" of Yupno everyday life.

There are differing behavioral norms for men and women with respect to the singing of the *koñgap* melodies (one's own or somebody else's). Transgression of these norms does not cause illness but is deemed to be "improper." Normally, a man (or a woman) sings somebody else's *koñgap* when approaching his or her garden land or bush area. By doing this, one proves to be "in the know," that is, a friend, and also announces one's arrival. This is the most frequent use of the *koñgap* melody. When one walks through Gua garden land during the daytime, these short precise melodies, also sung by children, can be heard from all directions. A man would not normally sing his own *koñgap* melody in the presence of others during the day, lest he be regarded as boisterous or arrogant. It would be an extraordinary event if somebody acted in such an egotistical, immodest way (or were permitted to do so), thereby elevating himself above the "ideal middle position" (see below). For example, this could occur in the case of a man who had been constantly put down with gibes but is somehow now able to contribute substantially to the raising of the brideprice for his own wife, thus proving himself to be a "real" man; or if a man has stolen a small part of somebody else's *moñan* ("breath spirit") (which may have stuck to the remains of a betel nut) with the intention to cause illness or to kill, or if he comes back to his village victoriously after a fight where he killed somebody from another village, he would be permitted to sing his own melody as a sign that he has defeated others. Such an occasion, called *mbɨdok koñgap*, "letting out the hidden feelings by singing the *koñgap* melody," simultaneously raises the singer over others and puts them down and shames them. It is always thus an act of status degradation, since it involves the defeat of somebody else.

There is only one "normal" occasion when a man may sing his own *koñgap* melody: during the night of the traditional *nsaguo-koñgap* dancing feast when the men, decorated with earth pigments and leaves and with a *nsaguo* wheel of feathers in their midst, dance around in a circle for hours, accompanied by drums, and reach a trance-like state by singing their own short melodies again and again without interruption.

A man may sing the *koñgap* melody of his brother as a sign of sympathy and pity if the latter is staying far away or has died; however, it is not fitting to sing one's father's *koñgap* melody for no reason, but would be appropriate only if somebody else were to destroy something one's father has erected or planted. Similarly, men do not sing the melodies of their wives or of other women, lest this be interpreted as an attempt to flirt, which would cause shame to the man and make him the subject of public rumors. When a man wants to call his wife from a distance, he sings the *koñgap* melody of one of their children.

The rules are somewhat less strict for married women, who may sing the melody of their husbands or other men without raising any suspicion that they are attempting to flirt.[5] They may also sing the melodies of other women whom they meet in the garden or with whom they have worked and are now farewelling with their melodies. Young girls, however, will be careful not to sing the melody of an unmarried youth in public, lest rumors about a possible affair ensue. Were an unmarried young man to sing a girl's melody, he would have to pay compensation to her kinship group because of his misdemeanor. This personal *koñgap* melody accompanies people all their life and may be sung by the relatives as a sign of mourning or in memory after the death of the owner. However, since it is indissolubly connected with the personality of its owner, it cannot be handed down or transferred.

2. The Ideal State

I

Three concepts define the state of a human being:[6] *tepm* ("hot"), *yawuro* ("cool"), and *mbaak* ("ice-cold"), which are dependent upon one another and form a continuum. The "ideal state" of a human being is *yawuro*, which lies midway between the two extreme positions, "hot" (*tepm*) and "ice-cold" (*mbaak*), and actually means "lukewarm" or well tempered: neither hot nor very cold, but rather cool. Because of the pejorative meaning of the word "lukewarm" in English, and in order to render the three interdependent concepts adequately and comprehensibly, I gloss *yawuro* as "cool," keeping in mind that *yawuro* means exactly the undesired state "neither-nor," the lukewarm condition in English. For the Yupno, however, this is the ideal condition. "Cool" (*yawuro*), which is used as a thermal term as well as a symbolic one, is found in compound nouns like *yawuro yawuro amïn*, "one who cools down" and is linked with other qualities. In the social sphere, it means a state of "being in the center," socially integrated and in harmony, just as in *mbït yawuro*, "to have cool, harmonious, unanimous feelings."

"Hot" (*tepm*), in contrast, is an "extraordinary" state, one of the extreme positions. *Tepm* means hot, fast, pain and, like "cool" (*yawuro*), is used as a physical term (as e.g., "the body is hot," "to have a fever") as well as symbolically. It also designates bodily disorders like headache or toothache. In the social sphere, *tepm* connotes "to be above"; an angry person, for example, is "hot" and has "raised" himself or herself above "the midst of the others." In the realm of illness concepts, "hot" (*tepm*) is an undesired, dangerous state, so every therapy aims to "cool down" the "heated up," to bring him or her back to a "cool" (*yawuro*) state.

The third important concept in this context, the other extreme position, is *mbaak*, meaning very cold, ice-cold. It is only used symbolically, not thermally, and refers to the state of people whose "vital energy" (*tevantok*) or *moñan* ("breath spirit") was intentionally frozen with certain "ice-cold" objects, rendering them incapable of actions or reactions. They become "frozen out" and "below," having sunk from the "ideal midst," and are speechless and in social seclusion. An act to bring the victim into a "cold" (*mbaak*) state can prevent certain reactions like revenge or hate (as the consequence of a theft or the discovery of a grave misbehavior). "Ice-cold" (*mbaak*), like "hot" (*tepm*), is an undesired state since a person thus afflicted has moved away from the "ideal" middle and the "cool" state yet is not thought to be "ill." In the context of concepts of illness, this state does not play a part but is used as a prophylactic measure against people who are potentially "heated," i.e., furious, scornful, or "dwelling above." *Mbaak* is also the term for a prophylaxis, a combination of various ingredients thought of as "ice-cold" and employed against possible "hot" activities of the bush-spirit *sindok* (see Chapter 5.3.).

II

The three states "hot," "cool" and "ice-cold" are changeable. In manipulating these states, both the initial state and the desired result are crucial variables. Men, and above all the older men, possess the encompassing knowledge regarding these manipulations of states, though there are a few exceptions in which women may perform them. For the change of states, some form of contact is essential: somebody who is in the ideal, "cool" state can be "heated up" or made ill (*sit*) with "hot" objects. Similarly, through contact with "cool" substances someone who is "heated up," an ill person for example, can be "cooled down" to the ideal state. With "ice-cold" objects, someone who is "cool" is totally "frozen out," and with "cool" components somebody who is "frozen stiff" or "ice-cold" can be "warmed up" again. There is only ever one degree of change: from "hot" to "cool" or from "cool" to "cold" and vice versa, but not from "hot" to "cold" and the other way around. The two states "hot" and "cool," as well as manipulation of them, are crucial for the concepts of illness presented here.

The goal of the manipulation is the "vital energy" (*tevantok*) of a person. In a healthy, socially integrated human being, this energy is in a "cool" (*yawuro*) state. However, when brought into contact with "hot" or "cold" objects,[7] that is with objects that possess much or little "vital energy" (*tevantok*), these objects act as agents and transfer the "heat" or "cold" respectively to the "vital energy," and as a result, the person gets ill or recovers. Knowledge of these "hot" or "cold" qualities of objects varies widely; some are known to everyone, equally well to men and women, and are used in "home remedies," whereas some are specific to the clans, and others (above all, "hot" or "cold" objects that are used in conjunction with certain "hot," secret formulae) are known only to those who specialize in either causing or healing illness. Common to all "hot" and "cold" objects, however, are certain characteristics:

- "hot" objects are red or black (like the red earth pigment *mañot*, the "very hot" paste *kowa*, the black earth pigment *noñgum*, red or black plants, the black stone *tip pilin*, the conical stones *sulek*—"heated up" with red earth pigment), and include all esoteric objects used for rituals and initiations belonging to men's cults like the *sindok kirat*, the "bone of the bush-spirit *sindok*," and the *kokop kirat*, the "strength-holder of the settlement" (see Chapter 3.1.), and the longish and round bowls important for the institution of the partner clans *ngapma ngapma*. Also "hot" are young, virgin men and women (not yet having "cooled down" via sexual intercourse), menstrual blood, dry, thorny, stinging or sharp-edged plants or leaves, spicy food and things that are above (like the eagle). For the Yupno, somebody with negative feelings like rage, hate, jealousy (see Chapter 5.2.c.) is also "hot," since he therefore has risen "above" (the others) and his feelings may manifest themselves via the transfer of "heated" *moñan* ("breath spirit"), causing illness in somebody else.
- In contrast, objects that are "cold" or suitable for "cooling down" are white (like the white earth *kuak* or whitish, light green plants and leaves); water and all the plants growing near water or in swampy places; living creatures (like the frog *meñgak*); objects that contain a lot of moisture or sap (sugar cane, oranges, all the leafy vegetables that lose a lot of moisture in cooking); and persons who have (or had, as in the case of old people, particularly) frequent sexual intercourse.

If people or their *moñan* ("breath spirit") who are in an ideal "cool" condition are brought together with "hot objects," their "vital energy" (*tevantok*) is heated up, and it becomes "different" (*tilagi*). This "different" and thus exceptional "heat" condition can also be created intentionally and methodically. However, in order to perform very risky actions at all, such as the heating up the *moñan* of a victim, the agents themselves, the specialists, have to reach a "hot" state (and, in turn, must afterwards "cool down" again). If, in contrast, "heated up," ill people whose "vital energy" (*tevantok*) is "different" (*tilagi*) and who are in a "hot" state are given "cold" things to eat that cool the "heat," rub their skin with "cold" substances, they lose their "heat" and can return to the ideal "cool" *yawuro* state. The basic principle is always the same: each act aimed at causing illness and every therapy are based on this principle of, on the one hand, "heating up" and "lifting up" and "making different" from the middle position, and, on the other, the "cooling down," "taking down" to the ideal, integrated, "cool" state.

Yupno ways of thinking about "hot," "cool" and "cold," of keeping a balance between the different conditions or of attempting to restore the undesirable extreme states, can very clearly be termed a humoral system. As some recent studies show, humoral ideas are also found in different emphasis in many Papua New Guinea societies; for example among the the Duna and Melpa (Strathern 1996; Strathern and Stewart 1999).

3. The Life Cycle of an Individual: Development into a Complete Human Being

I

In a newborn baby, the *moñan* as well as its social relations are not yet developed but are present in fragments. The baby already possesses the *wopm* ("shadow soul") while it is still in the mother's womb;[8] it is looked upon as originating from the mother's kin group and as returning to this group at the death of a person (see below), again accompanied by gifts. Hence, for the Yupno, a baby is not a complete human being and does not become one until he or she has formed and is completed out of the "human being parts." There is no fixed date for this completion, but it is generally thought to occur when a child is able to talk, listen and walk (skills for which his or her *moñan* is responsible) and can be experienced by others as an autonomous personality.

A child is created out of the father's semen, which nourishes the child (thus, the father is called *nan*, "nourishing food") and is responsible for the formation of its flesh and its bones, and the blood of the mother. One single act of intercourse does not suffice for the conception of a child, so the father has repeatedly to "feed" the embryo, *monji kuaap*, with his semen.

Experienced people detect a woman's pregnancy—apart from her increasing girth—from other signs as well: the mother's eyes "turn inside," her facial skin becomes lighter and her body "sturdier," the pelvic bones *sambek* (which, in contrast to those of a man have not grown together) start to separate, to open up. Newly married and hence "potentially pregnant" women, especially, are closely watched by the men who substantially contributed to their brideprice, since their future child, as the "product" of the brideprice, will "belong" to the clan and partner clan of the husband. To prevent a possible abortion, the pregnancy of such a woman formerly was publicly proclaimed as soon as possible: one night, all the men of the husband's clan and partner clan would together perform a *koñgap*-dancing feast in front of the woman's house.

Yet abortions were and are common, especially in pregnancies resulting from forbidden sexual relations, above all a concern of unmarried younger women. A widespread abortion technique (applied by the women alone) consists of tying the belly tightly with a piece of string. The (male) abortion specialist, called *mɨndak mɨndak amɨn*, one "who cuts out," practices another technique for a fee. The pregnant woman receives a small piece of *maam goman*, red, that is "hot" ginger; she eats one piece, but only chews another (to which her *moñan* ("breath spirit") will stick) and then hands it to the child's father. He in turn gives it to the specialist, who cuts down the soft parts of the "hot" *bumat* tree (these have little thorns on them, which are said to be the food of the bush-spirit *sindok*) and extracts a liquid from them. In the act, he says: "*monjiyok bakok*," "throw the embryo out," calls out the name of the bird *singeñ* (a "hot," high-flying, sky-dwelling bird of prey that stands for the bush-spirit *sindok*) and turns to it: "come on down and get this, carry it away and eat it up." He boils the liquid and the chewed piece of ginger together with the ("hot," belonging to the realm of the men's house) bullroarer *obip san*, puts the bullroarer back in its place in the men's house and gives the liquid to the pregnant woman to drink. Thus "heated," she will lose the child.

There are several, slightly varying "techniques," but the basic principle stays the same: the woman's *moñan* ("breath spirit"), adhering to any object she has touched or chewed, is brought into contact with certain "hot" plants or parts of them, and "heated"; then the specialist contacts the bush-spirit *sindok* (or one of its "representatives," such as the *singeñ*-bird) and asks it to "eat up" the embryo. Knowledge of religiously significant "hot" and "cold" objects plus those ascribed to the realm of the bush-spirit and the men's house (the bullroarer) is confined to the men, so it comes as no surprise that only men practice these abortion techniques. Women are more pragmatic: they simply bind strings.

II

Shortly before giving birth, the women are fed *ndamba*, a kind of fern growing near the water and possessing "cooling" qualities, as a prophylactic against the ("hot") labor pains. The birth of a child, *monji naknak altañ*, "arrival of the downy child," (traditionally) takes place in the family house. The mother gives birth, assisted by one or two experienced women who already have children of their own and who help her wash the child with the "cold" plants *mbañgam* and *kwebekal* (which grow beside watercourses). Since the baby has been in contact with the "hot" blood of the mother, which is like the menstrual blood, it is first "cooled" down with "cold plants." The father is excluded from this event, and cannot enter his house again until two or three days after the birth, or, and in the meantime, he stays with relatives. Before the woman cooks for the family, she has to wash herself and put on a new grass skirt; her *tevantok* ("vital energy") and her *moñan* ("breath spirit") can be transferred by touching and are dangerously "hot" for men—just as they are during her menstruation (see below). The mother remains in the house with her infant (*monji naknak*, see above) for approximately one week until she is able to walk around again: through the birth, her pelvic bones are thought to have become loose and must close again. For the first two to three days after the birth, a woman from the kin group wet-nurses the newborn, then the mother breastfeeds her child herself. During this first period, which is called *monji naknak yut*, "a downy child in the house," women from the kingroup or the neighborhood help out with water, food and firewood.

After this phase, which lasts about one week, the child was in former times carried for the first time in front of the house in a small ritual, featuring "hot" and "cold." This was meant to help the child to stay healthy, not cry too much or become stubborn, and, as a grown-up man, to be a good fighter and hunter, or, as a grown-up woman, a good gardener—in sum, a capable member of the kinship group. The ritual concluded with a big feast, which was held with the mother's relatives and the clan and partner clan members of the father. If the baby was a woman's first child, its maternal relatives were given strings of shell money to thank the mother's group for the new member of the kinship group.

Once a child is able to walk, talk and listen, carry a small string-bag or a small bundle of fire-wood or relay a short bit of news to someone, it is deemed to be a person capable of having social relations with other people, albeit on a small scale. It is now no longer a "downy child," *monji naknak*, but is called either *amin monji*, "little man," or *sak monji*, "little woman." Since its *moñan*[9] is developed, it is now an almost "complete" human being.

III

In former times, the initiation process for boys entailed passing through several grades, but today involves only a single grade, *nsaguo mbisap*, "the time of the *nsaguo*-wheel of feathers." It includes a big feast and dance where the young, nubile man for the first time wears this large wheel of feathers. His performance is watched with great interest by the young unmarried women of his and the other villages. In preparation, betel nuts, large amounts of food, new grass skirts, torches and fire-wood are readied, and a precise date is fixed. The matrilateral female relatives of the young man decorate themselves, rub their skin with pig fat until it shines, put on new grass skirts and, in the middle of the night, the man, decorated in the same way and rubbed with red ("hot") earth pigment, dances for the first time with the wheel of feathers (prepared by his father or father's brother) on a pole above his head. Singing his *koñgap* melody, beating an hour-glass drum and accompanied by his maternal relatives with torches, he approaches the main square of the village, where he is surrounded by the other men of his clan, who, likewise decorated with costumes made from leaves, are beating their drums and singing their individual *koñgap* melody. This dance, performed in a circle, lasts until another kinship group, with another wheel of feathers or a "smaller version" thereof called the *mbisoñ nda* (a dancing decoration on a bamboo pole carried above the head), appears in the village to join the feast and takes over from the first group. The organizers of the feast, the maternal and paternal relatives of the young man, together with their partner clans, use this interlude to eat together in the young man's father's house, consuming pork and marsupials, and afterwards they exchange betel nuts. The matrilateral relatives and their *ngapma* (as two partner clans) at this point break up betel nuts and give them to the patrilateral relatives and their *ngapma* (the other two partner clans) and vice versa.

I observed the feast, "time of the *nsaguo*-wheel of feathers," in the village of Kangulut in September 1987. It went on for a total of three nights between two o'clock in the morning and dawn, with three different groups from the neighboring villages of Gua, Uskokop and Taeñ appearing one after the other to assist the Kangulut dancers or take over from them. Notably, every dance group worked very hard to represent its village of origin to greatest advantage. All these groups were accompanied by spectators of several different kinds: older men for whom such a dance-feast was too strenuous (some of these older men, who in the village were called "weak and old and a bit frail," were so much gripped by the general mood and enthusiasm during this first night that they spent the following two nights as active dancers, some of whom reaching a level of "peak performance"); men who for different reasons did not feel like actively participating; younger men, who had not yet reached their own "time of the *nsaguo*-wheel of feathers"; and women and children. While the spectators were crouching around small fires to protect them against the cold of the night, periodically going into different houses in the village to warm up, get food and take short breaks for sleeping, the men danced untiringly on the village square. The performance of each group as well as individual performances were commented on and criticized for days later (one dancer broke his bamboo pole, and one singer ruptured the covering of his drum and then, in his frenzy, threw the drum away and simply continued to drum on his belly). All the participants, dancers and spectators alike, spent the days between these three nights resting or sleeping, since normal everyday life was suspended for the duration.

The "time of the *nsaguo*-wheel of feathers" makes a young man to an adult, competent person, a potential husband, and the young, unmarried women of his and neighboring villages pay close attention to his performance. Yupno women, however, do not undergo a protracted series of initiatory rituals. The sign that a woman is ready for marriage is seen in the swelling of her breasts as well as her menstruation *yagngap mbɨsap*, "time of the moon." During menstruation, she is thought to be "dangerous" to men, since her *moñan* is "dangerously hot" and can thereby cause illness, *keaknok*, which manifests itself by increasing weakness and shortness of breath and for which (traditionally) there is no cure. Accordingly, she is not allowed to fetch water at this time or cook (except for herself) or plant taro or yams. The name given to the young unmarried girls is *sak ngok*, "star woman."

IV

The next important stage in the cycle of life is the wedding (see "brideprice" in Chapter 2.3.). Newly-wed people are *amɨn kamam* and *sak kamam*, "new man" and "new woman," grown-up (married) men *amɨn amdi* (sometimes shortened to *amdi*) "real men," grown-up women *sak amdi*, "real women."

This point in life is deemed to be the best time, the zenith, of a trajectory of growth and decline that is thought of as a curve. *Amdi*, the "true people" are those socially most valued, who have many social connections and children, are full of knowledge and are experienced and competent in everyday life.

Old people are called *amɨn pilañ*, but if one wants to make a gender distinction, an old man is *amɨn pilañ*, an old woman *sak amɨn pilañ*. A freer translation of *pilañ* means "somebody who earlier (socially understood) was big or significant and who is now in decline." To identify someone as *pilañ*, changes in physical capabilities are adduced: a decrease of physical strength, or an incapacity to carry heavy loads and cover long distances; in addition, there are bodily changes, namely white hair, a bent back, and "bodily disorders" (loss of teeth, deteriorating eyesight, runny eyes or blindness, impaired hearing or deafness, shortness of breath, frequent catarrh and stiffness and pain in the knees) which appear more frequently in older people. Concepts like dementia and senility[10] are not connected with the term; the Yupno terms for "mentally disturbed" (*wulawula*) or "handicapped" (*kadɨm*, "mad," see

Keck 1999) do not form part of the "old age" complex. One's chronological age is irrelevant, and one is thought of as old (*pilañ*) when there are changes in physical capacities or looks. So although two men of the same age (in their forties, say) may think of themselves as in the same generation, one may seem visibly aged and thus be deemed "old" whereas the other is not, and in any case would vehemently deny this status.

People who are *pilañ* are looked after by their relatives (mostly their children). The care of old people is influenced by the concept of what makes a human being: as already mentioned, vexed "ghosts" or ancestors spirits (*koñ*) may become pathogenically active. Thus every Yupno will try not to annoy his old parents or relatives[11] lest he or his family are later deemed responsible for his behavior by their "ghosts" and punished with illness. Therefore everybody will look after their old relatives and cater to their needs, procuring food, fire-wood and water for them and—should they require help—taking the old parent(s) man or woman into one's own house and physically looking after them. Body care, such as washing them and removing excrement, is the work of the women.

In addition to this concept of the "ghost," which regulates behavior towards old people, there is the idea of delayed reciprocity, wherein repays one's aging parents for the care which one received from them in infancy and childhood. Therefore it is important to the Yupno people to have children of their own as insurance against neglect in their old age. The situation is more difficult for childless old people, who are looked after by relatives; such cases of childlessness, however, are rare.

These two concepts, of illness-inducing ghosts and delayed reciprocity, constitute a sort of frame or social norm that regulates the everyday needs of old people for the most important goods: food, firewood and water. Among the Yupno it would, traditionally, be therefore impossible to let old relatives starve, or to neglect them without consequences. Within this system, the kind of relationship between parents and children varies significantly. In some families, the elderly are taken care of "on the side" and are felt to be a burden, especially if they are physically incapacitated, whereas in other families they are integrated, and do small everyday chores like looking after children or peeling coffee beans. Even though their physical capacities decrease, respect for an old person does not change merely because he or she is now thought to be "old." Those adult "real men" or "real women," who were influential personalities, well versed in mythology, skilled in hunting, blessed with many healthy children, successful as gardeners and raisers of pigs, will in old age, too, retain their high social status. They will be respected people whose advice is sought and whose opinion in cases of litigation or other matters is taken seriously. It is also characteristic of old age among the Yupno that everyday life goes on as normally as possible, but a person retreats more and more from village affairs and takes an interest in events predominantly occurring within one's own clan.

Yawemu, an old woman from Gua, explains her situation:

> I used to live in Taeñ; my father's brothers brought me here [to Gua] and married me off here, to Gua. Now I have become like a woman from here and always stay here. Do you hear my dialect? I do not speak Gua, but Taeñ, I have not forgotten my language.
> I know well how to talk but my eyes are bad. I do not really go any-where else, I am just here, in the house. I have four children, two sons and two daughters, but one daughter died, only three are alive today. In former times, when my eyes were alright, I went to the garden or somewhere else, inside here [in the area around Gua], but now I do not run around anymore or go to the garden, I am only here in the house. Nanjañne [her son] and his wife give me food and fire-wood and water, they bring it to me and give it to me and then go to Kamk-wam [where their garden house stands] to sleep. Sometimes they sleep here with me, then they leave me and go off again. When I lived with my parents [was still unmarried], I did not do anything wrong [being unmarried and having sexual relations with a man], and when I was with my husband, I never said anything bad to the others. I lived peacefully and now I am quite well and I have grown old. And many others of my generation were headstrong, acted wrongly and they have all died.

A normative concept of growing old pervades Yawemu's narration: if one lives properly, without fights, trespasses, without raising oneself "above" oth-ers or getting into "hot" states, that is, if one is "adjusted" and hence in the ideal "cool" state, one lives to an old age. In contrast, anger, tensions, and transgressions are full of risk, since they may lead to pathogenic "oppressing problems" or vexed "ghosts" and can create enemies, who might "heat up" a person, causing illness or even death.

V

With some exceptions, such as the death of a baby (not yet a "complete" human being) or of a very old, feeble person (whose curve of life has arrived "at the bottom"), no case of death is looked upon as "natural" but is always held to have been caused by an agent. Signs of death are the discontinuation of breathing (and also the cessation of the heart beat), which indicate that the *moñan* ("breath spirit") has left the body.

A recently deceased person is called *amɨn koñwak,* and somebody who has died some time ago is *amɨn komakmbe,* "the finally departed." In former times, the dead were buried on scaffolds in trees or at inaccessible places, but today they are buried in a coffin in the cemetery. The more important and older a person, the longer he or she had therefore been part of the community and the more extensive his or her networks of social relations, the bigger and more elaborate the burial. At the death of a small child, of an "incomplete human being," the burial, in contrast, takes place in the bosom of the family. In his or her house, or, should this be too small for the many people expected for the burial, in another, larger house, the deceased is wrapped in a new piece of cloth leaving the head free. While relatives and acquaintances in far away villages are informed, for example, by singing the dead person's *koñgap* melody as "news" that is transmitted across the valleys, the preparations begin. Large amounts of food are collected by the relatives in one place, pigs may be killed, and betel nuts are organized. After these preparations, and when people from the other villages arrive laden with food, the joint mourning begins. This is conducted mainly by women, while the men gather in smallish groups in front of the dead person's house and sing, unadorned and rather discreetly, their own *koñgap* melody. The women, in contrast, enter the house in groups (each comprising women from the same village) while rhythmically dancing towards the deceased and singing the *koñgap* melody of the deceased as well as those of his male relatives, living or dead. (In case of a deceased female, the women sing the *koñgap* melody of her husband.) Thus while, for example, the women from Devil village as a group mourn the deceased, which takes between half an hour and an hour, the group of women from Uskokop have already pushed into the now overcrowded house, so the women from Devil dance in retreat to make room to the newcomers. After several hours of this mourning song, all the participants are invited to a communal meal. Later on, or on the following day, the corpse is put into a coffin, with few people present, mostly only the pall bearers and a few spectators, and then it is carried to the cemetery, located above Gua in a bamboo grove. An evangelist or pastor recites a few prayers and the coffin is lowered into the ground. Later on, a small wooden cross may be erected on this spot.

During the following days, the deceased's clan members give to the clan of the mother of the deceased, the *pek* (see Chapter 2), a "payment," *amɨn ngop,*[12] "human wrapping," consisting of a few piglets or money. This prestation should facilitate the return of the "ghost" from the father's clan (to which he in fact belongs) to his mother's clan, the place of origin of his *amɨnwop* ("shadow soul"), which at his death had changed into a "soul of a dead person" (*koñwop*), and where he or she therefore feels at home. "Death spirits" that are dissatisfied and wander around among the members of the patriclan are potential agents of illness. The burial is now over. During the following weeks, the time of the *guyam* (no translation), the closer relatives of the deceased (his brothers and their families) will live with the latter's family members to help them cope with their loss. Directly after the death, the "soul of a dead person" (*koñwop*) may at night dwell in the places where the deceased often stayed (in his or her garden or house). Several people told of such encounters, which frightened them very much when they spotted the "dead soul" as an "image" of the deceased, or noticed noises caused by it. If somebody walks around at night and hears a noise, he or she asks into the darkness: "*aminbamo bo koñwop*, "[are you] a real man or a dead soul?"

Over time, the power of the "dead soul" decreases, as it grows tired of the nightly wanderings and, according to the traditional version, either swims down the Yupno River to the place in the sea where the other "ghosts" (*koñ*) are, or else, in the mission version, climbs up into the sky. To the living, it becomes a more and more anonymous "ghost."

VI

How can we place the Yupno concept of the person in ongoing discussions about the concept of person, self and identity in non-Western cultures? In the 1970s, anthropologists increasingly began to study concepts of "person," "self" and "individual," construing them as culturally defined and constructed. These three terms are ambiguous and quite differently defined and understood by various writers (Strathern and Stewart 1998).

In older definitions, frequently quite simplified and stereotypical dichotomies had been constructed, such as a "sociocentric organic" view of the non-Western self versus the "egocentric contractual" self of Western cultures (Shweder and Bourne 1984). The spiritual and material dimensions of the human being are played down in these dichotomies. The concept of the person appears to be disembodied, since in most human societies, including the Yupno, the concept of a person is closely connected with the ideas about the body and about substances and body fluids, such as blood and sperm. In addition, most of the societies understand the person as a psychosomatic entity, which is embodied and imbedded in a network of social relationships (Morris 1994: 194–95). Other elements that define personhood may be space and social affiliation, as Fajans (1985, 1997) has documented for the Baining; or names, as for the Iatmul (Wassmann 1991); or a melody, as in the case of the Yupno *koñgap*.

Instead of continuing the rather awkward juxtaposition of a Western concept of person with (very numerous, other) non-Western concepts, in short, "the West versus the rest," in the 1980s, anthropologists studied clearly emically oriented ethnopsychologies and folk theories of personhood (White and Kirkpatrick 1985) as well as emotions, feelings, sentiments and cultural identities (Linnekin and Poyer 1990) in various Pacific societies.

For the Melanesian concept of the person, Marilyn Strathern's notion of the Melanesian person as a "dividual" rather than an "individual" (M. Strathern 1988), one that it is "defined by relationality rather than individuality" (Stewart and Strathern 2000: 17), became crucial and influential. In his chapter "People as Social Beings," Morris (1994) analyzes studies among the Gahuku-Gama, Bimin-Kuskusmin and Ifaluk. In all three societies, the person is conceptualized as an essentially social being, but recognized as well are "the individuality and idiosyncratic aspects of the personality" (Morris 1994: 166). Individuality is for him a ubiquitous phenomenon and not a Western privilege.

This is certainly the case among the Yupno, among whom the concept applies to a relational individual, a form of personhood in which elements of both relationality and individuality coexist (cf. Stewart and Strathern 2000: 17). The two spiritual elements, *moñan*, "breath spirit," and *wopm*, "shadow soul," together with the unique *koñgap* melody, are clearly individual aspects of a Yupno person. Emphasizing the relational dimension, social relationships are tantamount, and their quality is decisive for the mental state and the ideal position of a human being—that of a cool person in the midst of others.

Chapter 4

The Case Study: Nstasiñge

1. The Illness of the Little Boy, Nstasiñge, from the Point of View of his Mother and Relatives

The first part of this chapter is based on the detailed account elicited from Mayu, the mother of the baby, an analysis of discussions that went on for many evenings about the child's illness, and on interviews with relatives and people familiar with the family situation. Talks with the mother took place in August 1988, about one and a half years after the child's illness began; the emotional and temporal distance to the events can be felt in the rendering of her story. It was impossible to talk with the mother during the acute phase of the baby's illness (February 1987–July 1987); and in any case, these events occurred at a very early stage of my research, so I understood little about what was going on. In addition, the women, especially, were afraid of me and it took some time to develop closer contact with them. Mayu herself was at that time preoccupied with worry about her child and with how to cope with imputations of guilt coming from her relatives. Given this heavy burden, her reluctance to talk to a recently-arrived outsider was understandable, let alone having to deal with a completely new situation (including conversations recorded on tape and interviews about her child). The eventual discussion about the possible causes of the illness, here rendered in detail, was tape-recorded in Yupno and translated into Tok Pisin with the assistance of an interpreter. All the initially vague issues, such as kinship relationships and the past histories of single acts, were subsequently clarified with the actors in question during lengthy conversations. In some parts, I interrupt the remarks with short excursi that explain the subjects mentioned and make them comprehensible within the particular context. The possible causes of illness are only cursorily stated here, as are others not discussed in this case, since these are analyzed more comprehensively in the description of the Yupno medical system given in Chapter 5. The letters in brackets refer to the participants presented in Chapter 4.1.a), and the numbers in brackets indicate the suspected causes of Nstasiñge's illness as outlined by Mayu or her relatives; they are placed against the background of social relationships in Figure 2. Relevant Yupno language terms are in brackets and translated in the glossary.

a) The Participants

To begin, I present in concise form the persons participating in the events surrounding little Nstasiñge 's illness (or mentioned in the story), their positions in the kinship system and their network of relationships.

In the course of the illness, the social space changes; the more threatening the child's state of health becomes, the more the social environment expands (within the traditional system). More and more persons join the therapy managing group,[1] swelling the number of participants in the discussions and potential agents of illness.

The participants in the order of their "appearance":

a) **Mayu,**   the mother of the little baby Nstasiñge, a young woman, originally from the Tangoman clan from Uskokop;

b) **Nstasiñge,**   her little son and first child. He was born on 11 July 1986, and so was six months old at the beginning of his illness in January 1987. Like his father, Tanowe, he belongs to the Tuwal I clan;

c) **Susune,**   the mother of Mayu's husband Tanowe, therefore the grandmother (*owa*) of the baby on the father's side. A vivacious, quick-witted woman, originally from the Talam clan in Uskokop, she was married to the late Mañnau, a man from the Tuwal I clan from Gua. Susune (as a now-widowed older woman), Mayu and her husband Tanowe, and the baby Nstasiñge, form a household. They live in a house in Gua no. 2, the largest village sector of Gua (see Chart 1, house D), in Kaparɨkandom, the "hill of the *kapari* sweet potatoes," which extends up the mountain behind the church;

d) **Erarape,**   a sick old man from the Tuwal III clan in Gua. His house stands close to little Nstasiñge's house. As he is at home almost all the time, his house had become a popular meeting place for the men; Tanowe, the child's father, often visits. Erarape, as a neighbor, friend, and competent older man (and also as a distant relative, since in certain critical situations the Tuwal clan, although subdivided into three clans, is still looked upon as a unit), closely followed the baby's illness right from the beginning.

e) **Tanowe,** the father of the baby, Tuwal I clan, Gua. The young man seemed to be overtaxed by the illness and escaped from the situation by frequent absences. Since he had lived with his father in Rabaul for some years, he had problems with the level of social conformity demanded by life in the village and appeared to be unhappy with his situation.

f) **Virin,** an eloquent man from the Komin clan, Gua, who works as an assistant police officer at Teptep Station. As the sole male Komin representative, he associated with the Ngandum clan and the Kapbaga clan (both small in number). Tanowe's clan Tuwal I and his partner clan, the Umban, are also small in numbers, so they unite for important activities (such as brideprice transfer) with the Tuwal II clan or its partner clan (Komin, Kapbaga, Ngandum and, in this case, Umban), respectively. Virin thus assisted as a member of the temporary partner clan in raising Mayu's brideprice. Since he lives in Teptep, his house is a favorite address for people from Gua who come there to stay at the health center.

g) **Megau,** belonging to the Ngandum clan, Gua, and 'komiti' (officially elected village head) of Gua, Megau is a quiet, thoughtful "big man" (*amdi*) whose clan substantially assisted in financing Mayu's brideprice (therefore has a claim to the interest earned by that brideprice, namely, the baby); it also acts as partner clan to Tuwal I and II (which sporadically united due to the lack of male members; see f, above).

h) **Mian,** a young, unmarried girl from Uskokop village, who is distantly related to Mayu on the mother's side and sometimes spends the night at Mayu's.

i) **Nañgut,** an older man from the Tuwal I clan in Gua, former 'luluai' (a village head appointed by the government). Owing to his profound knowledge of acts that cause illness and of techniques to divine the causes, and also because of his generally unfriendly, aggressive manner, he is not popular in the village and is feared by some, but respected as well. He was *opmot* (a kind of adoptive father) to Tanowe when the latter's father was living in Rabaul. There is a persistent rumor in the village about a love affair between him and Susune (c).

k) **Kan,** from the Tuwal II clan, Gua, Nañgut's (i) second wife, Kan has for a long time allegedly been jealous of Susune (c). Her position in the village is quite isolated, because many villagers remain sympathetic to Nañgut's first wife, Praie (x), from whom he separated, at the mission's insistence, when he married Kan.

l) **Jurenu,** Megau's (g) younger brother, a man from the Ngandum clan, Gua. His house is close to Nstasiñge's house, and he also contributed to Mayu's brideprice.

m) **Saop,** a younger, unmarried woman, daughter of Nañgut (i) and his first wife Praie (x), with whom she also lives.

n) **Marope,** an old, frail single man, originally from the village of Kewieñ, for many years a mission worker in Gua who does little other than maintaining a close watch on all that happens in his village sector (Gua 1).

o) **Tsarau,** belonging to the Tuwal I clan, a brother of Tanowe's late father Mañnau (y), who, following disputes, has been living for years with his family in Bameleñ (the fieldname for the region Tapmañge). His son, Nstasiñge, is the older "namesake" (*wau*) of little Nstasiñge.

p) **Tinko,** Jurenu's (l) wife, a neighbor of Mayu (a) and Susune (c).

q) **Manau,** an older man from the Kawɨliñ clan, Uskokop, who today lives in Gua with people from the Ngandum clan; his house is close to that of Nstasiñge.

r) **Mapte,** an old and strong-willed "traditionalist," Ngangalbuk clan, Gua.

s) **Peloñ,** wife of Kewenu, a son of Mapte (r) who at the time was staying in Madang.

t) **Sauno,** the old evangelist of Gua (originally from Kewieñ). Responsible for the services on Sundays as a 'wokman' of the

Figure 2: Nstasiñge's Social Space

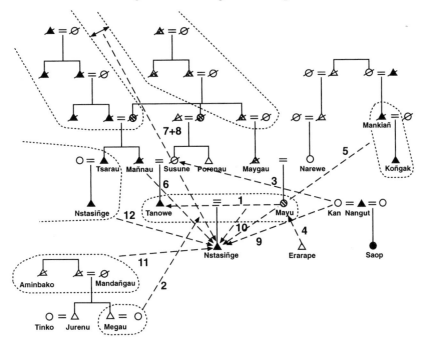

▲ ●	Tuwal 1 clan	
△ ⊘	Tangoman clan	
△ ○	other clans	
....	groups of people	
– – →	"oppressing problems"	

church but with little else to do; he rarely misses anything going on in his village, and is present at every invitation.

u) **Narewe,**   Mayu's (a) mother, originally from the Nyimal clan, Uskokop; she was married to Mayu's late father, Maygau, Tangoman clan, Uskokop.

v) **Mankiañ,**   Narewe's (u) "little father" (*nanjok*, FaFaSiSo), deceased a long time ago, a man from the Tuwal I clan.

w) **Koñgak,**   Mankiañ's (v) son, who, because of his father's contribution to Narewe's (u) brideprice, has felt left out of the brideprice for Mayu (a).

x) **Praie,**   Nañgut's (i) first wife and Saop's (m) mother, a *kumbu amɨn* (a person receptive to powerful dreams, a kind of medium) and a renowned interpreter of dreams.

y) **Mañnau,**   Tanowe's (e) late father, originally from the Tuwal I clan, Gua, but later moved to the Kapbaga clan, Gua.

b) The Child's Mother: "I Thought the Little Boy Wanted to Play a Trick on Me…"

Mayu, the mother of the little baby Nstasiñge, tells how she notices the first changes in her baby on the way back from a visit to her natal village, Uskokop:

> I thought the little boy [b] wanted to play a trick on me and that he was thumping me [he was tied to her back with a piece of cloth] because he wanted to be breastfed. I went on down a bit further, I heard him breathing heavily and got him out [of the cloth he was carried in] and I felt his body was completely hot [*ngodɨm tepmtok*], like fire. I went to my garden, sat down, and I saw that his eyes were all red [*ndavɨli goman*]. I saw his skin was trembling [*ninimoktak*], and he wanted to die, and what was I to do?
>
> I saw Susune [c, her husband's mother], she was busy digging up sweet potatoes, and I called out to her: 'hey, no time to dig up sweet potatoes now, get yourself up, you hold on to him!' I held him, and she also took him into her arms, he was not well, he was close to dying. He wanted neither his grandmother [*owa*] nor me. I had not walked far away with him and something was on his skin, and I became afraid, and I left the sweet potatoes [which Susune had dug up] behind, took the baby and came down [to the village of Gua from the garden land Gomevɨlka, see Chart 1, no. 2].
>
> I came, looked in my house, nobody was sitting inside, and I went into Erarape's [d] house and I talked to my husband [who was sitting there at the fire], and Tanowe [e] got up, lit *bumbum* [reed-like stalks] and came into our house. The baby was sitting, was sitting comfortably, but he was screaming all the time. Even when his father was holding him and then left, he screamed all the time and we gave him pancakes [*plaua*[2]] and all kinds of things; he did not want them, he screamed and screamed, he was still ill, and I saw, his skin was all hot, and I got up and took him to Teptep, at night. I looked into the house of the 'dokta,'[3] I knocked, and at that time a

small boy from Tapmañge had also fallen ill and slept in the ward [in the house with two rooms for stationary patients, built by the Yupno themselves out of bush material], and I sent this boy to go and look for the 'dokta.'

He came then, carried him [the baby] into the treatment house [the outpatient department] and examined him, looked at him and said: 'at what time exactly did he get sick?' They asked me, and I answered: 'only just now.' And they lit the lamp and poured water into a basin and lay him in this basin [bathed him] and he was not afraid nor did he tremble, he made no sound, he lay in the basin as if dead. 'Tomorrow morning, you bring him back here,' the 'dok-taboy' told me. And I got back to Virin's [f] house, lit *bumbum*-stalks, and [at night] went back to Gua.

Excursus: "Natural" Disorders

The first signs of a disorder Mayu noticed in her child were bodily changes, problems with breathing ("I heard him breathing heavily"), raised tempera-ture and shivering fits ("his body was completely hot," "his skin was trem-bling") and an altered appearance ("his eyes were all red").

The Yupno do not attribute great importance to the bodily symptoms alone (fever, colds, diarrhoea, wounds, and so on) as long as they fade away or dis-appear after a few days; that is, the disorder proceeds in a way felt to be "nor-mal"[4] and does not incapacitate or severely endanger a person. They may be felt to be *tepm* (hot, pain, fast), a "hot" disorder of the physical well-being (the "cool" ideal state), and are not called by the term for illness (*sit*) but explicitly with the appropriate term for the symptoms. Initially, they are treated in the lay sector with home remedies such as special prescribed foods, commonly known phytotherapy (plant medicine), rest or massage. Should these treatments have no effect, a "cooler" is consulted (somebody who brings the affected "heated up" person down to the proper "cool" state) or a traditional herbalist who treats the disorder with ablutions and certain plants thought to be cold. Alternatively, peo-ple increasingly resort to Western medicine, provided by the health center in Teptep and by different aid posts. Above all, the younger people (like Mayu) ac-cept biomedicine in case of bodily disorders, and modern pharmaceutical prod-ucts are increasingly replacing the therapy administered by traditional "coolers."

The sudden onset of physical disorders combined with the behavior of the child ("he wanted to die," "he screamed and screamed") scares her ("I became afraid") and at first makes her feel helpless ("what was I to do?"). When all attempts to calm down the child fail, she goes to the Teptep Health Centre because she no longer interprets his condition as a "natural" harmless disorder that originated "by itself" in the infant and would also pass by itself, or is curable by her. There, she hopes that biomedicine will take away her baby's bodily symptoms. She feels the state of the child becoming more and more life-threatening ("he lay in the basin as if dead") and she begins to look for possible causes for the illness; in other words, she now interprets his behavior as "ill." She does not exclude herself as a potentially illness-causing person: "I had not walked far away with him." This sentence must also be understood as a justification vis-à-vis her husband's Tuwal I clan and its partner clan, who together raised her brideprice and therefore hold a claim to the child and hence expect her as the mother to watch over her baby (the "product of the purchase" and a new member of the pair of clans). A mother who walks about alone over a great distance, that is, leaves the control of the village, is not behaving "properly," because she risks illness or death from "sorcery" (*mawom*), or at the hands of the bush-spirit (*sindok*), angered by her intrusion into its realm.

During this first phase of the baby's illness (from afternoon until night), the social space was confined to the household and the nuclear family (mother, child, father and grandmother). Since all the home remedies and attempts to mollify the child (with tidbits) failed, Mayu made the decision to take her child to the Teptep Health Centre to seek a cure for its bodily disorders. In this case, the decision was made easier by the proximity of the Teptep Health Centre (about three quarters of an hour by foot). In addition, Mayu is a young woman who favors biomedicine as an alternative to traditional cooling-therapy, so, had she and her baby lived in a village farther away from Teptep, they would have looked for help from either an Aid Post Orderly (APO),[5] if available, or from a traditional "cooler." For the latter's therapy, however, preparations lasting at least several hours (collecting certain leaves and plants, getting water from certain streams) would be necessary. Initially, then, her action seems aimed only at her child's exceptional bodily condition.

c) A Relative of the Child to the Mother: "Why Did Your Child Get Such a Serious Illness?"

So I went back to Gua and reached my house and saw that Tanowe [e] was sitting there, and I yelled at him: 'where have you been hanging around? Now you are sitting here and I am having such a hard time!' That is what I yelled at him and I told him: 'I think he has got a *njigi* ["oppressing problem"] [1][6] from you!' This is what I said and I was very angry with him. But Tanowe did not give it a thought, he did not think of the baby, he left us and disappeared, and it was very hard for me to watch the baby the whole night.

The next morning, when I woke up, I was still very angry at Tanowe [who had come back]. The others, Megau [g] and his wife, came, and they were both very furious about the two of us [Mayu and Tanowe]. 'We do not know anything definite about you, where have you been hanging around and [thereby] killed him!'[2]. That is how they talked to us. Megau [g] added: 'I cannot really tell you off now.'

And the two of us, the baby and I, went to the hospital. The baby did not think of his *mbawo* [grandfather, here: Megau] or anything else, he only thought of me, glued himself tightly to my skin and did not drink anything, just sat there and screamed and screamed.

I sent Mian [a young girl, h] to Nañgut [i] to make him come and talk a bit to the baby, that is why I sent Mian. Nañgut [i] came; they boiled this piece of pork [which Mayu had received before-hand at a *pelok*, a brideprice return] and tried to give part of it to the baby but he did not want it; we ate it and the baby just looked on and went to sleep. The two of them, Nañgut [i] and Mian [h], came and stayed with us, Nañgut's wife, Kan [k], also came and said: 'Susune [c], you have a *bɨmjɨt* ["oppressing problem"] [3] which stands at the wayside in Mbɨvɨka ["the place of the broken-up ground," see Chart 1, no. 1]' [where Nañgut's [i] house is situated] and she added: 'Susune, do you not see the *bɨmjɨt* and you are hiding and you go inside my fence [the fenced-in area where the house is]! And you, old man [addressing her husband Nañgut, i], why have you again come [here]?' Nañgut's wife then got very upset and was furious. 'This big fight of yours is there!' [it is unresolved], she said, and she was standing there at the door and was furious with us. Kan [k] grabbed a *bumbum*-stalk from me and made a fire outside and sat there and insulted us and talked. And Nañgut [i] got up and did not say anything, he only listened and he did not talk to his *mbawo* [grandson, the baby, b]; he was furious with his wife and went out and disappeared. 'I am leaving you now!', that is what Nañgut said and left.

And the baby lay there like dead. Everybody was yelling and they left. 'We cannot think of the baby now, that is something that concerns everybody. Whatever he is going to do [whichever "sign," *tauak*, he is going to give], we will see it.' This is what they said, and I grabbed a cloth and held him and the two of us slept. I felt him kicking again and I got up, and said: 'Mian [h], my child is dying; come quickly and hold him!' The two of us were busy holding him and Susune [c] thought of all kinds of relatives, where they might be right now, and she ran around looking for them and told it [the news that the baby was ill] to everyone.

Jurenu [l] and Saop [m] came and held the baby, and they brought the baby to Erarape's [a neighbor's, d] house. [...] Erarape started a fight with me [...] he yelled the following: 'why did your child get such a serious illness?' [4], and I did not say anything. They were all holding him and everybody's eyes closed and they wanted to sleep and they went to sleep all over the place, and old Marope [the mission worker, n] was sitting there and watched over the two of us. I got up and told Saop [m]: 'my backside is hurting, my back is all crooked and everything hurts. I am going to give him to you now.' I gave him to Saop, Saop was holding him, I stretched myself out. Saop was ill, too, and how were the two of us to hold him? It was very hard for the two of us to hold him, [but] this way we managed; my eyes wanted to close and I only slept lightly. Saop was holding the baby and the two of them were sitting there and Saop saw that he wanted to die and she woke me. 'Hey, Mayu, your child is going to die now!', that is what she said and shook me awake. Thus we spent the night until it was very late. Old Marope [n] also felt ill and said: 'I feel badly and that is why I am going to sleep; what are you two going to do? You both stay here.' That is what he said and he went into this house. 'Too bad if you do not watch out and he dies.' This is what he said and left.

And the two of us [Mayu and Susune, c] sent a message to Tsarau [o] and his relatives, and this group did not arrive. This is what we did and daylight came and it was also Monday, 'komyuniti de,' they came to get us, and everybody went off to work. Tinko [p, the wife of the neighbor Jurenu] got up and helped me, and the two of us took turns holding the baby, and Tinko was ill, too, that is what I felt. I said to Tinko: 'I feel like I am ill, too, Tinko, you hold the baby,' and Tinko held the baby, and I went outside, and I slept at the door of Manau's [q] house [which is very close], and I slept there. I slept very deeply, and they woke me up, and I got up, went into Jurenu's [the neighbor, l] house. Very early in the morning we had sent Mapte [r] to Bameleñ [Tapmañge] with the message for Tsarau [o] and his relatives, and they did not come quickly, they were all still running around outside, and late in the afternoon they all arrived, and they shook the baby's hand, and they went outside, and the baby was like dead, and Kewenu's wife, Peloñ [s], got up and said: 'oh, he has died.' This is what she said and went outside and disappeared.

I took water and poured it into the baby's mouth, and the water gurgled inside and came out again, the baby threw up, this is how I did it, and the baby became a bit livelier again. And old Sauno [the evangelist, t] went into the house and got a bamboo full of water and held it and poured water into the baby's mouth. This is how he did it, and at night everybody held a meeting and talked about some *bɨmjɨt* ["oppressing problems"] [5, 6] which concerned them, admitted their misdemeanor, *nduara*, and collected a 'kollekta,'[7] this is how they did it, and they all went outside and everybody in his direction and the baby was in Tinko's [p] arms.

Excursus: Social Misbehavior, "Oppressing Problems" and the Discovery of the Cause with the Help of "Signs"

The baby's illness is no longer interpreted as a harmless bodily disorder (see first excursus) but as a illness caused by *njɨgɨ*, by "oppressing problems." *Njɨgɨ* (*njɨgɨ*: heavy, in the physical sense—a stone is *njɨgɨ*—as well as in a symbolic sense), the most common causes of illness, are unsolved, oppressing problems caused by voluntary or involuntary misdemeanors of one or several members of the kinship group.[8] They can be explained only with reference to Yupno social norms and signify a disturbance in the network of social relations. The "oppressing problem" can affect the person with "guilt" (*nduara*) directly or indirectly as when the injured party reacts angrily or feels insulted, that is gets into a hot state (*mbɨt kandap*, "the belly burns," "it boiled inside"), which then develops into an "oppressing problem" (*njɨgɨ*). The Yupno thus distinguish various forms of emotional states that are culturally (through culture-specific values) defined (see Chapter 5.2.c.). We can roughly characterize them in terms such as jealousy, insult, the suspicion of having been lied to or betrayed, and as reactions resulting from these emotional states (somebody yells curses, or rages, or "blows his top"). The *moñan* ("breath spirit") and the "vital energy" (*tevantok*) of the person thus affected hence becomes negative, "hotly" charged, and the victim will unload this hot, illness-causing state onto the agent or somebody from the latter's kinship group.

Njɨgɨ is the generic term for "oppressing problems" of all kinds. Should a Yupno fall ill because of a "ghost" (*koñ*), one also speaks of a *njɨgɨ*, an "oppressing problem," or more precisely of a *bɨmjɨt*, an "oppressing problem" caused by a dead person or his "ghost." "Ghosts" are able to wander around at night close to the village or even in the settlement itself (most often where their former owner stayed), and by taking possession of a living individual can thereby cause him or her to fall ill. The motive is revenge, retaliation: the "ghost" or its owner had become greatly annoyed when still alive, perhaps because of certain incorrectly executed brideprice transfers, or lack of care by relatives in old age, or because of having been made ill or killed by someone, causing a desire to wreak revenge on the alleged perpetrators. Very often, the "owners" of the "ghosts" have been dead for decades, so it is difficult to discover why these "ghosts" became so malevolent.

The basis of every therapy is thought to be the discovery of the "oppressing problem" (*njɨgɨ*). To achieve this, the patient and his environment are examined for "signs" (*tauak*) containing indications as to the causes of illness, which thereby make it possible for those present to formulate a diagnosis and become therapeutically active. Thus, at first, the miming and gesturing of the patient are closely studied. Should he or she repeatedly make signs or should certain animals scurry past and thus point to a certain person (brother, spouse) or a group of persons (the own clan, *nut*, see Figure 1) as the culprits, the relatives of the mother (*pek*) or the wife (*mbasok*), then the kinship group and partner clan in question will be invited to a lengthy discussion, during which potential problems will be voiced and misdemeanors will be disclosed.

The Yupno have at their command a very complex system of knowledge regarding all kinds of signs and their interpretations,[9] such as the right-left concepts (right: the hand that pulls the bowstring and shoots the arrow means the patrilineage *nut*; left, the hand that holds the bow, signifies the matrilateral kinship group *pek*), and the hot-cool-cold concepts, which are ascribed to the domains of men or women or identifications between humans and the things of nature (e.g., a butterfly stands for a woman) and many more. As an example, if a patient drinks a lot of water or asks for sugar-cane, the cause of his illness points to a woman (with whom, for example, he had illicit relations and whose enraged and "hot" husband now causes an "oppressing problem"), since water and sugar-cane are thought to be cold, belonging to the domain of a woman. At the same time, attention is paid to the dreams of the patient or his or her relatives, which are interpreted by a specialist and provide additional indications as to the cause of illness.

In the case of little Nstasiñge, there was soon an agreement that an "oppressing problem" had to be responsible for his illness. Mayu was the first to announce this suspicion to her husband (e) and accuse him ("I think he has got a *njigɨ* from you!") (1).[10] Megau (g) and his wife, representatives of the group that substantially financed Mayu's brideprice, first hold Mayu and her husband to be the agents for the illness ("Where have you been hanging around?") (2); Kan (k), motivated by jealousy, accuses Tanowe's mother Susune ("Susune, do you not see the *bɨmjɨt*?") (3); while the neighbor Erarape (d) blames Mayu ("Why did your child get such a serious illness?") (4).

In order to gain insight into the illness-causing "oppressing problem" by way of discussion, Tsarau (o), Tanowe's "little father" (*nanjok*, FaBr) and his family, as the closest relatives, were informed of the baby's illness and asked to come to Gua.

The first debate about the illness took place in Jurenu's (l) house on 10 February 1987. The therapy managing group had enlarged: apart from the family, members of the Tuwal I clan as well as people from Mayu's matrilateral kinship group (Mayu's *pek*) were present. Various people (Mayu, her husband Tanowe (e), the neighbor Erarape (d) and others) had earlier observed the baby's behavior, looking for possible "signs" (*tauak*). Mayu had given her child to different people (Susune (c), Tanowe, Jurenu (l) and others) to hold, in order to see how the child would react to these people; for example, if he stopped screaming, this would be a sign that this person was not responsible for his illness, or if he screamed even more, this would point toward an "oppressing problem" emanating from this person. The child had been taken into the houses of various kinship groups and clans, but no clear conclusions could be drawn from his behavior. Everybody concurred with the diagnosis of an "oppressing problem" because it was no longer possible to interpret the child's behavior as a passing, "normal" disorder, but the illness could neither be attributed to individuals (the baby acted the same with everyone) nor be localized in kinship groups (having tested different houses). In the meantime, the little child refused to drink milk and cried and wailed almost ceaselessly, a behavior that pointed to an "oppressing problem" in the maternal clan (that of Mayu, the Tangoman clan in Uskokop). Mayu and other women together tried to carry the baby and to hold him in such a way as to retain his *amɨnwop* ("shadow soul") and prevent it from slipping out of his body for good—which would have meant death. There was talk of a *pekno tauak*, hence a hint that the cause of the illness was to be discovered in the maternal kinship group of the baby (*pek*), so people began to think along those lines. Who in Mayu's kinship group could be angry and, in order to punish the parents, cause the child to be ill, and where could the reason for this resentment be discovered?

Narewe (u), Mayu's mother, thought she had found the cause. During this first debate, she told of her own brideprice transfer. At the time, when she was young (and still unmarried), she was made pregnant by Maygau, a man from the Tangoman clan from Uskokop. Her father, a man from the Nyimal clan, Uskokop, was beside himself with rage when he found out, so he beat up Narewe, dug two deep pits, then put Maygau and Narewe into them and left them to their fate. Koñgak's (w) father, Mankiañ (v), a man from the Tuwal I clan, Gua, a "little father" (*nanjok*) of Narewe (Narewe's FaFaSiSo) watched this, grabbed his bow and arrow, went to Uskokop, freed Narewe and Maygau and brought them to Gua. Afterwards, he paid a very high brideprice to Narewe's clan, and consequently the matter was formally closed; Narewe and Maygau lived together as a married couple and Mayu was born. When Mayu's brideprice was paid, Koñgak did not receive anything; he was "forgotten." Koñgak was very upset about it, since his father Mankiañ had substantially contributed to the brideprice of Mayu's mother Narewe and traditionally he could, by rights, have claimed (as Mankiañ's son) part of Mayu's brideprice. At the time, he let Mayu know that his father or his "ghost" (*koñ*) (the father had died) would do his utmost to prevent[11] Mayu from having children and that, should she bear a child all the same, his father's "ghost" would "eat" this child. Mayu's brideprice was already completed—all the brideprice transfers had been (absolutely correct according to tradition) given to Mayu's paternal clan (the Tangoman clan), its partner clan (the Talam clan) and the "special gift" to Mayu's mother—and nobody had been thinking of Mayu's maternal clan (the Nyimal clan). So this is how Koñgak came to be overlooked. (He was distantly related through his father to the Tuwal I clan, which had raised the brideprice and could only claim anything because of his father's unusual intervention in Narewe's brideprice). It was now believed that Mankiañ's "ghost" (*koñ*) had joined the resentment of his son Koñgak (5) and was causing the child's illness, hence creating a *bɨmjɨt*, "oppressing problem."

In the course of this discussion of illness, other people related their dreams. Several had dreamt they saw Tanowe's father Mañnau (y) together with the baby. In her dream, Praie (x), Nañgut's first wife and a renowned "dream interpreter" (*kumbu amɨn*), had seen Mañnau cutting down a bamboo in exactly the same spot where he had once planted it. This "sign" (*tauak*) indicates exclusively that a member of the clan concerned is going to die at the hands of this man or his "ghost;" the man destroys something he has planted himself (analogous to something he fathered himself), in this case a bamboo, a plant very valuable to the Yupno, which the Yupno River had originally washed up and from which the people came. The dream was locally interpreted as *mbawo tauak* ("sign of the grandfather") or more precisely as *koñ tauak* ("sign of the ghost"). The dream visions therefore pointed to Mañnau or his "ghost" (6).

Tanowe (e), the child's father, then revealed that his father Mañnau (y) had cautioned him shortly before his death that he should not get together with his relatives (*nut*), and especially not with his brothers (FaBr, *nanjok* or *wau*, Nañgut (i) and Tsarau (o)) when he went back to the village. At the time, Tanowe was living in Rabaul with his father, who was working there on a plantation. Mañnau had left Gua after a fight because he thought his brothers (*pe*) had sexual relations with his wife Susune during his absence in town. There were even rumors that Tanowe was the biological son of Nañgut (i). The father let the inhabitants of Gua know, that owing to these affairs, he did not belong to his clan Tuwal I any longer but to the Kapbaga clan. He even related this on a tape shortly before his death and sent it to Gua. But Tanowe did not follow his fathers warnings when he returned to the village after his father's death. Nañgut (a Tuwal I member, a classificatory father's brother), Tanowe's *wau* ("namesake"), became his *opmot* (adoptive father), and he and other men helped Tanowe raise Mayu's (a) brideprice. Mañnau's brothers frequented the house of Tanowe and Susune, and the baby was given—as a *wau* ("namesake")—the name of Tsarau's son, Nstasiñge.

Both "signs" (*tauak*)—the child's behavior when he stopped drinking milk (*pekno tauak*, sign of the mother's kinship group) and Praie's (x) dream (interpreted as *mbawo tauak*, "sign of the grandfather")—were looked upon as *koñ tauak* (since the two potential agents were deceased, "ghosts," *koñ*). Because it could not clearly be ascertained whether one or both the "ghosts" together were responsible (the "signs" after all pointed to two annoyed "ghosts"), the two were combined and people talked of a *bɨmjɨt*, a problem caused by a deceased or his "ghost," and so they staged a small *koñ mɨndak*, a ritual "expulsion of the ghost." The child was rubbed with lime (as a substitute for white "cold" soil *kuak*) by Nañgut (i), a *koñ mɨndak* expert, who put a small heap of lime on the baby's hand, bespoke it and blew it off so that, by analogy, the undesired "ghosts" would leave the child and the house. Additionally, the baby's name was changed, from Nstasiñge (a Tuwal I name, a name from the clan to which Mañnau (y) did not want to belong anymore), to Nanjañne (a Kapbaga name, a name from the kinship group newly chosen by Mañnau). Everybody present gave some toea[12] for a collection, and the total amount (K3.20) was paid into the account of the Tapen congregation (the church district to which Gua also belongs) at the Teptep branch of the Papua New Guinea Banking Corporation. After this, people continued to watch the baby and wait.

The child stayed ill and, when no improvement was to be seen, a (second) discussion about the illness was held on 25 February in Nañgut's (i) house at Mbɨvɨka, the "place of the broken-up ground." Tanowe's father Mañnau (y) or Koñgak's father Mankiañ (v) (or their respective "ghosts") obviously were not responsible for the baby's illness, since their "oppressing problem" had been "cooled down" at the preceding gathering and resolved, yet despite all this the child was no better. No new "signs" from which potential agents for the illness could have been inferred were observed. The gathering was marked by a certain helplessness on the part of all present. Without concrete leads such as "signs" or dreams, there was a somewhat vague debate whether, perhaps generations ago, a member of Tanowe's clan (Tuwal I) might have killed a member of Mayu's clan (Tangoman) by "heating up" (*sit*) (7), causing an angry "ghost" to be still hanging around Gua (instead of having gone to its place near the sea, like all the other "ghosts"). In fact, the Tuwal clan and the Tangoman clan used to be enemies, and two members (Tanowe, Mayu) of these clans had since married without the dispute ever having been settled. The opposite case was also considered: that a member of the Tangoman clan had once killed a member of the Tuwal clan by "heating up" (*sit*) (8) (at the time, the Tuwal were not split up into individual clans as they are today). Since nobody present had any knowledge of genealogies reaching this far back to discover such "ghost" and the cause of his anger, this also limited the therapeutic possibilities. People again collected money and paid it into the account of the Tapen church district.

There was no change for the better in the child's condition. Mayu now left Gua village with her baby and spent one week at Bameleñ (Tapmañge) with Tsarau (o) and his family, hoping that the child's condition would improve there, in a different social environment.

By the beginning of April, the child had been ill for two months, and people in the village feared that he might not grow up normally but would instead remain physically weak and mentally handicapped.

d) The Debate among the More Distant Relatives: "This is How You Have to Speak Your Minds!"

The third gathering to look for the causes of little Nstasiñge's illness took place in Erarape's (d) house on 12 April 1987. The discussion lasted for three and a half hours from 9.15 p.m. Twenty three persons were sitting on both sides of the long fireplace in the dark house, thick with smoke (see Chart 2, see also Chart 1; the house stands directly next to little Nstasiñge 's house on the "hill of the *kapari* sweet potatoes"). Only a small kerosene lamp gave off a faint light in the front part of the house.

The people present (who are given numbers for easier "identification," see Chart 2) and their behavior during this debate:

1. **Mayu,**   the mother. During the whole debate, she was holding her
                      child **Nstasiñge** (2) in her arms. At the beginning of the

discussion, she talked in a very committed way, but later she seemed completely exhausted and was close to tears. When her child started to scream and could not be quieted down, she left the house with the baby for about half an hour. She followed the remainder of the discussion in a tired and resigned fashion.

3. **Susune,**	Tanowe's mother. She was sitting behind Mayu and again and again helped her to calm the child. During the first part of the discussion, she participated actively, vehemently representing the interests of the household (to which she, Mayu, the baby and Tanowe belong), and she adopted a position against Nañgut, acting de facto as the head of the family.
4., 5.,	two women. Sitting next to Susune, remaining quiet and in the background, two young women from the Tangoman clan, Uskokop, relatives of Mayu, who followed the discussion without ever speaking.
6. **Kan,**	Nañgut's second wife. She contributed substantially to the first part of the discussion in a loud voice, but also judiciously as she defended her isolated position against her husband Nañgut and against Susune. Nobody assisted her.
7. **Mañwepe,**	originally from the Tuwal II clan, Gua, married to Uñgwep, Tuwal III clan, Gua. Without herself participating in the discussion, she listened in as a curious neighbor (her house is situated in the same village sector) who is always very well informed about happenings in the village.
8. **Tanowe,**	the father of the baby, Tuwal I clan, Gua. He let the discussion wash over him without contributing anything, and did not answer the numerous requests to adopt a position regarding the event.
9. **Milyam,**	a young man from the Tangoman clan, Uskokop, a good friend of Tanowe, followed the discussion as a spectator.
10. **Sauno,**	the old evangelist from Gua. As a 'wokman' of the church, he took on a peacemaking role by unflaggingly agreeing with all the parties.
11.	A man from the neighboring village of Gwarawon, a friend of Virin (see below) who at the time was visiting him.

Chart 2: The Participants in the Debate

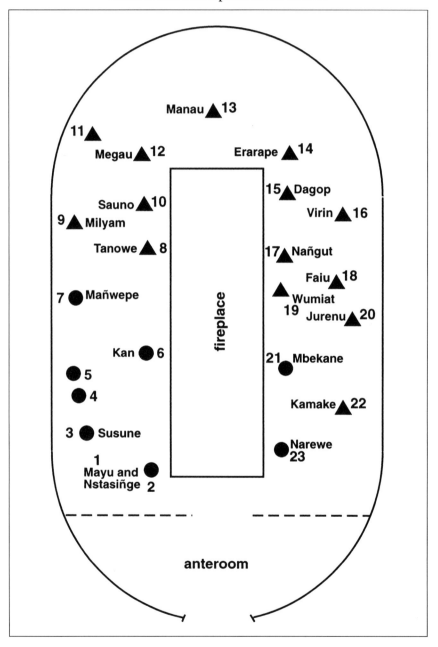

12. **Megau,**   a man from the Ngandum clan, Gua. At the time of the discussion, he was very angry at the inhabitants of Gua, who had shot two of his (the 'komiti's'!) pigs for invading another garden and felt that they were in the right. He slept more or less throughout the whole debate.

13. **Manau,**   as a neighbor, he silently witnessed the debate.

14. **Erarape,**   a man from the Tuwal III clan, Gua. The discussion took place in his house. As a neighbor and a friend, he had been following the baby's illness from the start.

15. **Dagop,**   a man from the Talam clan, Uskokop. He is in a cross-cousin relationship to Susune (*nok*; she is the daughter of his father's sister). He made no contribution but attended as a representative of Susune's clan.

16. **Virin,**   through his maternal kinship group (*pek*), Virin is well versed in the genealogical complexities of the Talam-Tango-man pair of clans in Uskokop. He intervened actively in the second part of the discussion and also tried to explain Tanowe's misdemeanor.

17. **Nañgut,**   during the discussion, he was convinced of the rightness of his behavior and seemed thus unwilling even to think about possible mistakes of his own.

18. **Faiu,**   the pastor of Gua, a younger man from the Kapbaga clan who had also contributed substantially to Mayu's brideprice. After he left the Tuwal I clan, Tanowe's father decided to join this clan. As an eloquent, considerate and educated leader of discussions, he is often called upon during litigation (about land, brideprice transfers and so on) and also represents the village in its dealings with outsiders (for example in front of the 'kiap'). His views are influenced by Christian morals, he possesses no secret knowledge, and he is not very well versed in the genealogical relationships obtaining within in the village, but he is nevertheless very popular with most villagers because of his commitment to their community, his sense of humor and his mediating manner.

19. **Wumiat,**   a man from the Tuwal I clan of Gua, Tanowe's clan, who followed the discussion as a spectator.

20. **Jurenu,**   a man from the Ngandum clan, Megau's (see above) brother. Since he stutters, he rarely speaks in front of a larger group (but makes up for this with floods of words in groups of two or three people), and in this case remained silent.

21. **Mbekane,**   a woman from the Tangoman clan, Uskokop, married to Erarape (see above), the owner of the house. During the debate, when not tending the fire or roasting sweet potatoes, she stayed in the background.

22. **Kamake,**   a young man from the Tuwal III clan, Gua, a cross-cousin (*nok*) and friend of Tanowe. Kamake is married to Erarape's daughter and is a spokesman for the younger generation, since he is the "youth group leader." Like all the younger people, he hardly ever speaks in the presence of older persons.

23. **Narewe,**   Mayu's mother. She silently followed the first half of the discussion — centering on Kan's misdemeanor — from her place near the door, and spoke only during the second part.

As usual, all the men were sitting in the rear "undisturbed" and warmer part of the house, and all the women in the front part; with the exception of Narewe and Mbekane, all the women sat on the left side of the fireplace.

Names mentioned in the discussion:

• **Tsarau,**   belonging to the Tuwal I clan, he has been living in Baméleñ (Tapmañge) for years, and is the brother of Mañnau, Tanowe's late father.

• **Mandañgau,**   the late mother of Megau and Jurenu, belonging to the Ngandum clan through her marriage. She could have claimed a part of Mayu's brideprice return (*pelok*).

• **Mañnau,**   Tanowe's father and Susune's late husband.

• **Aminbako,**   a deceased man from the Ngandum clan, Gua, who also could have laid claim to a part of Mayu's brideprice return (*pelok*).

Faiu [18] [who, being a skilled speaker, opens the debate]: We have now talked about all these problems [*njɨgɨ*] [he refers to the preceding, second discussion about the illness] but the little boy did not get well; I think that when the two old women [Susune, Mayu's mother, and Kan, Nañgut's wife] were fighting and took sticks and were hitting each other, he got scared and became afraid and lost his *amɨnwop* ["shadow soul"], and that is why he is ill. Therefore, we should now talk about it and see what comes of it.

Nañgut [17]: At the time, we were sitting together [in Susune's house] and the two of them [Kan and Susune] were fighting. When they were yelling and almost hitting each other, I got up and held Kan.

Mayu [1]: The two of us, I and the baby, we did not see her [Kan], we were sleeping, we were not thinking of anything but were sound asleep. The baby was sound asleep and I was just going to sleep; and I saw Kan coming to the door, she was talking, and I looked and heard her like in a dream. And this old man [Nañgut] was just picking up a bundle of *ndaga* leaves [chewed as a substitute for betel pepper], he was sitting at the top end of the fireplace. He was taking *awɨ* (lime) from his lime-container and wanted to chew *ndaga*. I talked with him for a bit, and I slept, like in the night, like almost in a dream I talked with him, and I was almost asleep. And I saw Kan as if in a dream and she started to hit me with a stick. I jumped up, grabbed the little boy by the hand and went to the back. I dragged the boy with me, he scratched my breast.

Nañgut [17]: I was sitting at the top of the fireplace and said to Kan [his wife]: 'look out what you are doing!' This is how I talked to her and I saw Kan hitting Susune and going to the front of the house and standing there. Susune was sitting at the fire and collecting the pumpkin skins lying around. I sat at the top of the fireplace and was just eating betel nuts, and Mayu and her baby were sleeping on the other side [of the fireplace].

Mayu [1]: I jumped up and gave the child to Nañgut and closed the door and stood at the door.

Faiu [18]: You?

Nañgut [17]: I had just taken some *awɨ* (lime) out of the lime-container and wanted to chew betel nut and *ndaga*. Kan positioned herself at the door and asked after Koki [a man from the Talon clan, Gua, whose wife is related to Kan]. I answered her: 'we have not seen Koki, it is only us who are sitting here.' Susune was sitting at the fireplace and gathering the pumpkin skins; I was just dropping in. And Kan did not come into the house. I thought she would leave the anteroom and would also sit down at the back, but she came and hit Susune. Susune became scared and went to stand in the corner of the house. I got up and asked Kan: 'why do you do that?', and I went to the middle of the house and held out my hand to her but Kan hit me on the hand. I pushed her with a piece of wood, she fell down and I held her arms tight. That was all. [He points to Mayu who is lying next to him, asleep:] Exactly like this Mayu and her child were sleeping, and Kan was hitting with the stick and I jumped up and told her. 'Calm down, tell us why you have come and are hitting about like this!' She did not answer and walked in the direction of the door and Susune ran past us to the back, sat down and held the baby. Kan jumped into the anteroom, I ran after her, held on to her and asked her: 'why are you hitting Susune? Tell me now, why?' She did not say anything, but put up fierce resistance so I let her go and she went outside. That was all. And we inside the house did not yell out or hit one another.

Faiu [18]: It is only because of this talk [*gen yuki*, gossip, untrue rumors, the rumor that Nañgut was having an affair with Susune, whereupon Kan hit Susune], that is why the little child is ill. Well, the old man [Nañgut] here should now tell us everything about this *njɨgɨ* ["oppressing problem"]. We have not gathered because of some chit-chat but because the old people have been fighting and hitting each other. I believe that is why the child is ill. At the time when you [Susune, Nañgut, Mayu and her baby] were sitting together, did Kan say anything or did she just start hitting? Did she also say something to the child? Speak up now and we will see. If she has provoked you and that is why you started to fight with each other, well then, that was just the anger [*mbɨt njap*], and you were yelling at each other. So then, if you really did it like that, then admit it now and the baby will get well.

Mayu [1]: I had inflamed eyes [*ndavɨlɨ goman*], and I could not see everything. I was just sitting there. I gave my baby to his *mbawo* [grandfather; she means Nañgut] and got up and saw the two [Kan and Susune] fiercely hitting each other. And I thought: if my eyes were alright, I would go and separate the two, but my eyes are inflamed. It would be bad if I tried to separate the two and they hit me. That is why I was just standing there and looking, and Kan came and jumped out of the anteroom and said: 'ah, the good woman from Uskokop here has really borne a marvelous child, indeed! Nobody is carrying him around! [Playing with him, caressing him.] Why did you actually give birth to him? He? Bring him in front of the house and I will break him like a piece of bamboo and throw him away!' That is how she insulted me. I answered her: 'I am a married [paid for] woman! You, you woman from Gua, are acting abominably and are talking a lot of nonsense to me. Go, catch a pig and give it to me! Why are you talking to me like that? I am neither a widow nor a woman who has been let down or is unmarried.' [...] This is how I talked to her and let her go. My eyes were almost swollen shut and I [turning to Kan] did not even see your skin and I was just talking. And she wanted to hit my child and said so. Thereupon I said to her: 'well, fine, you hit him, after all you have paid for the child. Well, you said, you wanted to hit him, you can take him and kill him. That is your business!' And I added: 'if the child is going to die because of someone else's *njɨgɨ* ["oppressing problem"], everybody will be afraid of you.' [Mayu's brideprice had been financed by the Tuwal I clan (to which through her marriage to Nañgut Kan also belongs), so she now belongs to this clan and the village of Gua, and the baby (as a "product of the purchase") also belongs to this clan because it is the "property" of those who have "bought" his mother.]

Nañgut [17]: Yes, that is how she talked. And Susune did not say anything to Mayu, no [did not help her].

Sauno [10]: You have told us this far, now tell us everything!

Nañgut [17]: That is everything. It is not a long story.

Mayu [1]: Yes, that is really all. Shortly afterwards, I saw Kan who had insulted me, walking around and I said to her: 'I did not steal your husband!' [with this, she alludes to the affair Susune/Nañgut] and let her go on. Later, I let her know she should come so the two of us could meet and settle our dispute and make up. But she did not come and I gave up and kept to myself.

Nañgut [17] [to Megau who has woken up in the meantime]: If I was to take a piece of wood or a stick and hit something in the anteroom, your *amɨnwop* ["shadow soul"] would get scared and leave!

Faiu [18] and **Megau** [12]: That is true! If you do something like this, somebody else will lose his *wopm* ["shadow soul"]!

Nañgut [17]: But this is not how Kan did it! She just went inside [into the house] and the two of them [Kan and Susune] did I do not exactly know what and I held on to Kan.

Kan [6]: Yes, that is true! I asked after Koki, that is why I came after all. And then I became so angry. I had heard the rumor [*murum gen*] and thus I went and I hit her [Susune] but not on the skin, I just hit her on her grass skirt.

Susune [3]: You did not hit my grass skirt, you hit my hip. After she had hit me, she came out and I said to her: 'I did not order Nañgut to come here.' [She points at Nañgut:] You just came and sat down beside me for a while in the house and she [Kan] came and hit me for no reason, I did not ensnare you or flirt with you. 'She is lying and publicly blackening my name and now she has to go and get a pig, buy betel nuts and give them to me. That is all.' That is how I talked to Kan and Nañgut. And when I came outside, I said the same thing as inside: 'she has to pay me back!' [Compensate her for the rumor.] We, we are always together [Susune, Mayu and the baby], we all sleep together in our house and we are also together the rest of the time. And I am not lacking a man, I have never called for you [Nañgut and Kan] to come so that we are together, I have never done that. I myself must know, I was there, and you [Nañgut] were running around wherever and sat down in my house. Kan came and screamed and hit me but I was only talking.

Sauno [10]: This is how you have to speak your minds!

Faiu [18]: This is why you were so upset [*mbɨt njap*] and spoke like this to Kan, that was all.

Mayu [1]: And I, I got up and said: 'I—and that is true—I am the wife of a young man, and why is Kan talking to me in this manner?' And, I admit it, I scolded her. And later I called for Kan she should come so that we could both cool our anger [*mbɨt njap*] but she did not come to me and I said: 'that is now your business' and gave it up. But now the 'doktaboys' have made me very much afraid [*mbɨt pasɨl*], my child may not get well again, and that is why I came to find out the problems [*njɨgɨ*], because my child must quickly get well again.

Kan [6]: I explained all this. I do not just hang around after all. I went up [to Tapen] where my *nanjok* ["little father," FaBr, Taminare, who is president of the church district] now lives, and he said there would be no more talk about it and told me: 'go now,' and I went. And I am no longer furious [*mbɨt njap*] because of this business.

Faiu [18]: You stop now and I am going to talk and you listen.

Nañgut [17]: You cannot talk about what Taminare said now. Leave that aside. We, we [the ones present] alone are going to talk now. At the time, Taminare was with you. Did you talk about the little boy or not?

Faiu [18]: They had the wrong ideas about the whole business and they railed. But that is finished now. At the time, we [even though Faiu did not participate, "out of courtesy" he includes himself in public mentions, as is the custom] did it like that, we scared him [the little boy] very much. 'Your *wopm* ["shadow soul"] has run off, it has to come back!' Talk to the baby like this and if you have a Kina coin, good, you have to take it and put it on a string and hang it around his neck. Tomorrow, we will examine him more closely and observe him and we will see how he is.

Nañgut [17]: We have already done all this.

Kan [6]: We have also already talked [like you, Faiu, are suggesting], but they [Mayu and Susune] just took the money to Teptep [where the child was at the health center for a short while] and brought it back and now I have it. And if you think so, well, then we will all touch it.

Faiu [18] [to **Kan**, 6]: You must talk like this: 'I went and grabbed a stick and put it on Nañgut's and Susune's skin. Well then, this child must come to no harm!' This is how you must talk, and put the money down. Because it is you alone who started with this *njɨgɨ* ["oppressing problem"]; call out his name, his *koñgap* [the baby's "melody"], sing it and say '*wupwup!*' to him [*wupwup*: come, come!, meaning: the "shadow soul" *wopm*]. That is all and then you put the money around his neck [the idea behind this: the money (as a valuable) entices the *wopm* ("shadow soul") to come back].

Kan [6]: When it was light, I talked exactly like this. 'You have to call me and you must take this money, talk to the baby like this and make a collection,' that is what I suggested. Why? I am not angry at the child. These two old people [Nañgut and Susune] talked nonsense to me and I reacted and now I am burdened with it. I think this is why the child caught his *njɨgɨ* ["oppressing problem"]. [She turns to Nañgut:] Now you are sitting here and they entrusted [*opmot*, a kind of adoption or namesake-relationship, since Tanowe's father had died in Rabaul; see above] Tanowe, this rascal, to you [Nañgut]. And his child is ill and why on earth did you make me so angry? Yes, only because of this did I behave like that. I think everything points to the fact that he got ill because of it. Well now, I talk about it, and I touched the money and sent it to Teptep [to the health center]. And I said, it [the *wopm* ("shadow soul")] had to return to its place. And now I am sitting here, too, while we are discussing our anger [*mbɨt njap*]. You talk about it, I do not talk about it. 'This child has to get well again,' this is what the two of us, Taminare and I, said, and we included it in the prayer.

Faiu [18] [turned to **Kan**, 6]: You must say: 'you must not be ill because of this business, we big people [adults] behaved like this and you must not start to be ill because of it or be in pain, and you must not behave like this' [scream, refusing to eat an so on], talk to him like this and hang the money around his neck, and we go then and the baby will find sleep in his house.

Nañgut [17]: We agree on this after all and we have also talked about the previous *bɨmjɨt* [the "oppressing problems" (5), (6), (7), (8), see above] discussed in the preceding meeting. Why has he still got a *njɨgɨ* ["oppressing problem"], why is he still not well? We can see it after all, he is still not well. And the two of them [Susune and Kan] are not fighting any longer or whatever, really not. The two of them agree and have made up. The two of them have talked about it and that is it.

Kan [6]: That is what we have just talked about, but if we walk around together, all the people will think: 'she has given another *njɨgɨ* ["oppressing problem"] to the baby.' 'I behave like this [I regret what happened], but you will walk around and talk about that [the "scene"] which made the child ill.' This is how I talked to Nañgut. I did not fetch firewood or once bring a little something to give to the child to eat. I do not even go to the door to his house, and what does it matter? I have not even seen him, do not know anything about him [meaning: she stayed away from the child on purpose].

Sauno [10] I can imagine that this could be exactly why he is ill [because of the lack of care from members of his clan, to which Kan also belongs].

Kan [6]: No! You, Nañgut, have talked about your *mbawo* [grandson, meaning: the baby] and you ran around and he got better, and he came here, and therefore I thought: 'the child belongs to me [to our clan], and I will see him later.' But Mayu never brought our baby, we never held him or caressed him, really not. What kind of a place is this where she is? We do not talk to her, no. I have scolded her, and the child felt ill, and this is why I do not go and visit her. I do not even think of it. I told everybody that and kept to myself.

Susune [3]: About what you just mentioned: we heard from other people that you said: 'oh, they [Mayu, Susune and the baby] may die or walk around and say whatever they want; it is their business alone and I could not care less!'

Mayu [1]: This is how you talked and we heard it from everybody else.

Kan [6]: It is only you who say that!

Nañgut [17]: Ah, stop it, you are spreading these rumors and I think that is why the child is ill.

Mayu [1]: Kan has often talked like this; we were watching her from a distance and we carried the child around.

Kan [6]: That has all been cleared up, that is what you told us, me and Nañgut. Everybody was talking like that when we were sitting in Mundagalgowañ and the others in Jurenu's house [the first discussion about the illness, see above]. I came and heard their voices and what they said. I heard it. We did not agree then, now we talk about it and want to put an end to the matter.

Nañgut [17]: Now I want to say something again. Taminare [Kan's "little father"] at the time saw the *njɨgɨ* ["oppressing problem"], I talk with him about it. Then, at that time, you did I do not know what and talked about it. I have seen it and I was all confused. Then, at that time, the baby was a bit ill, and Taminare after all was with us and saw us, and why do you begin with this matter all over again? Now I see, the two of you are here, and I want to talk about an important point. If you two married people [Mayu and Tanowe] know about any other cause, well, you have to speak up. And, by the way, the *pelok* [the brideprice return] which they [Mayu's relatives in Uskokop] gave—did you bring it here to Gua and show it to us or not?

Kan [6, for whom this whole matter starts to go on far too long and who wants to end the meeting]: You have talked about everything, okay, later we will hold the money.

Mayu [1, refers to the brideprice return [*pelok*] and addresses Nañgut and his clan]: Your child [she means Tanowe] has announced it [the brideprice return] and went [to Uskokop], and I called you that you should come so we could eat together but you did not come.

Nañgut [17]: Mayu, you are talking nonsense, let us forget this.

Faiu [18]: Now leave your former dispute aside.

Mayu [1, to **Nañgut**]: I went to your house in Mbɨvɨka [the "place of the broken-up ground," see Chart 1], and what did I say to you?

Nañgut [17]: I have already said it. You did not want to stuff everything [the brideprice return] into your netbag and take it to Mbɨvɨka. Tsarau [one of Nañgut 's brothers] and his relatives hid their anger and did not say anything; oh well, the child got their *mbɨt njap* [their anger] and now has the *njɨgɨ* ["oppressing problem"].

Mayu [1]: Recently, I went to Bameleñ [Tapmañge, where Tsarau lives] and I stayed there for a week and came down here again. Tsarau and his family did not do anything for me [e.g. talk about the "oppressing problem" due to the brideprice return, see below] to make the child healthy again, and thus I came down here again [to Gua].

Kan [6]: If you just keep to yourself, he [the baby] will never be alright.

Mayu [1]: Yes, that is what they [in Tapmañge] were saying, too. I went up and every single one talked with everybody else, and I came down.

Susune [3]: In Bameleñ [Tapmañge], everybody talked like this, 'cooled down' and 'took down' everything that had been said; everybody was sorry and applied *kuak* [white earth pigment which "cools"] to the baby's skin.

Nañgut [17]: I have only mentioned this [the brideprice return] so that everything may be clear; that is now done with.

Mayu [1]: There is no *njɨgɨ* ["oppressing problem"] on Tsarau's skin. I was there [in Tapmañge] for a week, the baby's skin was hot and painful and he screamed and we had a hard time with him, and we also cried. They tried to help me [which contradicts what she said before], talked, assisted me, everybody felt sorry for me, was full of sympathy, that is how it went, and it was not easy, everybody was trying. They cried for me and for the baby. [She turns to Nañgut:] Do you ever cry and talk like that? They talked a lot and cried hard at the time as if the baby was dead. And they did not stop crying and I became scared and said to them: 'you must not cry like that, you are crying and screaming as if the baby was dead!' And I was afraid and went and took my child.

Nañgut [17]: I wanted to name the cause and the two of you [Susune, Mayu] interrupted me.

Mayu [1]: What did you want to say? Say it now!

Kan [6]: I said to Mayu: 'Sister [meant as an especially cordial form of address], you cannot interrupt the discussion like that; the men who have something to say should talk alone.'

Faiu [18]: The two of you, Susune and Mayu, you cannot interrupt the meeting like that. He [Nañgut] now wants to name the cause of it all. We did not meet in order to just sit around like that. Mayu has a hard time with her child. I would like to voice some new ideas on that. Just sit still and talk and the matter will clear up [the discussion will go well]. Nañgut was [at the time, because of the brideprice return] furious [mbɨt njap], and I met him, and we talked. Stop thinking about all that now and come to the point.

Nañgut [17]: That is it!

Kan [6]: We have now talked about it, it is over, but everybody starts on it again, and the child is afraid, and Mayu is carrying him around. And the child was scared and lost his *wopm* ["shadow soul"]. After all, this is the only reason we are meeting. We finished the little dispute [she means the "scene"], and your *wau* [namesake, used here as a polite form of reference, meaning Taminare], Faiu, has finished that.

Faiu [18]: I think, his father [Tanowe] was playing cards ['laki,' a game for money], and that is why the baby got ill. [Argument: If somebody plays cards, he gets money from other people, and that is a kind of theft, at least for a Lutheran pastor.]

[Everybody is talking at once, vehemently contradicting Faiu's arguments...]

Faiu [18]: In case you [the baby's kinship group], you yourselves, say something bad to the child and cast him out, you thereby give him an enormous *njɨgɨ* ["oppressing problem"]. And about all this, it is true, we [out of courtesy he includes himself], were so furious [*mbɨt njap*] that we grumbled and defamed and got into a fight. The way you talked now, the child will find a way to get well, you will see.

Kan [6]: Tsarau and his relatives are still talking. Once they themselves say, 'Now it is enough and all is well,' that is it, then the child will get well. It is exactly this little sentence they should say, I tell you this.

[Everybody talks at once, fresh wood is put on the fire, some start to roast sweet potatoes...]

Faiu [18]: So far, so good, let us now stop this. We only talk in order to say everything clearly. We listen, and then we put an end to it.

Narewe [23]: We are continuously talking on the surface only.

Nañgut [17]: We talk about how the two women were hitting each other and we have now discussed it to the end and I have talked about the fight and that is the end of it.

Narewe [23]: It is up to the two women to settle it and then it will be over.

Susune [3]: We have already done that, we are only talking about it now.

Nañgut [17]: That is true; as to the two women, their dispute is settled now, and I can see it from the back here, but I also saw how everybody started all over again and brought it up once more. Enough of that, I am not starting all over again, I am finishing with it.

Kan [6]: In the house down there [in Mundagalgowañ], they all said the following: 'the child will now get a *njɨgɨ*' ["oppressing problem"]. Faiu, your brother-in-law [polite form of reference, meaning, Nañgut, her husband] has said that. 'Later, you [Mayu] will have a hard time with the child,' this is what he said, and now the child is ill and she is having a hard time with him. You have done it and now the *njɨgɨ* sticks to everybody [everybody knows it] and it is here and does not go away, just look, if everybody leaves me alone and only I see the *njɨgɨ*, then all the talk about the *njɨgɨ* which I have caused, will be finished, but you have blocked my way, and I was like beside myself in all I said. And you go and collect arguments [*mbalgerk*: to tie leaf to leaf] and talk an awful lot about that. You tie up this *mbalgerk* and make it into *njɨgɨ* and the rumor continues. That is not right. The child is not ill because of all kinds of people. I am like I was before, I wanted to see the baby, to end the rumor, you yourselves took up the rumor and spread it. I had stopped it and you must not take together some of the things I did and do it like that. You are talking complete nonsense. I know what I have said and I did say it. I dreamt a few dreams, I want to sum them up and tell them and you listen to them. We always follow the dreams in what we say and decide then. I thought Nañgut had gone to his woman [she means Susune and alludes to the affair Nañgut—Susune] and I was so furious [*mbɨt njap*] and was raving, and that was why the child lost his *wopm* ["shadow soul"]. And now I think, we are really talking so much and she [Mayu] is annoyed and carries her child outside, ah? [Mayu takes her screaming child out of the house]. Ah, no.

Nañgut [17]: They [Mayu's relatives in Uskokop] did so much to give the two of them [Mayu and Tanowe] pleasure. The two of them took it [the brideprice return *pelok*], brought it down [to Gua], and what did they do with it? Nstasiñge [the *wau*, older namesake of the baby, Tsarau's son], Tsarau and I, we checked it, it was not just a little. That is what I want to talk about now, but those two [Susune and Mayu] interrupted me, and I held my tongue and sat there. That which they gave to them [Mayu and Tanowe] and half of the money we have looked for and did not find. In the night, I was sound asleep, and Tsarau and his child woke me up. We set out to look for the money. We emptied out all the netbags, dumped everything on the floor but could not find anything. At the time when the two of them [Tanowe and Mayu] received the *pelok* [brideprice return] and brought it to Gua, they took the money and it [the money] went. I think this is the only reason we are so angry [*kwindañ*] at them and threw them out [Mayu and Tanowe were excluded from the kinship group because of their conduct]. I want to talk about it, and the two of them [Mayu and Susune] have interrupted me.

Virin [16]: Where is Susune? Is she here?

Susune [3]: I am here!

Faiu [18]: Listen, Susune…

Susune [3]: Yes?

Faiu [18]: Go down there; the two [Mayu and her baby] are annoyed [*teak ndapndap*] and went down there, you go now and call the two of them back again!

Susune [3]: No, the child was screaming, that is why she took him down to the house where we were sitting beforehand.

Narewe [23]: No, she just said he is screaming and carried him outside.

[*Everyone is talking at once: 'we had been sitting very comfortably down there, but after we came up, the child started to scream.'*]

Sauno [10]: Stop that now and talk. We are not sitting together here in order to insult each other, we must be peaceful and agree and talk.

Erarape [14]: The sweet potatoes which we are roasting there are not done yet.

Kan [6]: Go and get down some *bumbum* [reed-like stalks used as "lighters"] and make a bigger fire and they will be done faster.

Nañgut [17]: Well now, afterwards I checked it [the netbags] and I did not find the money; he [Tanowe] did not want to give me the money, and why? 'I took the money out and put it in your wife's netbags,' that is what he said to me, and where did he really put the money, and where did it go? It is not just some trifle which you [he turns to Tanowe] were throwing around, I can tell you!

Sauno [10] and **Faiu** [18]: Yes, now you talk about this point.

Susune [3]: This is not just one point. Everybody said to us, 'We have thrown you out [of the kinship group *jalap*, i.e.: 'you do not belong among us any longer'], we do not want to have anything to do with you anymore!', that is what they said to us.

Nañgut [17]: Finish talking about the two of them [Mayu and Tanowe] now; now I am talking and you listen for a change! In the middle of the night, we went up and got the netbag that Mayu had put there, we took it down and went through it, the money was not there, and we got biscuits, grass skirts, all these things out of it, we searched, we turned everything upside down and I myself saw that the money was not amongst it. And the pieces of cloth which everybody had folded and stuffed into it, those we also took down, searched and searched, it was not there. Tsarau started a fire at the time and he looked towards us. That was in the middle of the night. We searched, without success, gave it up and slept. The next morning, they [Tanowe and Mayu] did not see [ignored] us and cut up the pigs and distributed them. And when it was dark again, Tsarau and his child left. And they [the Uskokop villagers] had cooked the pigs to give us pleasure and they were running around and told us about it and Tsarau and his child had already left. If only you [Tanowe] had told the two of them [Tsarau and his son Nstasiñge] at the time and gone and got them and distributed the pig! Ah? I looked the two of them [Tanowe and Mayu] in the eyes and they took the pig and brought it back to Uskokop and sold it. That is what I was thinking of, and that is what one of my dreams is about. And I wanted to tell it, and why did you two [Susune and Mayu] stop me? You two know exactly and wanted to restrain me because of that?

Sauno [10]: That was because the child was screaming and they took him outside and everybody was talking at once.

Nañgut [17]: Yes, exactly, Sauno, we have mentioned a point which goes deeper and a *yupmo* [female kinship term] of yours was very angry about it [*teak kandap*] and she [Mandañgau, 25] died. And I wanted to tell the dream and the two of them [Susune and Mayu] were talking nonsense. And I became angry [*kwindañ*] about the two of them and almost left.

Sauno [10]: Forget it and talk, that is only women's gossip.

Nañgut [17]: Megau and Jurenu, the two of them did not see us, no. Mandañgau, [25, the late mother of Megau and Jurenu, who could have claimed part of the brideprice return], this *yupmo* of yours, Sauno, said: 'Why have the two [Mayu and Tanowe] left us and taken the pig and sold it, sold it on the market at Uskokop?' Mandañgau was very angry [*teak tevan*] about it and died. I think this *njigi* ["oppressing problem"] is here, and it grows and we make it grow all the time. And that is why I talk like this. [He turns to Mayu and Susune]: I have had great pains [*ngodim ndapndap*] and I talked and talked; why on earth did you talk such nonsense? You look like you are going to beat me up now, ah?

Virin [16]: Food, betel nuts, pigs and everything else they put into their own netbags. And the *njigi* ["oppressing problem"] from it you [the people from the Tuwal I clan] now have.

Jurenu [20, who wants to peel a sweet potato]: Have you seen my knife, which I put down there?

Faiu [18]: Saop [Nañgut 's daughter] had a dream, and what you have now said about Mandañgau, Nañgut, points in the same direction.

Sauno [10]: That is what we are talking about now, and now it has become clearer to us [meaning: Mandañgau's anger].

Nañgut [17]: I found a *njɨgɨ* ["oppressing problem"], it did not go away, and when the two women had been hitting each other, I slept here, and I had a dream and went to Mundagalgowañ...[he stops]. All I want to tell is the business with the two women who were hitting each other and that we looked through Mayu's netbag, that is what I want to talk about, and that is all.

Faiu [18]: That is right. Good, if you own up to all your own problems and do not think of the baby's *njɨgɨ* anymore [meaning: thereby settling the "oppressing problem"]. But it is bad, if you are all furious at each other [*teak kandap*] and the child gets ill. Now, talk about all your problems and come to an agreement, settle it and talk about it so that the child gets well [*nɨmantusok*].

Kan [6]: Tanowe and his wife heard what was said against them but they did not react, and Mayu and her child went up [to Tapmañge, to Tsarau and his family], and they all talked with her about superficial things only.

Faiu [18]: And Jurenu and Megau were the first to pay the brideprice for Tanowe. This old man [he means Megau, who has fallen asleep again] is sleeping; he is afraid and prowls around and is just watching us. Jurenu simply forgot it and is just walking around, that is what it looks like after all.

Virin [16]: Jurenu was certainly not pleased when his mother died, and why should he have been? He paid the brideprice for Tanowe, and everybody gave it back, and Tanowe did not give anything from it to the [now] dead mother. All these gifts [*ngaok*: betel nut; here: collective noun for brideprice], pigs, betel nuts, grass skirts, money, went to Tanowe; he did actually bring it down [to Gua], but did not give it to them [the people who had helped him pay Mayu's brideprice, the *tinyikabɨ*, "some good" (people)]; Tanowe himself ate it and squandered it.

Nañgut [17]: *Tekop erap* [to poke the embers, to light the fire anew, "dispute"], that is what she [Mayu] did. It is bad, she did it, and we are angry and that is why the child is ill. And we will find out what was there. And we talk…

Faiu [18]: That is not the proper way. She brought it [a pig from the brideprice return] up and cut it up in the woman's house [that of Mayu's mother, Narewe, and her late father in Uskokop], that is *tɨlagɨ* ["to be different," forbidden, taboo], they did *tɨlagɨ*!

Narewe [23]: That is true! It is true, that is *tɨlagɨ*. And I made everyone afraid; they got everything [again] out [out of her house in Uskokop], took it down [to Gua], turned back and went up again.

Sauno [10]: *mao, wao, mao*, everybody turned their back [acted in an insulting way towards the others], turned back again and carried it up!

Erarape [14]: Why did the two of them act like that?

Virin [16]: The reason is the following: if this Mayu dies, she cannot be buried in Uskokop [where her mother comes from and where Mayu's "dead soul" (*koñwop*) should go back upon her death]. When she dies, she will be buried in Gua [because she was chased away from Uskokop owing to her conduct]. That is why. And they all [Tanowe's relatives] paid her [her brideprice *añnok*] well, and later they [Mayu's relatives] paid it [the brideprice return *pelok*] back and thought it would be distributed in Gua to those who had helped with the brideprice, who had really tried so hard and helped him [Tanowe] to buy her [Mayu]. They [the Uskokop people] thought, they [Tanowe and Mayu] would bring it down [to Gua], and everybody would sit together and distribute the *pelok* [brideprice return], that would have been much better, and the child would not have fallen ill.

Narewe [23]: She [Mayu] did not want to get it and bring it down and talk to everybody and laugh and tell them to distribute the pig and to quickly hand her the knife. She did not want it like that. If she had just said then: 'now you cut your share for you!', all would have been well.

Nañgut [17]: I have smoothed the way for them. 'Get a piece of the pig they have prepared so as to give us pleasure, and everybody will cut it up, cook it and eat.' That is what I said. But they left this piece of pig lying there and it remained where it was. At the time, we were all sitting together, and he [Tanowe] went outside and left altogether. And that night we, Tsarau, his child and I, searched all the stuff but it [the piece of pig] was not there, and we went to sleep. The next morning, Tsarau and his child went again [back to Tapmañge]. And we let the matter rest and separated. Some of us have died in the meantime, and some are still here.

Virin [16]: Jurenu came up and said to me: 'a brother [Tanowe] and his wife have acted wrongly, we talked about it and that is it. And now we cannot help the two anymore.'

Faiu [18]: Saop was dreaming, I will tell her dream, and you will listen. Have some people already told it to you? I do not know. Shall I tell it or not?

Virin [16]: Go ahead and tell it, the thoughts of the men are clear [we all concentrate].

Faiu [18]: Nañgut is shaking his head, therefore I cannot tell it.

Virin [16]: Tell your brother-in-law [*mbasok*, polite form of address, meaning: Nañgut], it is good to tell, and you two hear it.

Faiu [18]: Well, I look at him, and he shakes his head. I cannot tell it.

Virin [16]: You two feel now if it is good to talk about it; well, think about it and decide.

Nañgut [17]: It is bad if it is not a good story and you [Faiu] tell something that burdens me in front of all the others, and I hear it and just sit here.

Faiu [18]: No, no, she was dreaming about Mandañgau who died.

Nañgut [17]: Mandañgau was very angry, I already said that.

Faiu [18]: You have now mentioned her name and I will now tell that dream.

Virin [16]: So she [Saop] dreamt about the mother [of Megau and Jurenu]. And we will now sum up the various points. Formerly, everybody said to a *pelok* [brideprice return]: 'very good' and they were very pleased and their belly was cool [in the "ideal" state, meaning: there was no resentment]. And 'luluai' Nañgut was sitting there, too. Now we just fool around, just fool around. And if the 'luluai' Nañgut does something hot [a large social transaction like a brideprice] and it [the *pelok*] comes back to him, he will say: 'I, an important man, am sitting here.' And he will rejoice and talk and laugh.

Nañgut [17] [to **Virin**]: Child [signifying: you small man], do you believe I am pleased about what they did?

Virin [16]: I now want to come to the central issue. This 'manki' [Tok Pisin, not yet grown-up, not fully responsible, ignorant young man] Mañnau marries a woman, but he does not marry a woman from another kinship group, no. Mañnau actually marries his sister [*tumot*, MoSiDa, Susune, see also Chapter 2.3. and Figure 1], and his child [Tanowe] they married to her [Susune's] little sister [*ngwa*, MoBrSoDa to Susune]. *Kettak* [kinship term] of Mañnau is Tanowe [which is not really true, since Tanowe, even though the son, is at the same time the husband of Mañnau's *kettak*, Mayu. [Here Virin wants to emphasize the impossibility of this complicated kinship situation; since it is forbidden to have a relationship with a *kettak*.] That is it. Did I tell it wrong? Is it true, Susune? And you, Mayu? Are you Susune's little sister, eh?

Susune [3]: Yes, Mayu is my sister.

Virin [16]: That is what I was getting at. Well then, Tanowe is your *mbasok*, yes?

Susune [3]: Yes [quite an unusual kinship relationship, Tanowe is Susune's son and at the same time, since he has married her [classificatory] little sister, as the latter's husband her *mbasok*. This breaks some of the rules about the relations between people in certain kinship positions].

Virin [16]: Now this baby, has he been born by a woman of the same clan?…I am now telling the whole truth!

Susune [3]: It is right, he has common ancestors [Mayu's grandfather on the father's side and Tanowe's grandmother on the father's side are siblings, see Figure 2].

Nañgut [17]: That is how it is done in modern times; you do not know anything about the essence of the speech, you want to hide a lot. Well, I also want to mention one of the main points. I am not a small child, after all, who sits here, really not. I will think about what you have said and watch you. Here now, in modern times, Tanowe has used up the netbags and everything just like that, and we wrote him [Tanowe] off, we cast him away.

Faiu [18]: That is true; old Nañgut once said that very clearly and I heard it.

Virin [16]: Me, too, I heard it, it is true.

Nañgut [17]: We do not say that simply without reason, I want to start in on it now.

Sauno [10]: You have now mentioned something new, and I heard it.

Nañgut [17]: At the time, Mapte [an old man from the Ngangalbuk clan, Gua] and Mandañgau [Megau's mother] and I were talking about the pig [which they did not get], and we decided: 'later, we will not think of Tanowe anymore,' that is how we talked and we parted. Virin is alluding to that time, now I have understood.

Erarape [14]: That is right!

Faiu [18]: That is how you have talked and have thrown Tanowe out [of the clan]. Now talk about that.

Nañgut [17]: You cannot say we are going to throw him out now, say: 'we have already thrown him out.'

…]

Nañgut [17]: At the time, we separated and went in all directions; they hauled the pig to Uskokop and cooked it.

Erarape [14]: The two of them carried it up and made a market with it [sold it for money].

Virin [16]: Tanowe and his wife did it like that; they were head-strong and guilty [*nduara*, something that remains from a misde-meanor, "guilt"], but you did not only write off the two of them, no, you cursed the child.

[…]

Virin [16]: You [Nañgut] called Tanowe, and we were very angry at him. He is a 'manki' [a little boy], he does not know how it is done properly and neither does he claim: 'I know the way' [the tradi-tion], and he tries to ruin his situation. But you did not notice this, you old men and women, you just sat there and your backside was sore and your mouth was sore. If you had told him, he would have given you the food and the betel nuts. […] He is a 'manki,' he did not learn how it is done properly and he was probably thinking: 'I am doing it right,' but he did it completely wrong and gave you a *njɨgɨ* ["oppressing problem"]. Do you not see that?

Nañgut [17]: He did it like that, and he and his wife did not come to us, and the pig they had cooked in our honor was ready. And the two of them just ran off, prowled around and I think that later on they ate it, or what? And later, the others said: 'the two of them have made a market in Uskokop,' and we heard it.

Faiu [18]: That is not such a big *njɨgɨ*!

Naṅgut [17]: And that is why we said, later on those two [Tanowe and Mayu] will not fare well, we told them like this. That is how we thought and we parted. Time went by, and now it has happened, I think that is why it is like this [meaning: the child is ill], and I say it openly.

Sauno [10]: That is true, go on talking.

Virin [16]: It is right, you are telling the truth.

[...]

Virin [16]: Aminbako [the brother of Mandañgau's husband, a member of the Ngandum clan] and Mandañgau were very angry [*mbɨt kandap*], and they both died [in a state of anger], do you not see that?

Sauno [10]: Well, yes!

Faiu [18]: And his [Tanowe's] *ngapma* [partner clan] decided together with the other men: 'later he will not fare well!' That is what they decided, that is a *tɨlagɨ gen* ["forbidden talk," "curse"]. That is why he [Tanowe] now got the *njɨgɨ* [meaning: that is why Tanowe's child is ill].

Kan [6]: You were there at the time, Mapte said '*ko!*' [go!].

Virin [16]: Yes, Mapte said '*ko!*' to you.

Sauno [10]: Yes, yes, that is how it was!

Kan [6]: '*kalapno kooo!*', said Mapte ["in the name of my ancestors, go!"].

Narewe [23]: They said '*ko!*' and some have died, they uttered this curse and that is why the baby's *wopm* ["shadow soul"] is gone forever.

Kamake [22]: The *ngapma* [the Ngangalbuk clan, the partner clan of the Tuwal III clan and, especially, the traditionalist Mapte, who also had a claim to the brideprice return (*pelok*)] said: 'I have thus decided and that is it.' That is why he said '*ko!*'.

Kan [6]: Mandañgau, Naṅgut or whoever were sitting down there [in another house] and thoroughly talked it over and said: 'the two of them [Tanowe and Mayu] have behaved like this' and everyone was beside themselves with rage and told this to Mapte and Mapte got up and said '*ko!*' and went outside.

[...]

Virin [16]: If we talk about it so openly, it is good. Tanowe should come here and sit down here together with his wife, we will all sit together and talk, then it will be well. Tanowe, so where are you?

Several people: There he is!

Virin [16, directed at **Tanowe**]: 'My *wau* [namesakes], my brothers [all the male members of his own and the partner clan], you have tried very hard and prepared betel nuts, money and everything [brideprice] for me. I have not given it back to you, that is true. I have done you wrong and acted wrong. Yes, I have done it wrong,' talk like that, and everything will come to an end!

Narewe [23]: He should get up and say why he acted like that!

Virin [16]: Hey, brother [Tanowe], get up and talk, answer!

Narewe [23, to **Tanowe**]: You have to say: 'for this and that reason I behaved like that!'

Virin [16]: That is right. 'My fathers, my brothers, my relatives, I have behaved like that and that is why I got this *njigi!*', if you talk like that, everything will be well!

Narewe [23]: You have to say: 'for this or that reason I was so angry [*mbit njap*], for that reason alone,' talk like this!

[...]

Sauno [10]: Yes, child, do it like that!

During the further debate, the same topics were repeated. Tanowe could not be moved to explain his conduct concerning the *pelok* (brideprice return).

In the above discussion of the illness, two possible causes of the baby's illness were aired:

1.   Kan, Nañgut's second wife, had for some time been jealous of Susune, Tanowe's mother. Because of the rumors brought up again—not least because of the first discussion of the illness (Mañnau's anger at his brothers)—that Tanowe was in reality Nañgut's son (who as a "namesake" (*wau*) and adoptive father (*opmot*) initially had also to a great extent taken care of Tanowe), Kan was very furious, and one day came to Susune's house, met her husband there sitting with Susune, which confirmed her suspicion, so she screamed out, grabbed a stick, and hit Susune. By making such a scene, she scared the sleeping baby's *amin-*

wop ("shadow soul") so much that it left its body. At first, people therefore assumed that the cause of the illness or the loss of the baby's "soul"
was a *njɨgɨ* ("oppressing problem") of Kan (see Figure 2, [9]), which
in turn had been caused by Kan's emotional state, "tormenting jealousy" (*teak tevan nda añakdak*), which came about through the continuous taunts, and her "obsession" (*nandak nandak yuki*) about the
alleged affair between Nañgut and Susune.

2. Mayu's brideprice return was discussed as a further cause. The *añnok*,
i.e. the payment to Mayu's relatives (to the clan and its partner clan as
well as to her mother), to which Nañgut (hence the Tuwal I clan to
which Tsarau also belongs), Megau and Jurenu (Ngandum clan) and
Faiu (Kapbaga clan) contributed substantially, was uneventful and sat-
isfied everybody. But the *pelok*, the repayment to the relatives of the
husband Tanowe (to his clan, partner clan and to those who helped him
with the brideprice, i.e. Nañgut, Jurenu, Megau, Faiu, Virin et al.) had
not—from a customary point of view—been performed correctly.
Tanowe and Mayu collected some of these *pelok* gifts in Uskokop,
Mayu's natal village, an act that already was not customary since normally the whole *pelok* should be fetched in one piece by those concerned
themselves. They brought it first to Gua, but did not distribute it there
to Tanowe's brideprice helpers, as would have been correct. Since he felt
left in the lurch by them and possibly also because, as a result of his
long absence from the village, he did not know the rules too well—a
point Virin mentioned in the discussion—he carried the pig back up
to Uskokop again and butchered it in the house of Mayu's mother
Narewe (which was also *tɨlagɨ*, "forbidden," as a *pelok* pig may only be
distributed in the house of a member of the husband's clan), then sold
the individual pieces of meat as if he were in a market. He spent the
pelok money and the proceeds from the sale of the pig on himself.

There was thus no certainty in the discussion as to whether the misdemeanor
of Tanowe and Mayu had caused their child's illness ("oppressing problem"
[10]), whether it was the anger at Tanowe of the people who had not received
the *pelok*, such as Mandañgau and Aminbako, who had died angry, hence two
"ghosts" ("oppressing problem" [11]) or if the decision of the injured person to
expel Tanowe and Mayu from the clan ("*ko!*": "go!", [12]) had led to a *njɨgɨ*
("oppressing problem") and made the child (as Tanowe's child) ill.

Tanowe could not be moved to admit publicly his guilt in the failed *pelok*
(brideprice return), so the discussion made no headway and most of those
present went to sleep one after the other. Faiu, with the agreement of the oth-

Illustration 7: A Kina coin is hung around little
Nstasiñge's neck, April 1987

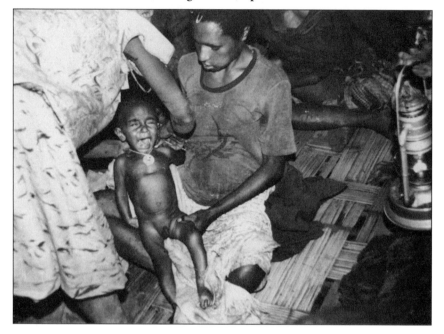

ers, decided to end the discussion. Kan again publicly regretted her behavior, appealed to the baby's *wopm* ("shadow soul") to return to its place (in the baby). She called the baby's name, sang his *koñgap* melody and called "*wup-wup*" ("come, come!"). After a prayer recited by the evangelist Sauno in the Kâte language, a small bowl of water was prepared and then consecrated with a short prayer. Afterwards, all the relatives touched a Kina coin, which Kan put around the baby's neck, and Mayu gave him a spoonful of this consecrated water to drink. With that, the discussion was over, and people went home hoping for an improvement in the baby's condition.

The Kina coin touched by all symbolizes reconciliation, the unanimity of all the participants; nobody has a *njïgï* ("oppressing problem") "on his skin" anymore, everybody is balanced "cool" (*yawuro*), and this ideal state should transfer to the coin and thereby to the "hot," ill child. Once positively "cooled," the coin should signal to the child's *wopm* ("shadow soul") that it may safely return to its place in the child; also, as a valuable, the coin should speedily entice it back. The consecration and administration of water (something "cold") constitute a new form of therapy that replaces the traditional cure, involving the incantation of a certain formula over a patient and the rubbing of the body

Illustration 8: The little boy, Nstasiñge

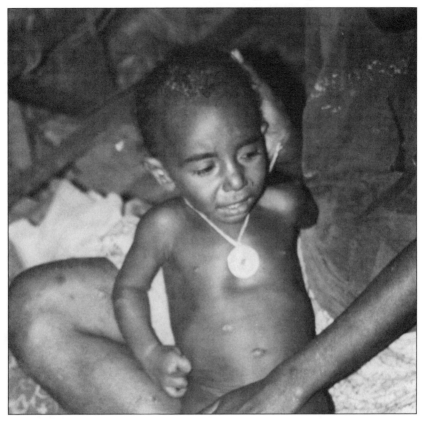

with the "cold" white earth *kuak*, as it happened at the house of Tsarau and his family in Tapmañge. Depending on the case and the context (presence of church representatives, degree of Christianization of the patient and his relatives), the Yupno choose one or the other form of "cooling down."

e) A Suspicion: "I Thought Somebody from Yupno Valley Had Made Him Ill with the *Mawom*-Technique"

The mother Mayu reports what happened after this debate:

> And I got up [the next morning], got my things ready, the two of us were ready, and we went to the hospital.

> The 'doktaboy' examined the baby, did not find anything, and they poured medicine on a piece of cotton wool and rubbed it on the

Illustration 9: Mayu, the mother, gives Nstasiñge, the child, "consecrated" water to drink

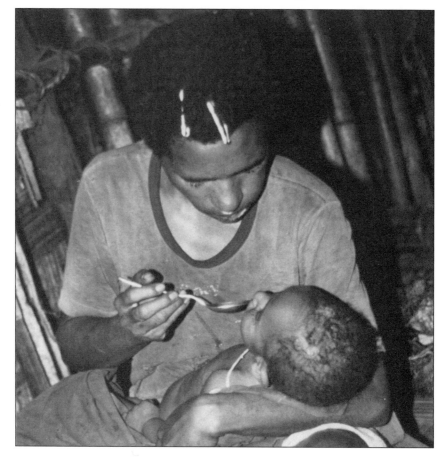

baby's back, they rubbed and rubbed and gave him an injection. They pumped blood and water into his skin, and water and blood they pumped out, and they said: 'the baby is not going to die!' That is what they said to me. 'You have no reason to be afraid and you should not think about it that much, go without worries and watch over him, go and take good care of him.' That is what the 'dok-taboy' said to me. I came to the village and I did not follow the ad-monitions of the 'doktaboy,' I saw, my skin was afraid, and I did not put the baby down to sleep, I held him all the time in my arms. I did not wash myself, I stayed dirty, and I sat down and held him.

His eyes came out and he just looked, and like that he spent the whole night, and the sun came, and he just looked.

[She went again to the Teptep Health Centre.] That is how the baby behaved, and the 'dokta' went and tickled him and he laughed at the 'dokta.' He was babbling to himself now and he was laughing with them, and Saop [a younger woman who had accompanied Mayu] held him and carried him around outside. In the night, I took him again, and he screamed again, and we came again to the ward, late at night, and I held him until very late. That is how we did it, and we said: 'people have died in this house, and many koñ-wop ["souls of dead persons"] are therefore here, and the koñwop are holding him and that is why he cries, and we took him to Virin's house.' We came and slept in Virin's house and went back [to the Teptep Health Centre], to get the medicine; three nights we slept, that is how we did it, we were slowly getting fed up, and his illness was not over, it was still there, and 'he will become [and remain] like a little boy' [he will be mentally handicapped], we were completely exhausted and talked like that. We talked like that and came back to the village.

We came [...] and they [her relatives] held further discussions, and they all talked about a njɨgɨ ["oppressing problem," she means the fight between Kan and Susune], and they all admitted their nduara ["guilt"], and they all did it like this.

When the child was so ill, I did not think some man could possibly have carried and dropped him, since only I carry him around. I thought he would die, he was so ill, or somebody from Yupno valley had made him ill with the mawom-technique [a kind of "pathogenic technique" that is thought by the Yupno to be the worst cause of illness for the Yupno; see below], that is how I thought and was afraid of my own thoughts, I only thought of mawom. I thought they [the mawom-men] would kill him or do whatever with him and I was scared and carried him around. This is how it went for the whole time, the baby did not get well, we had discussed to the end all the rumors and njɨgɨ ["oppressing problems"], without success, he did not get well. We went back to the hospital.

Excursus: The Worst Causes of Illness, Sɨt and Mawom

Exceptionally serious, often fatal, illnesses are caused by human actions. We have to distinguish two kinds: sɨt (in Tok Pisin called 'poisin,' "leavings sorcery") and *mawom* (in Tok Pisin 'sangguma'). On the one hand, the Yupno use the term *sɨt* for what passes for "illness" in our culture. *Sɨt* is not only the generic noun for "illness" but also signifies a certain cause of illness[13] which in anthropology is often paraphrased with "black magic." Literally translated, *sɨt* means "I burn, heat, cook." Outside of the context of illness, people say e.g. "*kandap sɨt*," "I burned wood, I made a fire." The term is also found in sentences like "*sɨt asat*," "I am ill," "*sɨt njɨgɨ*," "I am seriously ill," or "*sɨtni mi*," "I am not ill."

To injure another person, one takes an item containing some of his or her *moñan* ("breath spirit"), like a piece of chewed skin of betel nut, a carelessly thrown away piece of sugar cane which had been chewed, or something similar, then hands it, together with a fee, to a specialist, the *sɨt amɨn*, the "burner." He will then, in an extremely secret gathering, supervise young, unmarried (hence "hot") men, who wrap this particle with special leaves and ritually burn it. This technique is based on the idea that the small stolen *moñan*-particle (hence the "breath spirit") also entices the *amɨnwop* ("shadow soul") of the victim. The victim (the owner of the "breath spirit") will shortly afterwards fall ill (become "hot") and (without "breath spirit") die from it.

The person who falls ill through this *sɨt*-technique will show certain typical symptoms like sunken eyes, a totally dry nose and mouth, hot cheeks and a whitish tip of the nose. These are interpreted by specialists as *sɨt tauak*, "signs of the *sɨt*-technique." As a cure, there are various measures, often called "divination" in the literature, aimed at finding out who stole the *moñan* ("breath spirit") and, far more important, who wants to destroy it. These acts and various methods are performed by different specialists (see Chapter 5.4.c.).

The inhabitants of the upper Yupno region are very much afraid of *mawom* (no translation), a different kind of pathogenic act which is practiced only by people from the lower half of the valley. The customer of *mawom* conveys the name of the victim to the specialist, the *mawom amɨn*, the "*mawom*-man." He in turn will supervise young men who have ritually made themselves "hot" in order to get close to the victim on the sly; they then shoot a special arrow at the victim, who becomes momentarily unconscious. They remove the arrow, close the wound with soil and fix a day on which the victim will die. The victim goes back to his or her house but is unable to report what has happened. Within the shortest time, he or she will fall gravely ill since his or her *amɨnwop* ("shadow soul") is already about to leave the injured body, and only in delirium will the victim tell what has happened. The only cure consists of a coconut picked in a special way and then eaten. There is danger of *mawom* when, for example, strangers are seen in the village. No inhabitant of Gua would then leave the house on his own.

Detailed knowledge of *mawom* procedures is confined to just a few specialists. Since women (like Mayu) and younger men do not know anything definite, and hear only about the (mostly lethal) results of this technique, and know no cure against it, they feel *mawom* to be the most threatening. It is a totally unfathomable, incomprehensible affliction that "comes from outside" and thereby breaches the boundaries of their customary social environment. The term *mawom* is thus employed rather confusingly for all serious illnesses and death where no other cause can be found, without concrete reference to the procedures and techniques of *mawom*. Bodily disorders can be treated by "cooling down," "oppressing problems" (*njɨgɨ*) can be cleared up with talks and settled with gifts that mollify, and loss of the *amɨnwop* ("shadow soul") from fright or as a result of the *sɨt*-technique can all be reversed by specialists in the village, and so are culturally manageable causes of illness for which there are solutions. This does not, however, apply to *mawom*, because it comes from "outside," and is mysterious and therefore not amenable to treatment.

Mayu's mention of *mawom* expresses her helplessness and her serious fear for her child. Despite all the solutions to the various "oppressing problems" proposed during the long debates, her child does not get well, and the cause of his illness is therefore not to be found in her social environment. The "threat," therefore, must come from outside.

Her thoughts about *mawom* are not shared by her relatives—or at least not followed up. On the one hand, the course of the baby's illness was evidence against it: victims of *mawom* survive their illness for a few days at the most, but the baby had at the time already been ill for two months; on the other hand, it is highly unlikely (even though theoretically possible) that someone would take considerable payment to a *mawom*-man to kill a six months' old child, an incomplete human being, that is not yet a valuable member of society.

f) The Journey into Town: "Where Would the Two of Us Go?"

Mayu, little Nstasiñge's mother, continues her story.

> We went to the hospital [to Teptep]. Everybody accompanied me and then they left me and in the afternoon the baby was screaming again; he urinated and excreted. And Saop [a younger women who had accompanied Mayu] cleaned everything up, and we sat there. The first 'doktaboy' [the highest in rank because of his better training and status as head of the health center, a Health Extension Officer, H.E.O.] was playing badminton, but later he came and looked

and said: 'oh man, this child here I have not seen yet, did only the 'doktaboy' [his subordinate male nurses] treat him?' This is what he said, felt insecure and was biting his fingernail. He called for Triope [another 'doktaboy'] and told him: 'the 'kiap' [district officer of the Teptep subdistrict] has not gone home yet, so go quickly to the office, write his [the baby's] name on the list [of the airplane passengers] and send [by radio] a message to the big hospital in Madang [the provincial capital].' Triope ran, wrote the name on the list and sent a message to the big hospital.

I did not see anyone from Gua and did not send a message here [to Gua]. Old Jowage [a man from Gua] was just tearing down the house of Mbasa [his son who owns a vegetable storage house in Teptep]; he came, and at the same time Praie [Saop's mother] also came. The first 'doktaboy' said to us all: 'this woman here and her child will take the plane tomorrow.' This is what he said and left.

It was still night when we got everything ready to go to Madang. The next morning, they all came to see us and walked around [in Teptep]. At the time, I was afraid, where would the two of us go and with whom? And the two of us [she and her child] were thinking a lot. It is not good if I alone take him there and something happens to him. Everybody will be mad at me then. Or, if I take him there and something happens, what am I to do then? I was scared. So the men came [from Gua] up here [to Teptep] and talked about accompanying me. The 'doktaboy' told them: 'no, no man can go with them, since nobody looks after them and only the two of them are here.' [Mayu had so far always come alone to the health center with her child, so she could also go alone to the hospital in town; the H.E.O. was taking a passing shot at Tanowe who, in his opinion was neglecting his wife and his child.]

This is what he said, and I just looked into his eyes. And the others [who did not understand this allusion to Tanowe and thought it was aimed at them] said: 'if it is not possible, she will go together with Tanowe.' And Tanowe had already gone out [of the ward] and was carrying the baby around outside. Saop went and told him: 'I do not want to kill you, so, hand over our child!' This is what she said, took the baby, and we were there, and a plane arrived.

I packed everything up and came out, and the men said to me: 'no, this is not the plane on which you will go,' and I went back into the house [the health center]. I therefore went back into the house

again and wanted to roast a sweet potato and was just busy with
that. And the plane [the right one] came flying in over the mountains. Well, I took the child, gave him to the first 'doktaboy,' I did
not carry anything at all, and Praie brought our netbag, and we
went. And the first 'doktaboy' said: 'in case some men want to
climb into the plane with you two, I shall throw them out, well
then, leave them all behind and sit down in the plane!' Well, I now
climbed into the plane, the others [some men] unloaded its freight,
and afterwards the other passengers got in, and we started out. We
landed in Sisiak [Madang, Sisiak is the name of the small settlement quarter of the Yupno who live in Madang, for Mayu the only
place known from hearsay and therefore synonymous with
Madang], and they had already called the hospital, and we left the
other passengers behind, and the driver of the ambulance asked:
'where are the patients from Teptep?' and I said: 'here we are,' and
we went to him. We [she and her baby] said to Kwañbe [a school-
boy who happened to fly with them from Teptep and who goes to
high-school on the Rai Coast]: 'we have never driven in a car and
do not know the way, well then, you come with us.'

Well, we got into the car and took off. We got to a street and saw
Mañnau [one of Tanowe's relatives], he was at the market. I waved to
him but he did not see us and we drove by him. We got to the hospital, Kwañbe said good-bye and said: 'go and tell them your names,
then you go into the house, into the house where all the children and
babies are. I will go and see his grandfather' [the above-mentioned
Mañnau]. And Kwañbe left. At the same time, the 'doktaboy' got the
baby's card ready [filled it in], and we went to the sleeping-place [to
the ward].

There was a man from Urop [a neighboring village] with his wife
[who had accompanied her ill son to the hospital], and the two of
them said: 'put your netbag here, at the place for netbags.' I put it
down and went to the office. And they examined Nstasiñge; this
took a long time, and they did not know what was wrong, and they
thought about it. And I thought now he would die and I was very
scared. And they sent us back to the bed, and there we stayed. And
they brought the sick boy from Urop there where people are cut up
[to the operating theater]. The 'dokta' wanted to cut him up and
examine him, and his anus was all closed. They cut up his belly and
cut in the middle of it and stuck a plaster on it to close it. And they

cut off a piece of plastic and fixed it to his behind. And they put his behind into the plastic and all around it they tightly fixed plaster. They brought him back to the ward. He was talking and eating, and at the same time his excrements were running into the plastic like water. When the plastic was full, they carried it outside, threw it away and fixed a new one, that is what they did all the time. And we were very close to that. And during all that time, Kwañbe was with us. He was with us for quite a long time, and then he had to go to school on the Rai Coast.

Well, Mañnau came and took his place. We were quite well, and then they said they wanted to cut up the baby. I was afraid and told them: 'only if I give you my permission can you cut him up.' And I stopped them. Because it was at the same time that they were fighting for the life of the boy from Urop, and he died. And his relatives begged the 'dokta' to enable them to return to Urop [to pay for the plane ticket]. The 'dokta' said: 'I have no possibility to send you to Teptep, if you want to buy your own ticket, okay.' This is what he said. And at the same time I got scared. I told them: 'my child did not get well, there-fore you should send him back to the village.' This is what I said to them. 'It will be bad if he dies and I have no possibility to take him back. I did not come with a husband, I brought the baby here on my own, so please send him back.' And the 'dokta' said: 'we think he is not going to die. There is no sickness in his body, it is only on the skin, we are trying very hard, and you, do not think so much about it, you stay here.'

This calmed me down, my feelings were 'cool' [mbɨt yawuro], and I stayed there. The 'dokta' took blood and water from his back and sent it to Mosbi [the capital Port Moresby] and to other places. And the 'dokta' examined this water and blood. [...] We were sent to a different ward, time passed, and he did not get well, and again they sent us to a different house.... So there we were, and the first 'dokta' came and said: 'this is your last week here, next week you will go to Teptep!' This is what the 'dokta' said. During this week which we still spent in Madang, we washed our clothes and visited the town, then it was time for us, and I was very much looking forward to going back to the village. They told us that we had to go to the airport when it was still the middle of the night.

We were waiting at the roadside, the hospital ambulance picked up all the people and at the very end it picked us up. We were [in the

meantime] hungry and told the cook [of the hospital] to give us
something to eat, and he gave us something, and we ate. While we
were eating, the car came for us. We climbed in, the car dropped us
at the airport, and we waited. The plane first went to Goroka [a town
in the highlands], there it stayed for a very long time, and we got
bored. Then the plane came back, we got in, we landed at Saidor,
and there the plane made us wait, it went to Long Island [Arop], and
we stood and waited and we had enough, it was getting to be afternoon and then late in the afternoon it came, took us on and let us off
here [in Teptep]. And we came back here again [to Gua].

In Mayu's report about the decision of the Health Extension Officer to send
her to Madang to the Modilon Hospital with her child, the central themes
were her thoughts about how the clan members and members of the partner
clan would react to the eventual death of the baby, and her fear of these reactions and of the blame that would be laid on her ['It is not good if I alone take
him there and something happens to him. Everybody will be mad at me
then']. Her fear is reinforced when she witnesses the death of the boy from
the neighboring village of Urop and the problems his parents had in getting
back to their village. That she has difficulties in making decisions on her own
in this totally new social environment becomes obvious. Being in a strange
town, among unknown people, hardly able to communicate, since she knows
no Tok Pisin—all this makes it hard for her to decide if she should go back
to the village with her ill child or if she should wait to see whether the baby
gets well again. Here, there is no therapy managing group akin to her relatives
in the village, which could make decisions together with her and take collective responsibility.

Mayu's reflections about the illness of her child, and her decisions and actions correspond to the basic pattern presented here in a simplified way of how
the Yupno deal with an illness episode and how they determine the therapy.
Initially, they assume a more harmless disorder (caused naturally), which is
treated with home remedies (or increasingly with Western pharmaceutical
products). Then, after a trial and error procedure (or using the principle of
exclusion), attempts to find the cause (such as the search for "oppressing problems" in discussions and through the interpretation of "signs") and the therapies connected with this, they turn to the worst causes of illness, sɨt or
mawom. For this, the symptoms of the patient do not necessarily have to
change, the same complex of symptoms can be followed back to different
causes. In Nstasiñge's case, the traditional possibilities had been exhausted, so
Mayu now places her hopes on the biomedical therapies at Madang hospital

(far superior to the small Teptep Health Centre), from where she returns to Gua village after about three months.

2. The Disease of the Little Boy, Nstasiñge, from the Biomedical Point of View

The interpretations of the disease of the little boy Nstasiñge from the viewpoint of biomedicine form the focal point of this chapter. The analysis of the clinical report was undertaken on the basis of his file from Modilon Hospital in Madang,[14] which was photocopied by the physician Sandra Staub (who was working there). This analysis was supplemented with interviews I conducted among the staff at the Teptep Health Centre as well as a later discussion of the case between Dr Staub and Dr Flueler, the Assistant Medical Director of the University Children's Hospital in Berne, Switzerland.

a) Symptoms of a Cerebral Inflammation

On 3 February 1987, the little boy Nstasiñge was taken by his mother to the Teptep Health Centre; he was at that time almost seven months old (date of birth: 11.7.1986) and weighed seven kilograms.

As can be seen in the letter of transfer from the Health Extension Officer (H.E.O.), Bokung Wenani (see Document 1), the boy showed symptoms of a cerebral inflammation, which pointed to meningitis. For clarification, a lumbar puncture (a tapping of the brain-spine-liquid) was performed, which confirmed the diagnosis of a bacterial or tubercular meningitis. The child was thereupon (as stated by the H.E.O.) treated for two weeks with Chloramphenicol, a broad spectrum antibiotic, then a second lumbar puncture was performed and resulted in a clear fluid, whereupon the child was discharged.

According to a (Papua New Guinean) nurse in Teptep, the child had arrived at the health center with the typical symptoms of meningitis, his fontanels (seams of the skull) were sunken, he was sleeping too much and between times screamed loudly ('hai spid krai'). Over the course of several weeks (the H.E.O. mentioned two weeks), he was treated four times a day with Chloramphenicol injections which, however, did not improve the child's condition. In the nurse's opinion, a 'hevi' (heavy, an "oppressing problem") between the parents was responsible for the child's illness and had marred the efficacy of the drugs. This nurse was not originally from the Yupno region but from the Rai Coast; her opinion shows how widespread the concept of "to-be-weighed-down-with-problems" is as a cause for illness. Her statement also indicates that male and female nurses do not give up their traditional cultural etiologies in their dealings with illness, even after being biomedically trained, but supplement it by integrating biomedical knowledge. The non-Papua New Guinean physicians in the towns (for the most part Australians but also Europeans and Japanese) tend to dismiss traditional indigenous concepts of illness as "humbug," often without ever having investigated them. Not surprisingly, then, the medical-pluralistic approach of the indigenous personnel tends to be concealed. Various nurses and medical orderlies of the Modilon Hospital, when sick themselves, will very discreetly visit a local 'glasman,'[15] a specialist who can see and thereby clarify the cause of illness rather then merely treat the symptoms with drugs. The higher the level of training (and correspondingly the position) of a biomedically schooled indigenous staff member, the stronger he or she hides his or her own traditional concepts of illness, or else discards them altogether.

I could not definitely establish how many lumbar punctures were performed on the infant, but this method of examination requires considerable experience and it carries some risk. Such a procedure would be feasible in Teptep because it has the necessary technical equipment and the requisite level of employee training (see the following excursus: "The Teptep Health Centre"). Also, Mayu's sentence ("they pumped blood and water into his skin, and water and blood they pumped out") can be interpreted as a lumbar puncture, although several nurses employed there told me that they would not perform this examination in Teptep since they had too little experience with it.

It thus remains at least questionable that the child would have been treated four times per day with broad-spectrum antibiotics over the course of two weeks. Mayu's fear of a prolonged stay at the Teptep Health Centre (because of the presence there of many souls of dead persons, koñwop) led her to spend the night either with Virin in Teptep or to return to Gua village; also medical staff did not try to prevent her absences. An announcement by the H.E.O. to all the patients, which is displayed in the ward, reads: "Examination days: Monday, Wednesday, Friday, time 10 a.m. All the patients have to be in their beds [then]." According to Mayu's story, the Health Extension Officer, the "boss" of the Teptep Health Centre, never once saw the baby during this alleged stay of two or more weeks ("…this child here I have not seen yet, did only the 'doktaboy' treat him?"), and with an average of only two or three patients per night he should at least have noticed the child during his rounds.

On 13 April 1987, the mother again went to the Teptep Health Centre with her baby. In his letter of transfer (see Document 1), the H.E.O. described the condition of the boy: without fever, but with stiffness in his neck, back, feet and hands, staring eyes, loss of weight and signs of malnutrition. To calm the child down, he received Phenobarbital, an anti-spasmodic.

The H.E.O. could not diagnose more exactly, but assumed that the boy had a "big problem in his head": malnutrition, brain damage, mental retardation, TB meningitis, encephalitis (inflammation of the brain) or a tumor. Since he could not do anything more for the baby with this "complicated illness," on 24 April 1987, eleven days after the mother had again (for the second time) gone to Teptep Health Centre, he admitted him to the Modilon Hospital in the provincial capital of Madang. Why he sent the child to Madang only after eleven days, even though there are six flights a week, remains unclear. According to Mayu's story, she only spent one night at the ward before her flight to Madang, so the child was probably not an inpatient at the health center during these eleven days. In the letter of transfer, the H.E.O. stated the child's age as seven months ("ZAZINKE [the Kâte spelling of Nstasiñge] TAHANUWE [Tanowe, the father's name] M/7 MONTHS"); in fact, the baby was nine months old in April 1987, but now only weighed 5.5 kg.

Excursus: The Teptep Health Centre

Biomedicine is provided in the form of a health center at Teptep, the government station, and—on a somewhat reduced scale—by several local aid posts. The Yupno call this little health center *nimantok yut*, "house where nothing remains hidden," *marasin yut*, "house of medicine," or *sut yut*, "house of injections."

The first aid post[16] at Teptep was established in 1963, then in 1979, this small health station was extended into a Health Centre. In 1987, the health center consisted of five buildings.

The actual "main building" (A), a modern house with corrugated iron, has eight rooms. Rooms 1, 2, and 3 function as outpatient department. Room 1 is the outpatient ward, where patients are registered and examined: it contains several chairs, a couch, a table and various posters giving information on how to brush one's teeth properly and which foodstuffs offer optimum nutrition,[17] and these fixtures provide a waiting-room atmosphere. In Room 2, the dressing room, the patients receive their medicine or dressings. Room 3 is used as a storage room, and contains a large refrigerator filled with drugs, as well as frozen chickens, sausages or pieces of lamb (sporadically flown in from Madang), the sale of which pays part of the license fees of Teptep's Social Club (really a bar). During their storage time, the drugs are simply stored somewhat less cool outside the fridge. Room 4 functions as the office of the Health Extension Officer, the head of the health center. Room 5 is the family plan-

Document 1: Letter of Transfer

Teptep Health Centre,
F.H.B.S Teptep,
Madang.

24th April, 1987

The Admission Officer,
Madang Hospital,
P.O. Box 2030,
Yomba.

Attention: DR PHILIP WATT (SMO) PEDIATRICIAN.

Subject: ZACINKA TAHANUNG M/7 MONTHS

Dear Doctor,

I would like to bring to your attention about the condition of above small boy. He was admitted to Health Centre on the 3 rd February, 1987. With signs and symtoms of cerebral inflammation.

I thought he may had meningitis therefore did LP on him. It was cloudy. The diagnose was confirmed therefore commenced him on chloramphinicol for two weeks. Repeat LP was done with clear CSF. With this satisfaction of improvement he was discharged home after two weeks.

How-ever he was re-admitted again on the 13th April with similar signs and symtoms. This time without fever, stiffness of neck, back, feet, and hands. Made worse when irritable on disturbance. Has starring eyes, weak, losing weight, and becoming malnourished. He is being getting phenobarb only to calm him down a little bit.

It is most likely that he may has a big problem in his head. I thought it could be malnutrition, brain damage, mentally retarded, TB meningitis, encephalitis, and may be a tumour.

I can't do much for him here with this complicated illness therefore decide to send him down to your hands for advance care.

Yours sincerely,

BOKUNG WENANI
OFFICER INCHARGE.

ning office, where talks on the subject are meant to be given. Rooms 6, 7, and 8 comprise the delivery ward. In Room 6, the maternity station, there are four wooden stretchers for the women. Room 7, used for women in labor, contains one stretcher, a pair of scales and several instruments for examinations

Illustration 10: The Teptep Health Centre

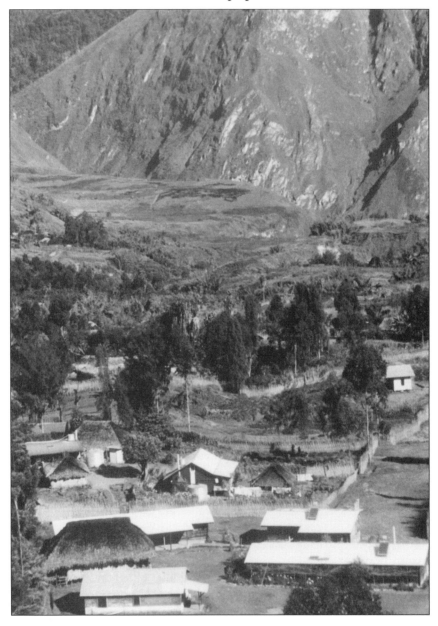

(a speculum, a suction pump for babies, oxygen apparatus, various catheters, disinfectants, and so on). A shower and a toilet are installed in Room 8.

Chart 3: The Teptep Health Centre

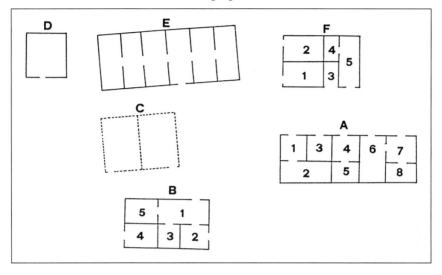

The older building (B) is used as a little store. It is the best-stocked shop in Teptep, offering an "urban" choice (tinned cakes, syrup, 2-minute noodles ('harriap noodles') in various tastes, several cosmetic articles and much more) and is used mainly by station employees. The profit from the shop goes towards new purchases for the health center. In Room 1, the goods are kept; Room 2 is the actual 'stoa,' the sales room, where items are sold out of a window-like opening; dressing material and other provisions are stored in Room 3; Room 4, the workshop, houses all kinds of odds and ends (such as a bed, and drums of kerosene), and Room 5 is used as an office.

Building C is a house built in 1986 by the Yupno during many 'komyuniti de' (days of communal labor) in the traditional manner (out of bush material), 'haus kunai,' "grass house," and serves as a ward. It consists of two rooms (one for women and one for men) with a large fireplace each. In house D, a workshop, building-material (sheet metal, faucets, and so on), tins of paint and four lawn-mowers are kept. The large modern building (E), which has six rooms, was built as a ward, but today stands empty, apart from twenty more or less intact wooden camp-beds, since it proved to be far too cold at night and could not be used by the Yupno without blankets. House C took over its function. Building F, with five rooms, serves as the cooking and ablution building for the patients. There are two toilets and wash-rooms (for women and men, 1 and 2), a washroom open towards the outside with four basins (3), and a kitchen (5) with a kerosene cooker and two old drums in which (like in a fire-bowl) a fire can be lit. Room 4, the pantry, is empty. The rooms are supposed to be kept in order by the employees, but they are rarely ever used and actually hardly usable.

The health center has two solar cells for the generation of hot water and electricity and is linked to the outside world by a radio in the office of the Sub-District Officer.

The catchment area of the health center, which comprises about 6500 to 7000 inhabitants, stretches from the upper Nankina region (Bambu) via Kewieñ, Isan, Nokopo (the upper Yupno Valley) down to the lower Yupno region, to just short of Tapen. The health center is financed by the provincial government of Madang and is subordinated to the Health Department. According to a the H.E.O., the budget is adequate.[18] Five aid posts, in Nokopo, Tapmañge, Bambu, Gwarawon and Isan (which, however, is financed by the Morobe provincial government), are subordinated to the health center, Tapen gets its medicine from Teptep, but is financed and controlled by the Lutheran Mission.

On average, the Teptep Health Centre has eight permanent employees, a Health Extension Officer (H.E.O.), who is the head of the health station (also called 'namba wan dokta'), two Aid Post Supervisors (A.P.S.,) who are responsible for the aid posts and are suggested to visit them regularly but mostly work at the Teptep Health Centre, three nurses,[19] and two Aid Post Orderlies (A.P.O.). The employees live in four modern houses close to the health center and are paid every two weeks.

The main task of the health center is care of the population along Western medical lines. Apart from curative measures (diagnosis and deciding the therapy of a patient), it also carries out preventive[20] activities like patrols within the catchment area of Teptep, vaccination campaigns, infant care in the baby clinic, family planning, care of pregnant women and training of village assistants ("voluntary village health workers"). The H.E.O. is responsible for these preventative tasks. Every two months, the patrols are supposed to reach the more distant villages (like Kewieñ, Nokopo, Kwembun, the Nankina region) and control and advise the aid posts, visit the villages struck by epidemics and treat patients. Some patrols are combined with vaccination campaigns. The baby clinic is supposed to be held every month[21] in the villages of Taeñ, Uskokop, Gua and Kangulut, where the babies are weighed and recorded on a baby-card (a sort of "health pass" which every child should have), vaccinations should be given (against polio, tuberculosis, diphtheria, tetanus, whooping cough and measles), wounds are bandaged and, if needed, drugs administered.

Family planning addresses itself to the married couples who, in a half-hour talk, are jointly advised on the possibilities of contraception. Two kinds of contraceptive pills are offered: Microlut (28 tablets) is given to women with babies less than one year old, hence to women who are breastfeeding. Neog-ynon Ed Fe is given to women whose children are older than one year and who want further children. The failure rate of the contraceptive pill is very high since the women are not used to a regular intake (and since it is probably not always in stock at Teptep). Women who want no further children are given a three-months-injection of Depo Provera 150. All contraceptives are handed out free of charge. Prophylactics are not distributed; they are said by the med-ical staff to be unpopular. No contraceptives are given in Teptep to single or younger, unmarried women for whom an illegitimate pregnancy would be so-cially precarious and who, in this case, would undergo (perhaps forcibly) an abortion (see Chapter 3.3.). They could get a prescription from a physician in Madang and have it filled at the pharmacy for money, a possibility which in practice no Yupno woman can exploit. The family planning office is mainly visited by women from Teptep, mostly of whom are wives of station employ-ees; on average, six women per month ask for contraceptives. The family plan-ning program, which was established by the government but then came under pressure from the Christian missions, restricted the distribution of contra-ceptives to married people. Because of this major compromise, the program fails to meet the needs of the Yupno population.

There are annual courses in midwifery, lasting a week, for women from the villages, who are trained by the H.E.O. via Tok Pisin in the basic skills of mid-wifery and may then assist births in their villages. During the time of my stay (1986–1988), only women from the Nankina region took part in this course; according to the H.E.O., the women from the villages around Teptep lack the motivation ('ol i stap les': "they are lazy"). Their non-participation, in my opinion, owes less to their laziness than to the fact that—except for some younger girls—no woman speaks Tok Pisin and therefore would not have been able to follow the course at all. The women from Nankina (above all, from Bambu village), however, do have sufficient knowledge of Tok Pisin.

Every Friday morning, there is a course for pregnant women attended by two to three women, again almost exclusively from the station. Births by Yupno women at the health center are rare; they go there only if a previous examination has indicated possible complications or if a woman's labor is un-duly protracted. For the most part, educated women or those who are living away from their usual environment (such as most of the wives of the station employees) come to the health center to give birth. Should there be compli-cations at birth that cannot be treated at Teptep, a plane can be chartered and the woman is flown to Modilon Hospital in Madang.

The Primary Health Care-system includes the training of individuals whose village does not have an aid post. The one-week course is annually refreshed and expanded. The goal of this measure is that the "voluntary village health worker" (VVHW,[22] also called voluntary village health aid, VVHA) is able to treat simple diseases in the village (the village assistant is allowed to inject penicillin, for example), and that no patient has to walk for more than one hour to get (bio)medical help; the more seriously ill patients should be sent by the VVHWs to the nearest aid post or directly to Teptep. For a treatment, the villagers pay 10 toea, which the VVHW may either keep for himself or deposit into the village account. Since the Teptep Health Centre can be reached from the villages of Gua, Uskokop and Kangalut within one hour, no man from these villages took part in the training course.

Compared to other such institutions in Papua New Guinea, the health center is medico-technically well equipped and, with eight employees, overstaffed (measured against its utilization by the local population, see Chapter 5.1.c). Three times a week, the H.E.O. does a round of the ward. He is responsible for the work-schedule of the employees, the organization of the preventive measures already presented, the ordering of drugs and purchasing of technical instruments. He also oversees the budget and the further training of staff, and he decides which patients have to be evacuated to Madang. The employees are on 24 hours rosters but need not be present in the health center the entire time; they can also stay at home but are "on call" and should be reachable. When on duty, they have to administer medicine to inpatients and should work in the outpatients' station during the day. However, in 1988, for example, the outpatients' station was open only on weekday mornings for two hours, and wounds were dressed only every other day ('de long pasim soa'), so many patients came to Teptep in vain. This restriction of services offered by the outpatients' station remains unfathomable.

The following procedures can[23] be performed: lumbar punctures for the diagnosis of meningitis or cerebral malaria, ear examinations (but the apparatus was broken in 1987), and flushing of the ears, eye examinations, installation of infusions in the veins, checking the status of hemoglobin by way of the Sahli method, and analyses of blood for malaria and tuberculosis (the blood is taken with finger pricks and the slides are then sent to the laboratory at Madang). The health center has instruments for examinations and medical-technical equipment like a speculum for vaginal examinations, plaster-forceps for removing plaster, sterilizing apparatus for syringes and needles, a children's tubus (for intubation, i.e. artificial respiration), an autoclave, an oxygen-bottle, dressing material, various syringes and needles, fever thermometer, clamps, sterile thread, infusions, and so on.

Treatment of diseases follows the official manuals for medical personnel in Papua New Guinea, one of which is aimed at the treatment of adults, and one for children.[24] The patients are told about the kind of treatment "as far as they can understand it" (statement of the H.E.O.). A report is written for each inpatient, consisting of a piece of paper on which the drugs administered are written down, the Admission Report (of the initial examination), the current observations of the H.E.O. (three times per week), a list of the various examinations and diagnoses, and possibly also the transfer to Madang as well as the discharge.

The outpatients are written down in a book with the date, name, place of residence, diagnosis and therapy, unless they were admitted for a very minor problem. This outpatient treatment costs twenty toea, and for inpatients there is the single payment of two Kina, which includes the examinations and drugs. The transfer to Modilon Hospital in Madang (including flight and treatment in Madang) is free of charge apart from an admission fee of two Kina.

The following drugs are used for biomedical treatment in Teptep:

orally administered (in form of tablets, capsules, drops or syrup):

Chlorpromazine:	neuroleptic, against psychoses and various psychological nervous conditions;
Phenobarbital:	against epilepsy, also as a tranquilizer; a drug little Nstasiñge also received;
Chloralhydrate:	(for psychiatric diseases), tranquilizer, soporific;
Promethacin:	antihistamine (against allergic reactions) and neuroleptic;
Diphenhydramine:	antihistamine, against allergic reactions;
Salbutamol:	antihistamine;
Amoxycyclin, Chloramphenicol, Oxytetracyclin, Clotrimazole:	antibiotics;
Chinin, Chloroquine, Amodiaquine, Primaquine, Fansidar:	against malaria;
Probenecid:	for the treatment of gout, in addition, it raises the concentration of penicillin in the body;
Ferrosulfate (iron):	against anaemia;
Folic acid:	vitamin (against anaemia), for the formation of red blood cells;

Mebendazole, Pyrantel:	against worms;
Aminophylline:	against bronchial asthma;
Polyvitamin:	against vitamin deficiency;
Digoxin:	for heart problems;
Aspirin:	pain-killer ("blood thinner");
Paracetamol:	pain-killer;
Metronidazole:	against amoebae and other protocea;
Pyridoxine (vitamin B6):	against nervous disorders and as an accompanying drug in the treatment of tuberculosis;
Rifampicin:	antibiotics, especially against tuberculosis;
Isoniazid, Sulfadimidine:	against tuberculosis;
Dapsone:	against leprosy;
Aluminum Hydroxide:	against heartburn (dyspepsia);
Nystatin:	against mycosis;
Stomach-mixture (syrup):	against stomach upsets;
Cough-mixture (syrup):	against colds;
Codein[e]:	against cough.

Subcutaneously injected or **intravenously** infused are:

Chloramphenicol:	antibiotic; little Nstasiñge was also treated with these injections;
Oxytocin:	administered during labor;
Procaine-Penicillin-vials:	antibiotic;
Streptomycin-vials:	antibiotic; especially against tuberculosis;
Chinin-vials:	against malaria;
Inferon-vials:	iron medication;
Paraldehyde-vials:	spasmodic, soporific.

Rubbed in or **dabbed** on are:

Salicylic acid:	against grille (tinea imbricata), a fungal skin infection;
Benzoic acid, Cristal violet:	disinfectant;

| Scabies-lotion: | against scabies; |
| Acriflavin, Savlon: | an antiseptic cream. |

b) The Diagnosis at Modilon-Hospital, Madang: Meningitis, Possible Meningo-Encephalitis and Suspected Tuberculosis

Mayu and her child arrived at Modilon Hospital in Madang on 24 April 1987. The results of the examination at admission for the anamnesis as noted on the first page of the patient report,[25] in relation to the history of the disease: loss of weight (from 7 kg in February to 5,5 kg at the end of April), status after meningitis ("had meningitis 3/2/87"), status after convulsions ("had convulsions"), tuberculosis unknown in the family ("no known TB in family"). The latter statement resulted from interviews of the child's mother, and remains uncertain because Mayu does not speak Tok Pisin and could not answer a question like this, even if asked by an interpreter. There is no tuberculosis (or 'tibi' in Tok Pisin) as a cause of illness in the Yupno traditional medical system. The physical disorder *keaknok*, "to continuously cough up and swallow [phlegm]," which is often linked with shortness of breath and which comes closest to the symptom of a case of tuberculosis, can be caused by a number of things: a (vexed) "ghost" (*koñ*) or an incorrectly performed *sit*-act, or (in men) through contact with a "hot," dangerous *moñan* ("breath spirit") of a woman during her menstruation or directly after giving birth. This vast complex of notions about *keaknok* cannot therefore simply be answered with "yes" or "no," as happened at the interrogation. Since it is linked with misdemeanors of the most varied kinds, and Mayu herself, throughout the earlier discussions in the village, had been pondering repeatedly the most diverse "oppressing problems" (*njɨgɨ*), her thoughts were thus totally occupied with possible transgressions and problems, she definitely could not have answered this question spontaneously and so replied in the negative, probably also to protect herself.

The examination at admission revealed: the boy would be about ten months old, looked alert ("eyes alert"), showed stiffness of the body ("has stiff posture") and an opisthotonus (spasm of the neck and back muscles, with backward bending of the torso) and appeared weak ("appears wasted"). Closer examinations showed the following results: the temperature was 36.5° (according to the temperature scale included, the child had a temperature of 37.5° in the evening, hence a slightly raised temperature), the pulse was 80 (and therefore normal), breathing frequency was 28, he weighed 7 kg (whereas on the included weight scale the same day he weighed 5.525 kg), was conscious, the fontanels (seams of the skull) were sunken, his reflexes too strong ("hyperreflexic"), there were retractions at the thorax ("chest en-drawing," "chest soft, not tender"), murmurs could be heard on the lungs on both sides ("bilateral creps"), his skin was afflicted with infected scabies and tropical ulcers and the turgor (water content) of the skin was reduced; the child did not seem apathetic ("no dull"). The child did not have any oedema (water deposits in the hypodermis), no cyanosis (bluish discoloring of the skin due to lack of oxygen in the blood), no murmur could be heard between the two heartbeats.

Based on these results, the following diagnosis was established: meningitis or possible meningo-encephalitis, brain damage after the meningitis ("child had meningitis. Now appears to have sequel of brain damage"), pneumonia, and suspected tuberculosis. Based on this, further, more differentiated examinations were scheduled, consisting of a blood-analysis to detect malaria pathogens, a full blood examination, a chest X-ray, a lumbar puncture and, three times in the row, an examination of the sputum (analysis of the phlegm coughed up from the lungs) to detect possible tuberculosis (more precisely: tubercular bacteria).

As an initial therapy, the following was prescribed: Chloramphenicol[26] 125 mg (an antibiotic to treat meningitis) four times per day (over a fourteen day period), by intramuscular injection (according to the "drug sheet," however, the child received this medication orally); drying out of the ulcers and treatment of the scabies; Phenobarbital (a hypnotic and anti-epileptic, which was sup-posed to suppress the child's spasms) 15 mg (half a tablet) daily (over a thirty day period) and physiotherapy (to empty the lungs). On the very same day—probably after the results of the blood test for malaria—half a tablet of Amodi-aquine, an anti-malaria medication, (daily over a thirty day period) was pre-scribed. As can be seen from the drug sheet, the next day the child also received half a tablet of Pyrantel, a highly effective anti-helminthic against different kinds of worms. The therapy so far corresponds to the standard therapy as suggested in the handbook ("Standard Treatment for Common Ilnesses of Children in Papua New Guinea") for all the physicians, H.E.O. and nurses and male nurses.

During the first week, the child received vaccinations against diphtheria, tetanus, whooping cough, polio, tuberculosis and measles. The suddenly-ap-pearing disturbance and agitation of the child during the night were treated with Chloralhydrate(a soporific). The blood tests, which were frequently re-peated, indicated an inflammation but did not lead to a definite diagnosis. The lumbar punctures, too, were initially repeated almost on a daily basis but were often traumatic, i.e. at the puncture of the spinal fluid, a blood vessel was hit and thereupon accurate assessment of the obtained fluid was no longer possible. At the few successful punctures, the results, which were based on the detected standards of sugar and protein, were normal. No pathogenic agent could be found.

The course of little Nstasiñge's disease changed very little over the weeks. Almost daily, his temperature was taken[27] by the nurses and male nurses and recorded (it lay between 35.7° as the lowest and 37.8° as the highest result, and was higher in the evenings than in the mornings). Every three to four days, he was weighed (his weight slowly increased—interrupted by some minor decreases—from 5,525 kg on 24 April via 5,9 kg on 18 May to 7 kg on 30 June) and he regularly received the prescribed medication. The notes in the patient report read again and again: "neck still stiff," "fever," "feeding o.k.," "condition much the same." On 8 May, he is transferred from the "A-Ward" (the station of the acutely ill patients) to the "B-Ward" (the station of the convalescents), which Mayu also notes: "We were sent to a different ward." On 22 May, the nurse noted as the only reactions of the parents to the stay in hospital: "Parents want to take child back home for trial of village medicine." Mayu only briefly mentions this phase: "Time passed, and he did not get well." After that, there is no more entry that would, for example, point to a renewed attempt by the parents to return to Teptep with the baby. Tanowe, the child's father had followed his wife and his baby to Madang about two weeks later (Mayu did not mention this in her story). He did not live at the hospital but stayed with friends in the Yupno settlement, Sisiak, and only rarely visited Nstasiñge.

Tuberculosis therapy, following the pattern customary in Papua New Guinea, was not begun until 26 May, one month after the child's admission, and at the time when the parents wanted to return to Teptep with their child. Over a period of two months, each tuberculosis patient receives a fourfold combination therapy ("A-therapy"), which, in most cases, is performed on inpatients because of the daily administration of the medication. This "A-therapy" is followed by "B-therapy," where two medications (twofold combination) are taken twice weekly over a period of four months. Where possible, this "B-therapy" is performed on outpatients who remain at home and come to the nearest health center only to get their medication. In Nstasiñge's case, the long lapse of time between admission to the hospital and the start of the "A-therapy" can probably be explained by the fact that no tuberculosis pathogens could be found in his sputum, blood or bodily fluid. Thus it remains unclear whether he was suffering from tuberculosis at all. The treatment with Chloramphenicol was terminated. Following the tuberculosis "A-therapy," the child received Streptomycin, Isoniazid, Rifampicin and Pyrazinamide. One week after the beginning of this tuberculosis therapy, the child was also given Prednisolon,[28] but the reason why this additional medication was administered cannot be deduced from the patient's clinical report, though it was probably prescribed to treat a suspected brain oedema. The child also received Gentamun, which, as Gentamicin, is an antibiotic that is very effective "backup medication."[29]

During the following month, there were still no major changes. The child continued to have peak temperatures, weight gain was minimal, the stiffness of the body did not disappear, he cried a lot ("still cries a lot at nights") and continued to be very restless. He was again transferred to a different ward ("C-ward"), where the rounds are not made daily. (Mayu's comment: "And again they sent us to a different house.")

In the middle of July, after almost three months' stay at the hospital, an improvement was at last registered. According to the patient report, the child was now free of fever, had no more spasms, did not show any stiffness of neck and ate and drank well. From this time on, his condition was checked at greater intervals. The two months of intensive tuberculosis "A-therapy" were concluded, and the "B-therapy" was planned, along with the transfer of the little patient to the Teptep Health Centre. On 20 July, the male nurse noted: "Seen this am [a.m.], afebrile, eating and drinking well, repatriate to Teptep." Since the child no longer wanted to be breastfed, in the following week the parents were taught how to make M.O.F. (milk oil formula, a milk substitute). The entry on 22 July: "Await. repat. back to Teptep. cond. [condition] afebrile, eating/drinking well, refuse breast milk/wants M.O.F. only; father requested to get free supply at milk—told to buy his own milk; nurse to explain to parents how to make M.O.F. at home." The last entry, on 27 July 1987, reads: "seen by paed. [pediatrician] team. arrange repatriation, cont. [continuing] B Regime ["B-therapy"] cond. [condition]: no new problems, afebrile." On 31 July 1987, the child was discharged (without a final examination) and flew back to Teptep with his mother.

Two points are notable in this patient report:

1. The child received a large number of different, potent medications; in part, these were administered at the same time, in part (like with the tuberculosis therapy) without clarifying exactly whether the child really had tuberculosis. Treatment therefore followed an trial and error method. In addition, the child was subjected to very frequent (according to the patient report at Modilon Hospital, ten) lumbar punctures, during which, in five instances, vessels were damaged ("traumatic").

2. The evaluation of the child's condition was again and again reduced to the following four criteria: stiffness of the neck; fever; appetite and state of nutrition, and state of excitement.

After these four conditions had been successfully treated with biomedicine and—from a medical point of view—were satisfactory, the stiffness of the neck was no longer noticeable, the child was free of fever, ate and drank well, had gained weight and had calmed down, Nsatsiñge was considered "healed" and the therapy (with the exception of the planned continuation of the "B-therapy") concluded. He was now twelve months old.

From the various therapies performed at the Teptep Health Centre and at Modilon Hospital in Madang, as they noted in the patient report, some interpretations from a European-biomedical viewpoint[30] can be made vis-à-vis little Nstasiñge's disease. It can be assumed that, when first taken to the Teptep Health Centre on 3 February 1987, little Nstasiñge had bacterial or tubercular meningitis; the flocculent ("cloudy") appearance of the fluid that was obtained after a lumbar puncture (should this have taken place) points to this. According to the H.E.O., the child was successfully treated with Chloramphenicol, a broad spectrum antibiotic. In Switzerland, for example, bacterial meningitis would be treated similarly. Once the pathogenic agent (resulting from a lumbar puncture) was detected, an antibiogram would be made, to discover which antibiotic the pathogenic agent responds to, in order to adapt the initially "blind" therapy to the pathogenic agent, should this be necessary. Between 24 or, at the most, 36 hours after the start of the therapy, a control lumbar puncture would be performed.

If tubercular meningitis, which in Europe is very rare, is suspected, a special coloring or cultivation of the agent from the fluid would take place and, with proof of tuberculosis, subsequent therapy would be prescribed specifically for the tubercular agent. At seven months, little Nstasiñge was at an age where (in tropical countries) meningitis tuberculosae is not uncommon. The disease begins insidiously, with indisposition, vomiting, and loss of weight, then, after one to three weeks, the first signs of meningitis appear, such as stiffness of the neck, vomiting spasms, changes in the pulse, breathing disorders and fever.

The H.E.O. at the Teptep Health Centre on April 13 describes a "flare-up" of the tuberculosis which suggests that tuberculosis was suspected at the time of first admission on 3 February, in which case the administration of Chloramphenicol would have been of no use whatsoever. Methods of examination that could have detected a tuberculosis agent are not feasible at Teptep (see excursus: "The Teptep Health Centre"). The stiffness of the neck, the rigidity of the whole body, the staring eyes and the grave weight loss point to encephalitis, an inflammation affecting both brain membranes and the brain itself. This corresponds to a serious course of disease (meningitis developing into encephalitis). In Europe, tubercular meningo-encephalitis has a death rate between 10% and 20%; residuals, i.e. remaining damages after the disease affect between 20% and 40% of all the diseased persons. Therapy in Europe would be tuberculosis-specific, aimed at the healing the tuberculosis, and the symptoms of encephalitis could only be attacked symptomatically by treating individual symptoms like fever and spasms with the appropriate medication. In terms of medication, the little boy Nstasïnge's treatment in Europe would have varied only minimally. However, these considerations and interpretations have to remain speculative because of the missing proof of tuberculosis agents or any other agents of meningo-encephalitis. From the biomedical viewpoint, too, we cannot definitely identify the disease from which the little boy was suffering.

In little Nstasïnge's case, both forms of treatment, the traditional and the biomedical, failed. This failure was explained in different ways.

Following the traditional interpretation, too many "oppressing problems" (*njïgï*) existed between the parents, the situation was too highly charged with conflict, and in the end these conflicts had never been satisfactorily solved. Even though various "oppressing problems" (*njïgï*) (see Figure 2 [1–12]) had been identified during the discussions, the one that was responsible for little Nstasïnge's illness could not with certainty be specified and thus dealt with.

Biomedically interpreted, the child probably arrived too late at the Teptep Health Centre and then had not been treated correctly and regularly there (although the above-mentioned uncertainties in regarding the identity of the disease as a bacterial or tubercular meningitis have to be considered). The delayed start of the antibiotics therapy was probably decisive for the further course of the disease. The subsequent patient report shows that the child (at a weight of 5,5 kg) was heavily treated with medication of the most varied kind and had to suffer numerous critical examinations (like the frequent lumbar punctures), which are not without risk and, in case of incorrect performance, could cause lasting damage, such as paralysis. From a biomedical point of view, the definite cause of the disease, the specific pathogenic agent, could not be detected. From the Western viewpoint, the child was discharged as "healed," that is in a "stable" condition, which could not be further improved with medication.

In summary, the parallel application of traditional medicine and biomedicine proceeded as follows:

Little Nstasïnge's Sickness

Coping with Illness	Treating a Disease
2. 2. 1987: First signs of illness, "hot skin", continuous screaming, visit to Teptep Health Centre. The mother assumes illness caused by "oppressing problems" [1-4],	3. 2. 1987: **Admission** to Teptep Health Centre. Diagnosis: possible meningitis. Two weeks' therapy with broad spectrum antibiotic.

gives the screaming boy to other relatives and carries him into other houses, to watch the baby's reactions ("signs").

1. Debate of illness on 10. 2. 1987: the "signs" (*tauak*) of the child point to the maternal kinship group; dreams, on the other hand, point to the paternal grandfather. Problems discussed:

1. A distant relative of Mayu's mother Narewe and the "ghost" of his father felt left out at Mayu's brideprice, and their "hot" anger caused the child's illness [5].

2. The "ghost" of Tanowe's father (the baby's grandfather) was annoyed since Tanowe, against his father's admonitions, lived with his clan. Dreams are interpreted in which Tanowe's father had been seen together with the baby [6]. Performance of a ritual to chase away the two angry "ghosts". Consequence of the debate: the baby's name is changed, money is collected.

2. Debate of illness on 25. 2. 1987: problems discussed: 1. the clan of Tanowe (the baby's father) might possibly have killed members of the clan of Mayu (the mother) - both traditionally inimical groups - by *sit*-actions [7] or vice versa [8].

Consequences of the discussion: money is collected.
The mother and the baby spend a week at Bameleñ (Tapmañge) with her husband's kinship group.

3. Debate of illness on 12. 4. 1987:
two problems are discussed:

1. out of jealousy, a woman raged so vehemently in Nstasiñge's house that the baby got scared and his *amɨnwop* ("shadow soul") slid out of him [9].

2. Mayu's brideprice transfer was not performed correctly; many (also in the meantime deceased) people felt cheated and were angry [10-12].

Consequence of the debate: public regret over the jealousy and the resulting behavior; appeals to the *amɨnwop* ("shadow soul") of the baby to return to its place in the child; and collection of money.

13. 4. 1987: **Second visit** to the Teptep Health Centre. Therapy: Phenobarbital to quieten the child.

24. 4. 1987: **Transfer** to Modilon Hospital at Madang. Statement at admission: weight of child 5,5 kg, skin with scabies, murmurs of the lungs on both sides, turgor of skin diminished, sunken fontanels.

Diagnosis: meningo-encephalitis, braindamage at status after meningitis, suspected tuberculosis, pneumonia.

Therapy: drying of the ulcers, Chloramphenicol 125 mg (4x/d) during 14 d (meningitis), Phenobarbital 15 mg/d during 30 d (spasms), Amodiaquine 1/2 tbl/d during 3 d (malaria), Pyrantel 1/2 tbl 1x (antihelminthic).

During the first week, administering of missing vaccinations: diphtheria, tetanus, whooping cough, polio, tuberculosis, measles.

22. 5. 1987: The parents want to
return to Teptep with their child.

> After 26. 5. 1987: tuberculosis therapy
> with Streptomycin, Isoniazid,
> Rifampicin, Pyrazinamide.
>
> Discharge to the village on 31. 7. 1987

3. The Mother's Epilogue

During my third visit to the village, in autumn 1988, one year after the completion of the child's treatment, I again met Mayu. She was living in Gua with her mother-in-law, Susune, in a different house and had given birth to a little daughter, her husband Tanowe had left the family and the village and was living in Madang. The little boy Nstasiñge was now mentally and physically handicapped. She commented on her situation:

> I do not think about it much, I am not angry, I am well now. Really, he wanted to die, but I was torn this way and that, he almost wanted to die, but I felt so sorry for him, and I watched over him, I loved him and watched over him. I do not give him to anybody else, I alone walk around with him. If I want to go to the garden, I give him to his grandmother and I only go to get sweet potatoes and come back at once. If I go further into the garden, I carry him, the two of us go to the garden, I put him down, I do the gardening and look for sweet potatoes. I hear if he cries, I think, he is hungry, and I give him the sweet potatoes cooked beforehand and put him down again and go on digging sweet potatoes. That is how I do it, and when I have found enough sweet potatoes, I carry him, and the two of us go back to the house. This group of young girls here (who also sometimes spent the night in her house), they do not help me and carry him for a while, no. Sometimes I am angry because of it. That is all.

Chapter 5

The Yupno Medical System:
An Attempt at Systematization

1. "Natural Disorders" or the State of "Not Being Ill"

Symptoms thought to be "natural" or "harmless" disorders of physical well-being manifest themselves as cuts, fractures, infected insect-bites, catarrh, cough, headache, rheumatism, diarrhoea, and so on. As already noted, if such symptoms fade away after a few days or disappear, the Yupno regard them as normal, since they do not unduly incapacitate or endanger a person. Because they are based only on bodily symptoms that can be seen or felt, they are not called "illness,"[1] *sɨt* ("to heat," "to burn," "to cook") but disorders, so one does not say: "*sɨt asat*," "I am ill," but *ndol tepm*, "[I have a] toothache" or *kokɨlɨt*, "[I have] diarrhoea." An afflicted person suffering from one of these disorders, while no longer in the "ideal," "cool" state of well-being (*yawuro*), is "hot" (*tepm*) but not "ill" (*sɨt*).

These disorders accompany a state of illness (caused by an agent) as physical symptoms, or appear as a consequence of physical exhaustion (beating bark-cloth for hours on end, for example, causes pain in the shoulders) or of climatic conditions (the rainy season and cold weather may lead to chills), but the Yupno do not attribute any great importance to them, in contrast to "real illness" (see Chapter 5.2.). The Yupno way of coping with the bodily disorders (which are not thought of as "illness" per se so they pay little attention to them), may also be compared to the behavioral pattern of the Gimi, for whom they likewise do not belong to the realm of "illness" but are categorized as "minor ailments" having no socially significant cause (Glick 1963: 114, Glick 1967: 35). For the Yupno, however, these bodily disorders accompany "real illness" as "physical disorders," and various specialists exist to treat them, so they are significant and thus should not be neglected.

Traditionally, these disorders are treated[2] with certain food prescriptions, plant medicine, rest and massage. For example, certain kinds of dry bananas are eaten in the event of diarrhoea; wounds are treated with the application of certain leaves; for rheumatism, the body parts concerned are immobilized; and for a headache, the head is tightly bound or massaged.[3] Should someone regard his or her "disorder" as harmless, one turns to home remedies, resorting to a kind of knowledge possessed by every adult Yupno that remains within the popular or lay sector (cf. Kleinman 1980: 50). Should this treatment prove ineffective, one consults a specialist, a *yawuro yawuro amɨn*, a "cooler," who can bring the "hot" patient down to the proper "cool" state. Within this category, there are three specialists: the *kandap arap amɨn*, "heat extinguisher," the *ngesam amɨn*, "soother," and the *kamam kuok amɨn*, "restorer." All are representatives of the folk sector (cf. Kleinman 1980:59), herbalists who dispose of clan-specific, strictly kept secret, mythological knowledge and of their own herb- and "water"-recipes. Their therapy is based on the Yupno humoral concept that somebody suffering from bodily disorders is "hot" (*tepm*): so, to cure the patient, he or she has to be cooled down to the normal "cool" state with the help of special plants, or water from certain springs, that are thought to be "cold."[4]

All these specialists learned their skills from their parents. Normally, a father hands them on to his son, or less commonly, he teaches them to his daughter, who in turn instructs her son or her daughter. No exceptional status or particular prestige is ascribed to them because of their special skills alone. However, since they (above all, male representatives) at the same time possess extensive mythological knowledge, which is most often connected with skills concerning how to change the "condition" of a garden, influence social relationships, how to "heat up" an enemy and how to make a hunt successful, they are generally very well respected. Exactly like the other villagers, they fulfill their daily chores and duties. However, the "coolers" work for a fee, the amount and form of which varies according to the economic situation of the patient. Younger people who grow cash crops and therefore have money pay one to two Kina, whereas old people are more likely to pay in kind.

a) The Traditional Cures

The forms of treatment of the "coolers," the "soothers" and the "heat extinguishers" are now described in more detail.

Treatment by a "Soother"

I

The "standard therapy" performed by a "soother"[5] proceeds as follows: First, the patient (or one of his or her relatives) summons the "soother," who sets the date and the place of the treatment (most often the ill person's house) and then begins his preparations. He collects the following plants,[6] which grow in a variety of different places, in the bush, in the village or close to water, growing wild or under cultivation:

komupkomup	the flowers and fruit of the *komupkomup* resemble those of the *komup* plant, 'marita,' a type of pandanus from which the red liquid *komup* is obtained; hence the name, a plant with thorns;
ndamba ɨsip[7]	a plant that grows close to water and is thought to be "cold";
tapmat	a plant with small thorns;
nyaknkuak	a "cold," fern-like plant;
leaves of the *makum* tree	a tree with a thorny trunk;
amɨn tekok	a kind of grass;
amɨn sisap	a kind of grass;
mbok	a cultivated plant with red, "hot" leaves;
leaves of the *joñwijok* tree	a mythologically relevant tree with pale-green (Yupno: "white"), that is, "cold" leaves;
mbɨtkuak	a bush with leaves whose inner parts are pale-green (Yupno: "white"), "cold";
kokop amɨn kamam	a fragrant flower.

These plants share certain characteristics, being either pale-green (Yupno: "white," meaning "cold"), or else red, that is "hot," and are remarkably aromatic, fragrant, thorny, astringent, sour or stinging (a contra-irritant).

The "soother" lays the plants and leaves listed onto a leaf of the *petmbat* plant, a kind of pale-green, "cold" rib of leaf, and wraps it with *mbalgerk*, dried strips of the ribs of banana leaves, like a parcel. He then ties the leaves of the plants *mbañgam*, *kwebekal* and *numbun*, three "cold" plants that grow at watercourses, into another parcel with an *umban* leaf.

Afterwards, he chews a piece of the aromatic bark of the *ngwawan* tree, which smells of muscat, repeatedly chants over some water which he has earlier poured into a wooden bowl, "Ndondoro Panjewik."[8] Naming such powerful things (being full of "vital energy," *tevantok*) brings them into an exceptional state (*tilagɨ*); he then spits the pieces of *ngwawan* bark into this "activated" water. The patient lies next to the wash-basin. First, the "soother" splashes water onto the patient, then dips the bundle of leaves consisting of the three "cold" plants into the water and strokes the ill person's skin with it. He then puts the large bundle of leaves (the first one) into the water, takes it out again and repeatedly but lightly hits the patient's body with it. The whole procedure takes about one hour.

As a "soother" himself would say, he cannot heal the sick, that is, clarify the cause of the illness; he is consulted only for its alleviation, the soothing of the physical disorder (such as pain or fever) by cooling the heated up patient. His prescription consists of a balanced mixture of predominantly cold but also several hot components, which prevent the afflicted from lapsing into the other extreme state, which is ice-cold (*mbaak*).

II

Within the category "heat extinguishers," every single specialist has at his disposal varying specific possibilities of treatment that, in part, are prescribed for certain physical symptoms. I recorded therapies utilized by two "heat extinguishers," one by an old man and one by an old woman, which varied considerably in their structure. As a rule, for their therapy male specialists use paraphernalia of a more markedly mythological-religious importance, which is to be expected, since religion and mythology were traditionally the exclusively reserves of the men (and in part still are). The choice of these paraphernalia is furthermore strongly influenced by clan membership. Female specialists, on the contrary, have more pragmatic skills, and their clients are predominantly babies, infants and breastfeeding mothers.

Treatment by a Male "Heat Extinguisher"

The principle of the therapy of a male "heat extinguisher" resembles that of the "soother" since it, too, is aimed at soothing the physical disorders of well-being through cooling. His treatment centers on the water of certain streams, which, having been created by the Yupno River itself or by different culture heroes, are thought to be especially "different" or "exceptional" (*tilagɨ*).

The therapy of a male "heat extinguisher" proceeds as follows: First he gets water from different watercourses, which are all the property of his own clan, the Talon, and originate from areas on which it has a claim. The specialist pours the different waters into a coconut shell. Then he collects *boa*, a kind of moss, the two cold plants, *mbañgam*, *kwebekal*, and cuts a leaf stem of the banana *ngolda*, a "cold" banana. He dips the three plants into the coconut shell filled with water and stirs. In the meantime, he calls out the names of various streams from which he has fetched water, chews a piece of *ngwawan* bark and some *numbun* leaves and says[9]

> I chew *ngwawan* and *numbun*, they are in my mouth. I have taken from the Pangowañ a banana leaf stem of the *ngolda* banana, I have fetched Pan water, Nantjañon water, Tilak water, Mundogon water, Wumbokgowañ water, Kwengowañ water and collected leaves of *mbañgam*, *kwebekal*, *numbun*, have crushed it in the bowl, have fetched water from the Dalgowañ, ill person, I now take you so that you go into this water, I lift you up, so that you go into the water, I take you into it, to this cool place, I take you there, your skin gets cool, and you will sleep, and you will be well.

Then he spits what he has chewed (*ngwawan* bark and *numbun* leaves) onto the patient's body, takes *mbañgam* and *kwebekal* leaves, puts them on what he has spat out, and washes the afflicted by repeatedly splashing the water in the bowl with the *boa* moss onto the patient.

Treatment by a Female "Heat Extinguisher"

The (only) female "heat extinguisher" in Gua specializes mainly in the treatment of breastfeeding women whose milk dries up, and in weakened babies and infants. If a mother brings her baby in a weak condition or if the mother herself can no longer breastfeed her child, the "heat extinguisher" collects different leafy vegetables like cabbage, water-cress, 'pitpit,' 'krusako,' 'aibika,' *kwawɨl* as well as the leaves and the fruit of the pumpkin, which the Yupno regard as full of water and cool. She cooks them, together with the leaves of two bananas said to be very dry, *joñgat* and *ngambum*, with the ginger *maam si*, salt and sugar-cane *yaat* in a bamboo pipe of the cold bamboo species *ngavɨ*. The vegetable broth is trickled into the mouth of the baby, which is meant to grow rapidly like a plant shoot; at this stage, the baby's skin lacks fat and so sits firmly on the bones, but after drinking the broth the child will unfold, like a vegetable shoot after a downpour, and "shoot up." The mother eats the vegetables and drinks the liquid. The treatment is performed once or repeated several times.

The above-mentioned pragmatic knowledge of the female "heat extinguisher" manifests itself here: Yupno food concepts of cold vegetables having high water content are congruent with Western nutritional science perspective on optimal nutrition as rich in vitamins and protein. The addition of salt and sugar (in the form of sugar-cane), which is based on ancient handed-down experience, forms the Yupno counterpart to the "oral rehydration therapy," a mixture of water, salt, sugar and other minerals, that Western physicians widly propagate for dehydrated children with diarrhoea, it is administered at the Teptep Health Centre (see Kaiser and Kaiser [1986]: 12–7, 12–8; Werner 1983: 152). The traditional therapy of this "heat extinguisher" therefore corresponds closely to some of the most modern medical and nutritional science findings.

b) Individual "Disorders"

The following representation of physical disorders posed some problems for me. As already mentioned, the Yupno have no generic noun for the "bodily disorders." From the Yupno point of view, a classification which for our own Western medicine would be "logical" (cough, catarrh, nasal congestion, diseases for which an ear-, nose- and throat-specialist would be consulted, or skin diseases, for which we would visit a dermatologist), would make no sense since for them such a classification does not exist.[10] To avoid the danger of a biomedical classification (which this study emphatically tries to do), individual symptoms are simply listed in alphabetical order.[11] The bodily symptoms listed singly (for clarity's sake) could of course also appear as a syndrome, a complex of symptoms. In most cases, when the complaints are more serious and people have exhausted their home remedies, a "soother" or a "heat extinguisher" is then consulted. The people concerned or (as is always the case for children) the family as a therapy managing group makes the decision, which depends on subjective criteria: the feelings of the ill person, or his own skill with home remedies, his clan and his partner clan, his relationship and his kinship position with regard to a "cooler," his trust in traditional medicine and his acceptance of biomedicine.

In the following representation, the Yupno terms are listed in the left-hand column together with short notes regarding bodily disorders; also added are physical malformations, such as strabism (being cross-eyed), which do not count as an illness but are, as a "remarkable disorder," given their respective names. In the central column are the biomedical terms for the disease or symptom,[12] and in the right-hand column, the traditional remedies (if any) are listed.

Yupno term	Western term for symptom	Yupno remedy
amek ("swollen belly"), looks like a highly pregnant belly, afflicted can barely walk anymore, mostly caused through *sɨt*-act; an often terminal illness.	DD (Differential Diagnosis): acute abdomen, malignant abdominal disease, ascitis	None
arokarok, itchy skin disease, contracted by contact with dogs or pigs or from *elin* grass with small barbed thorns that prick the skin. Younger people call this disorder 'kaskas' (Tok Pisin for scabies).	Dermatitis as a generic noun, possibly scabies	None
mbisoñ tepm, "headache."	Cephalgia	Sleep, tightly binding the head with string, massage by pulling at the hair.
mbɨt madeptok, "swollen, inflated belly," in most cases counted among the complaints of old age.	Not assignable	None
mbobok, "belly swells," new term, used only by younger people.	Rectusdiastasis	None

Yupno term	Western term for symptom	Yupno remedy
mbook, "sniffles" (with runny nose). *Mbook* and *kaldok* (see below) can be caused by cold, running about in the rain, or the blossoms of certain trees or plants when their scent gets into the nose: *kunagat* (pandanus species), *rap silup*, flowers from *rap* tree, *kua*, a creeping vine, and *ngasu*, a kind of tree. *Mbook* and also *kaldok* (see below) are contagious, and according to the younger, educated people, are especially communicable through saliva. Therefore, these disorders are also called *sɨt yɨt namejak*, "he/she gives seeds of illness."	Rhinitis, allergic rhinitis	Home remedies: *kamam kuok* leaves are dried and crushed (today, also tomato leaves, since tomatoes are held to be "cold") and are rubbed on the afflicted person's skin. Preparation and drinking of a brew from water and crushed *paña* leaves or by boiling and eating the leaves.
ndakkok, "bloody diarrhoea."	Dysentery, colon tumor	Home remedies: "Dry" food, roasted bananas called *joñgat* (very dry and normally not eaten), *tɨmni kadɨm* and *ngambum*.
kokɨlɨt, "diarrhoea."	Watery diarrhoea, as in cholera, for example	As a home remedy and therapy of the "heat extinguisher," the two plants *kokmbɨsap* and *mbutndañgwan* are rubbed on the belly of the afflicted person, and the remains are afterwards hung over the fire; as they dry (substituting for the diarrhoea) so does the bodily disorder disappear.

Yupno term	Western term for symptom	Yupno remedy
ndakda nokndat, "the blood beats, stings me," often also called *njibu* (see note 3). The pain, for example, may start on the left at the ribs and spread up through the body. The blood is thought to be too thick, concentrated in one place and therefore blocking the veins and the arteries. Cause: Straining work, carrying heavy loads.	Not assignable	The *njibu amɨn,* a kind of masseur, kneads the affected part so that the blood "runs" properly again.
ndak yuki, "bad blood," the body part in question hurts or feels numb.	Not assignable	None for chronic disorders, a household remedy is minor blood-letting *pɨrap.*
ndavɨli dɨrɨñ, "to be cross-eyed."	Strabism	None
ndavɨli goman, "red eyes."	Conjunctivitis	Therapy of the "heat-extinguisher," who crushes *ndamba kuak* leaves, "cold," white leaves, then he puts this paste on the eye; the liquid stings at first, but the reddening fades. Alternatively: the leaves of the two "cold" plants, *mbañgam* and *kwebekal,* are fixed over the eye.
ndavɨli mi, "no eyes," meaning: "blind."	Amaurosis (blindness)	None

Yupno term	Western term for symptom	Yupno remedy
ndavɨli mpagmbe, "watering eyes," said to be a complaint of old age.	Keratoconjunctivitis sicca	None
ndavɨli pɨlɨnda, "bad eyesight"; generally, a condition of old people.	Loss of vision, pterygium or cataracts	None
ndel yamak, "bamboo splinter" (in the eye). If one sits too close to the fire and a bamboo cooking container bursts, small splinters of it fly around and may get into the eye.	Intraocular foreign body	Either the person affected or a relative tries to remove the foreign body with a little stick. Treatment by "heat extinguisher": he takes a blade of grass, turns the eyelid outwards and lightly cuts the inner side; the foreign body is washed out with the blood.
ndol tepm, "tooth-ache."	Dentalgia	For strong, long-lasting pain, a relative extracts the infected tooth with a string. Therapy of the "heat extinguisher": the tooth is smeared with a paste made of crushed *pobalok* leaves, sugar-cane and "cold" dew-liquid.
ndolɨ mi, "toothless," especially common in old people.	Toothlessness (Adentia)	No, people assert mastication by crushing the food (or the nuts when chewing betel nuts).

Yupno term	Western term for symptom	Yupno remedy
ngigngekno tepm namejak, "my ribs give me pain." Cause: if one sleeps all night on one side, for example. Often also called *manjɨt tepm namejak*, "the back gives me pain," or *manjɨt tepm tok*, "backache."	Not assignable	Waiting or else rubbing the affected part with nettle-like *yaal* leaves, a counter-irritant.[13]
ngodɨm mok, meaning: "to be only skin and bones."	Cachexia, in babies maybe exsic-cosis	For babies and infants therapy of the female "heat-extinguisher" (see Chapter 5.1.a.).
ngodɨm tepmtok, "the body hurts," "is hot," "fever"	Fever, general pain in the joints	• Crushing of leaves *ndankwɨt kasɨt*; a brew is made with water, which one then drinks. • The skin is rubbed with leaves of the *ngodɨm tɨraptok* plant.
ngom sɨt[14] "mosquito-ill-ness." Symptoms: headache, shivers.	Diseases spread by insects, like ar-boviroses, rick-ettsioses	Ablutions by a "soother" or "heat extinguisher."
ñuak madep tok, "swollen knees." Most often caused through neglect of certain norms of behavior vis-à-vis persons in certain kinship positions (see Chapter 2.3.).	Not assignable	None

Yupno term	Western term for symptom	Yupno remedy
kaandapno komokndok, "my gone-to-sleep leg." The other body parts are called, accordingly, for example, *kalañno komokndok,* "my gone-to-sleep-foot."	Paraesthesias, paresis (paralysis)	Movement
kaandap yukidak, "bad leg," name for injured, painful leg.	Not assignable	Depending on symptom (dressing the wounds, putting in splints, etc.).
kalañe kadɨmtok, "totally numb foot with no feeling."	Paresis, paraesthesias	None
kaldok, "cough," often with phlegm.	Cough with sputum	As a home remedy, *ndavieñ* leaves and young fruits of this variety of cucumber are cooked with water, then one drinks the concoction. Or: *ndavieñ* leaves and fruits are cooked together with *mbañgam* leaves, and the concoction is drunk to dissolve what is blocking the throat. Or: One crushes leaves of the *kalit sewak,* a cabbage (with thorns), that grows wild, then adds water, mixes the soaked leaves with food or drinks them.
kalsɨt nywok, "swollen loin." Symptoms: the afflicted feels cold. Often also called *aljoko pok,* "swollen armpit." Both can be caused by major wounds.	Lymphadenopathia	None, apart from dressing the wounds.

Yupno term	Western term for symptom	Yupno remedy
kandapda sañgamok, "burns." Major burns are mostly attributed to the bush-spirit *sindok* (see Chapter 5.3.).	Combustio	*kandap arap*, generic noun for a "heat extinguisher's" paste, made of various components: *mbomak* leaves, *miañmiañ* leaves, *kandap arap* leaves, *ngodan* moss, *ndamba isip*, and soot. This paste is applied to the affected body parts.
awida sañnamok, "lime has burned me," meaning: "burn in the mouth." The black wound often occurs when, during the chewing of betel nut, lime drops onto the tongue.	Cauterization	Therapy: with a small piece of outer bark of a young bamboo, which is still soft and flexible, the wound is stroked until it bleeds (and then heals).
kasiro wanpelak, "hand or arm fracture."	Fracture	Therapy: the "heat extinguisher" beats bark of the *kalo* tree that is still growing beneath the ground, until it is soft, beats the plants *kauak* (no translation), *popmdeñ* and *komupkomup* until they are pliable, ties them around the fractured part of the body and fixes them with a banana leaf or an *umban* leaf.

Yupno term	Western term for symptom	Yupno remedy
keaknok, "to continuously swallow what is coughed up." Shortness of breath, cough with phlegm. Cause: *keaknok* may be caused by a "ghost" (*koñ*), through a failed *sɨt*-act or (in men) through contact with menstruating women. Thought to be a frequent "disorder" in old age.	DD: pneumonia, chronic-obstructive lung disease, left-heart-insufficiency	None
kɨrarogen, "only skin and bones," "very skinny."	Cachexy	In babies and infants, treatment by a female "heat extinguisher" (see Chapter 5.1.a.).
kosum kalɨmdak, "blocked ear."	Cerumen obturans (ceruminal clot)	Therapy of the "heat-extinguisher": to collect the blossom of the *mbiawandat* plant, inside which there is a liquid which is dripped into the ear; it softens the earwax which is then removed with a piece of bamboo or wood.
kosum mi, "deaf." Old people are those most often afflicted by it; in younger people, this symptom is explained as a lasting consequence of illness caused by "oppressing problems" or by "ghosts."	Cophosis	None
kosum tawa, "festering ear."	Purulent otitis	None

Yupno term	Western term for symptom	Yupno remedy
kuapmo tepm namejak, "my shoulder gives me pain." Cause: over-exhaustion, carrying heavy loads.	Not assignable	Rest
moñan da añakndak, "to catch a gust of wind ("draught"), a complaint of old people that most often occurs in the afternoon.	Not assignable	No, one sits close to the fire.
mum ndakndak, "breast pain."	Mastitis, mainly puerperalis	None
mum darok, "no more milk," meaning: a lactating woman who has no more milk.	Hypo- or agalactia	Treatment by a female "heat extinguisher" (see Chapter 5.1.a.).
ninimoktak, "earthquake," "trembling," shivering fits, accompanied by "catarrh" (*mbook*) and "cough" (*kaldok*); see above.	Shivering fits	To sit close to the fire; also, one drinks "cough" (*kaldok*) ablutions from one of the two herbalists.
sit tevan, "serious illness." Symptoms: the wound is hidden (on the penis, in the vagina), but the afflicted walks with an unusual gait. The illness occurs mainly in young returnees from the towns.	Gonorrhoea, lues, generally sexually transmitted diseases (STD)	None
talbok, "runny nose," snotty nose.	Rhinitis	None

Yupno term	Western term for symptom	Yupno remedy
tapmɨmo mi, "weak, feeble." This symptom often accompanies *keaknok* (see above).	Not assignable	None
tɨmnɨ gorok, "blocked up nose."	Rhinitis	None
wam suok, "piercing pain in the stomach," "stomach cramps," also *wam tepmtok,* "stomach pains."	Not assignable	As with *kokɨlɨt,* "diarrhoea" (see above).
wandɨtɨt, "to vomit."	Vomiting	Sometimes, the afflicted eats *kalañ kuak,* a kind of ginger[15]. Younger people often eat a piece of 'rombo' (Tok Pisin for chili), which "cleanses" the body.

Yupno term	Western term for symptom	Yupno remedy
wuda (generic noun for wounds, cuts etc.), "wound." Depending on the kind, it is distinguished from *wuda bap*, "big wound," *wudawuda*, "many small wounds," "rash," *ndak wuda*, "bleeding wound," *wuda goman*, "(smaller), "open, bleeding wounds." Old people, especially, are prone to large wounds on their shins. Often, the part of the body with the wound is named, e.g.: *ndavɨl wuda* "wound in the eye." In most cases, the cause is stated, for example, people talk about *mandak nañ mandañamok*, "the knife has cut him."	Traumatic injuries Large traumatic injuries DD: eczema, pyodermitis Bleeding wound caused by trauma Not assignable Ulcera cruris	Not for small wounds. Personal therapy for larger wounds: • dressing with a leaf, to deter flies, or: • rubbed with a paste made from crushed *nyingwalmelbi* leaves and *mbomak* leaves, or: • rubbed with a paste from snail excrement and crushed *sukuak* leaves. Arrow-wounds are coated with chewed ginger *kalañ kuak*. Therapy of a "heat-extinguisher": he heats a leaf of the *manañgan* plant in the fire until it is soft and pliable, puts it on the wound and fixes it with a piece of string, raffia or something similar, and the wound later bursts open, then heals.

c) The Acceptance of Biomedicine

For these above-mentioned bodily disorders, that is, for complaints held to be "disorders" but not "illness," the Yupno resort in part to Western medicine. Before describing the present situation,[16] some historical remarks are in order.

I

Comments on matters concerning health and disease among the Yupno are to be found in the patrol reports of the Australian government officers. Their notes do not lead to epidemiological conclusions since they do not furnish any quantitative data (though, sporadically, some epidemics are mentioned); nevertheless, their statements are important since they give an impression of the Yupno population that at first glance remains the same today: the impression of a healthy people.

Thus in 1938, L.G.Vial (1938: 144), the first Patrol Officer noted: "An average state of health existed. I saw no signs of chest complaints, and at one village, Isan, the general physique was remarkably good for mountain natives."

Seven years later, in 1945, Rylands notes that the villages of Gua and Nokopo had been deserted; he blames this on a dysentery epidemic, but his impression, too, is positive:

> Natives are living in the bush and there is said to be dysentery....[Appendix A:] In general the health of all the mountain natives was good. Grille and Kas Kas had a lower incidence than on the coast although the cold does not encourage the natives to wash much...Crossing in the YUPNA, health is good at the two high villages (7,000') of KEWIENG and ISAN...No yaws or filariasis was noticed and little skin diseases....It can be very cold, especially when it rains and there are some horrible graveyard coughs but there does not appear to be a very high death rate from chest complaints (Rylands 1945: 3 and Appendix A).

In 1953/54, Steven (1953/54: 9) briefly notes: "The standard of health is very high..." Neal (1954/55: 9) also stresses the good state of health of the Yupno; his observations on washing habits are, however, not shared by any other Patrol Officer.

> The health of the people was very good with such ailments as grille, malaria and yaws appearing to be almost non-existent....the coolness of the climate seems to be conducive to good health among the people, coupled also with an apparent fanaticism for personal cleanliness.

The natives are exceptionally clean and daily indulge in a bath in the nearest icy cold stream (Neal 1954/55: 9–10).

In the following year (1955/56), Patrol Officer Hanrahan ordered three Yupno to undergo training as "medical orderlies."

The URUWAS and YUPNAS, particularly the latter, were generally found to be robust and of good physique and were the healthiest tribes encountered to date in the WASU area. These people do not appear to be so subject to respiratory complaints and pneumatic troubles so common in other mountain divisions such as the TIMBE and NABA. The extreme isolation of the two areas could perhaps have something to do with this.... The people are highly susceptible to malaria when they leave themselves open to infection on the coast.... At present, no medical facilities exist for the YUPNA people... With this in mind, three natives were selected from the central villages of KEWIENG, ISAN and MEK with a view to attending the native medical training school at MALAHANG (Hanrahan 1955/56: 8).

In 1959, Patrol Officer Muskens writes about an epidemic of influenza:

Recption [sic] at most villages was extremely poor. This, however, was undoubtedly due to the effect of the influenza epidemic on the people. [Appendix A:] The influenza epidemic, which was prevalent at SAIDOR... also passed through the villages in the Upper Nankina Tax District.... When the patrol passed through the latter five (5) villages, the influenza was at its peak; these villages were almost deserted upon arrival, most people having moved out into the bush near their gardens and water supplies. Considering that most cases of influenza were not medically treated... the death toll of 95 was comparatively low.... Villages effected [sic] most were: YOGAYOGA (5 deaths)... GUA (6)... (Muskens 1959: 4, Appendix A).

Shortly afterwards, Robins (1961/62) mentions an epidemic of whooping cough:

The general health of the people is quite high considering their lack of personal hygiene [sic]. The worst complaints are burns and ulcers. Every person in the area has burn scars on the shin and in some cases only a very thin skin covers the bone. This causes the slightest scratch to go bad and usually the worst sores are found on the legs. These burns are caused by the constant scorching of the skin at night when the people sleep huddled close to the fire. Prior to the last Medical Patrol to the area an epedemic [sic] of whooping cough swept through the area and claimed many lives. Most of these were in the one to four years age group (Robins 1961/62: 8).

Nixon (1965/66: 5) found the good state of nutrition remarkable: "Health in nearly all instances on the patrol was found to be of a high standard in spite of the peoples [sic] inherent dirtiness. The people are an extremely well fed group and this is possibly a contributing factor to their good health." Finally, Scarlett (1967/68: 8) remarks on the difference between the upper and the lower Yupno: "The villages of the upper Yupno support a much healthier population than the lower Yupno villages and very few cases of goitre were observed. The number of mentally retarded people was very small in this area."

From the foregoing notes, it is clear that, from the perspective of the various Patrol Officers at least, the state of health of the Yupno was very good, although probably these reports reflect an implicit comparison to the health status both of coastal populations and other mountain people. With the establishment of Teptep as a subdistrict government station in 1972, most patrols longer than several weeks in duration were discontinued. The local aid posts and the health center in Teptep (see Chapter 4.2., and 5.1.c.) have become primarily responsible for the (biomedical) health care of the population.

II

In the Teptep Health Centre, the common health problems are listed on a poster in the outpatients' department. They coincide with many of the symptoms that the Yupno concept classifies as bodily disorders. The frequency of certain bodily disorders of the Yupno also corresponds to the first three groups of illnesses listed at the health center.

In the first place, there are respiratory tract diseases, which comprise the viral and bacterial infections of the thorax and the respiratory system ("viral upper respiratory infections," "bacterial respiratory infections"), bronchopneumonia, chronic obstructive lung diseases, pneumonia, asthma, colds, cough, catarrh. They correspond, more or less, to the Yupno disorders *mbook* ("sniffles with runny nose"), *kaldok* ("cough"), *keaknok* ("to continuously swallow what one has coughed up," linked with shortness of breath), *talbok* ("runny nose"), *timni gorok* ("blocked up nose") as well as *ninimoktak* ("trembling") and *ngodim tepmtok* ("fever") as accompanying phenomena. Depending on their degree of "seriousness," these diseases are treated first with cough syrup, later with penicillin injections or tablets (capsules), possibly an infusion. Should this be of no help, Chloramphenicol (a broad spectrum antibiotic) is administered, and if it proves ineffective, Tetracycline is given. The therapies thus consist of increasingly potent (effective) drugs aligned with the particular course taken by the disease.

The second most frequent diseases are gastro-intestinal and manifest themselves as diarrhoea (without dehydration, with dehydration, with grave dehydration), dysentery (an infectious disease caused by bacteria or amoebae characterized by frequent bloody and mucilaginous diarrhoetic feces) or gastroenteritis (stomach-intestinal inflammation). The Yupno call these physical disorders by the names *kokɨlɨt* ("diarrhoea"), *ndakkok* ("bloody diarrhoea"), *wandɨtit* ("vomiting"), *wam suok* ("stomach cramps") and *wam tepmtok* ("stomach pains"), and the term *kɨrarogen* ("skin and bones") may also be used in this context. The Yupno do not know a corresponding term for intestinal parasites (protozea, "worms"), but practically everyone has them[17] and, per se, they are not held to be a physical disorder. In Teptep, there is an initial worm cure; the patient drinks a lot of liquid, then receives a sugar-salt-solution (the biomedical counterpart to the therapy of the female "heat extinguisher," see Chapter 5.1.a.). In more serious cases, antidiarrhoetics are (orally) administered, but should this not be possible, the medicine is given by infusion.

Skin problems are listed in the third position, among them cuts, injuries, inflammations, stings and sores as well as infections caused by mites and fungus. The Yupno terms *arokarok* ("itching skin disease"), *kandapda sañgamok* ("burns"), all the nouns formed with *wuda* ("wound") as well as *kalsɨt nywok* ("swollen loin") and *aljoko pok* ("swollen armpit") belong to this group of illnesses. They are treated with disinfectants or lotions, and afterwards covered with a bandage or plaster. For serious infections, antibiotics (Penicillin) are given.

The fourth main health problem in Teptep is malnutrition, especially among children and babies. According to statements of the health center, 65% of all the children in the Yupno region are malnourished. As it stands, this statement is certainly incorrect,[18] since American average standards (modified for Papua New Guinea) are taken as basic criteria. However, there is no standard especially adapted to the Yupno that incorporates their height, weight, nutritional habits, hence their own cultural determinants. Medical staff cite a variety of causes for malnutrition: The mother has too many children (often born in very close succession); lack of intact family conditions (father is deceased, mother is sick, and the child is left to itself); and small children "run around in the bush too much and forget to eat," indicating neglect. Staff also cite a cultural taboo, wherein, traditionally, children are only weaned and fed different food once they get their first teeth. This long lactation period (which, in most cases today, is no longer observed by Yupno women) contradicts widespread biomedical opinion that an infant should receive food other than mother's milk after the age of five months. However, the causes as stated by health center employees, who live in nuclear-family structures in Teptep, are not correct. Families in difficulties find help and assistance in their kin group (that of the wife or the husband); infants running around "in the bush" mostly play in the company of older children in the gardens, where they snack on wild fruits, tubers or small animals or get sweet potatoes or bananas from the women working in the gardens. By contrast, the children who go to school at Teptep go hungry; they are away from home all day, and unless they have money have almost no chance to obtain food while at Teptep.

For the controversial[19] biomedical complex of malnutrition there are only limited corresponding Yupno concepts, *mum darok* ("no more milk") and *ngodïm mok* ("to be only skin and bones"). Almost all Yupno children exhibit the inflated bellies cited by some physicians as evidence for ill-balanced, protein-poor nutrition; but the Yupno attribute these "fat" bellies to the exaggerated appetite of their children. Malnourished patients are treated indirectly in Teptep, by giving nutritional advice[20] to the mothers.

Neonatal infections (such as infection of the navel, for example) and complications at house-births ("B.B.A," "birth before aid mission") are subsumed under the rubric of fifth health problem. A corresponding Yupno concept does not exist for these.

Further illnesses treated in Teptep are: Malaria, including cerebral malaria (in people who have spent some time on the coast), urinary tract infections, venereal diseases, arthritis (predominantly in older people), broken bones (fractures), tetanus (through burns or pig bites), meningitis (rare), tuberculosis, leprosy (one case), anemia and vitamin deficiency, and psychoses (defined, according to the information of the H.E.O., as "any psychic deviant behavior which calls for treatment"). The Yupno concepts *ngom sït* ("mosquito illness") and *sït tevan* ("serious illness") correspond respectively to malaria and venereal diseases; since both are "imported" physical disorders for which there is no traditional cure, an afflicted person either does nothing or goes to the health center. In the Yupno language, fractures are called by the respective part of the body and the verb *wanpelak* ("to break"). Symptoms of tuberculosis may (under certain circumstances) be counted among *keaknok* symptoms ("shortness of breath"). Patients suffering from tumors, open or internal fractures (needing an X-ray), diseases of the liver, allergies and internal haemorrhages are not treated at Teptep but transferred to Saidor or Madang. Those who have more complicated eye-diseases go to the eye doctor in Madang, and for dental problems they consult an A.P.O.[21] at Saidor who specializes in dentistry.

The most frequent causes of death[22] as listed by the staff are meningitis, influenza, diarrhoea, pneumonia and non-diagnosed diseases (like a tumor or internal haemorrhages). Old people, according to Western interpretation, die most frequently of general physical weakness (they eat and drink too little), often linked to chronic inflammation in the thorax caused by living in smoky houses.

It is noteworthy that, despite the above correspondences and approximations between Yupno-defined disorders and biomedical concepts of disease, they belong to different systems of classification. However, there are some interesting parallels. Ndakkok ("bloody diarrhoea"), for example, contains in the noun (ndak, "blood") the biomedical definition for melaena ("bloody feces"); likewise, kokɨlɨt ("dripping feces," "diarrhoea") contains the biomedical definition for diarrhoea (which can also be assigned to dysentery) and therefore comes very close to the Western concept of (the symptom) diarrhoea and (the disease) dysentery; however, it is not classed as sɨt, "illness," but as a "disorder," whereas dysentery in biomedicine is a disease.

Furthermore, some of the physical disorders presented above that are named by the Yupno, and which for them are clearly defined disorders (like amek, "inflated belly" and others), have no correspondence in biomedical concepts, since for physicians they are too diffuse. The opposite also holds: For hernias (ruptures in the abdominal wall) or intestinal parasites like worms, there are traditionally[23] no Yupno terms, because these conditions are widespread and thought to be normal,[24] not a disorder. Likewise, all the sicknesses that can be detected only through blood-tests or other modern types of examination have no corresponding term in the realm of physical disorders.

III

The medical examinations[25] conducted by physicians Sandra Staub and Andreas Allemann among the people of Gua produced the following results: A total of 322 people (89.7% of all those present) were examined, 125 male and 197 female persons. The first question was about the subjective complaints of the Gua people; the spontaneous (first) statements were noted, and then questions were asked about specific symptoms.

As Table 1 indicates, fully 58.3% of the people spontaneously said they had been "healthy" during the last four weeks or did not have any physical com-

Table 1: The most frequent (i.e. first) remarks regarding the state of health during the past four weeks.

58.3%	healthy
12.1%	stomach pains
9.3%	back troubles
2.1%	colds
2.1%	ailments in the cheek-ear region
1.2%	skin problems
0.9%	shortness of breath
0.9%	eye troubles
0.6%	headaches
0.6%	pains in the thorax region

plaints. Other problems, such as eye affections, shortness of breath, toothache, and headache were mentioned only sporadically.

However, closer questioning about individual symptoms (Table 2) reveals an interesting discrepancy between spontaneous mention of a diagnosis and

Table 2: Answers to precise questions about certain symptoms

7.6%	cough
13.0%	fever
9.0%	diarrhoea
4.3%	vomiting
4.0%	haematuria

statements made after more precise questioning. It is difficult to evaluate this discrepancy, though various reasons might be cited for it:

- From an Yupno point of view on illness, such a symptom is either not taken to be illness or, as a physical disorder, little attention is paid to it;

- cough, diarrhoea or also other symptoms may be evaluated by the patient as normal because they are a frequent manifestation and thus are not thought worthy of mention;
- since four weeks is a relatively long period of time, some complaints may have been forgotten.

The most frequent pathological conditions detected (based on the examination) among the Gua people are presented in Table 3.

Table 3: Frequency of individual symptoms or diseases among the Gua population			
Symptoms		Persons	Percentage of population
mouth:	teeth with cavities	169	52.5%
	other	25	7.8%
skin:	tropical ulcers	85	26.4%
	mites	9	2.8%
	other	31	9.6%
abdominal diagnosis		81	25.2%
splenomegalia		17	5.3%
Hepatomegalia		15	4.7%
abdominal hernias		16	5.0%
eyes:	pterygium	34	10.6%
	strabism	7	2.2%
	lessening of vision	6	1.9%
	conjunctavitis	4	1.2%
	cataracts	2	0.6%
	other	16	5.0%
lung diagnosis		56	17.4%
enlarged lymph nodules		53	16.5%
skeleton:	joint problems	24	7.5%
	deformity	18	5.6%
	others	2	0.6%
kidney		18	5.6%
ears:	reduced hearing, deafness	9	2.8%
	otitis media	7	2.2%
	defect of the eardrum	2	0.6%
	other	1	0.3%

Table 4: Examples for the correlation of the anamnetic (stated at the questioning) evidence and the clinical diagnosis

Problem	anamnetic complaints (by people)	clinical diagnosis (of people)
toothache	1	194
skin	4	125
eyes	3	69
ears	1	19
lung	12	56
abdominal	39	81
skeletal	30	42

If the results of the questioning are correlated with the results of the examination (Table 4), the difference between illness and disease becomes very clear. Thus (in the questioning), only three persons spontaneously complained about eye problems, while in the examination, 69 were diagnosed with pathological evidence. Even more impressive are results of the dental examination (one person complained of toothache, yet 194 actually had teeth problems) and for the skin problems (four persons complained of skin affections, 125 persons showed pathological evidence). A close correlation between the questioning and the examination occurred only with respect to skeletal and abdominal affections.

The examination shows that, according to the clinical evidence, about 57% of Gua people examined suffered from one or several symptoms or diseases at the time of the examination.

IV

The statistics for inpatients in the year 1982[26] show that a total of 179 patients[27] had been admitted to the hospital in Teptep, with a monthly average of around fifteen. In July 1987, eleven patients[28] were admitted; for August 1987, the statistics count thirteen patients[29] as inpatients. If one bears in mind the statement of the H.E.O. that most patients come only during the dry season (July and August are the driest months), and if one compares the results to the annual average of 1982, the number of patients in the ward shows a tendency to decrease. Despite a lack of further statistical data that could confirm this trend, other support is available. First, it cannot be assumed that fewer people had fallen sick (since malaria and venereal diseases, especially, are on the increase owing to more frequent visits to the coast), or that the village aid post had multiplied its treatment of patients and therefore fewer patients were taken to Teptep, since the above-mentioned diseases cannot be treated by the local aid posts. It would thus seem that, despite a number of health campaigns and the presence of the health center staff, there was no improvement between 1982 and 1987 in the level of acceptance of Western medicine by the Yupno.

Various problems reported by both the health center's employees and the Yupno provide a possible explanation for this failure. Staff members say that their jobs are made difficult by a number of factors, which are sorted here according to the topic, but in fact most are interconnected (and in part are also cited by the Yupno):

Topography and size of the catchment area. The most distant place in the catchment area of the Teptep Health Centre lies six hours away by foot, and the journey is very slow for the patrols of the staff because of the bad, narrow and steep paths. Patients from the furthest villages almost only come to the health center during the dry season, which lasts from about May to October. For old people who find it difficult to walk or the gravely ill who cannot walk any more, the journey to Teptep is too far and too strenuous: They have to be carried by their relatives for several hours. Gua, however, is only 40 minutes walking distance from Teptep, and is very convenient. Also, the increasing spatial distance to Teptep correlates with an increasing feeling of unfamiliarity. A remedy, at least for the villages closer to Teptep, might consist in regular visits to the village by the staff during which they could treat the sick. By doing this, they would also gain closer contact with the population and thereby may become better able to judge the situation of Yupno daily life instead of condescendingly complaining about their "unsanitary conditions" (see below) and "malnutrition."

The employees find the **"conservatism" of the population** regarding sickness and birth to be a hindrance in their work. Patients often come to the health center "too late," since the traditional therapies are typically first sought.

Quantsañne, a traditional "soother" (*ngesam amɨn*) from Gua:

> If I go to the health center, then I can get medicine. And if I do not want to, then I stay here. That is not because I am fed up with the drugs, but that is how I think, I want to stay here [in the village], and then I stay here. Once when I was very ill, this is how I thought: 'Later, I will go [to the Teptep Health Centre]'. This is how I thought and I stayed at home. For example, if I am very ill, and I think, the *sindok* ["bush-spirit"] or whatever has made me ill, then I send a message to the *pieñ*-specialists ["anti-*sindok*-specialists"]. They do it, and I get *pieñ* [see Chapter 5.3.] and smoke it and stay here. That is how I do it, I get well and I stay here.

Illustration 11: A patient is carried on a stretcher to the
                  Teptep Health Centre

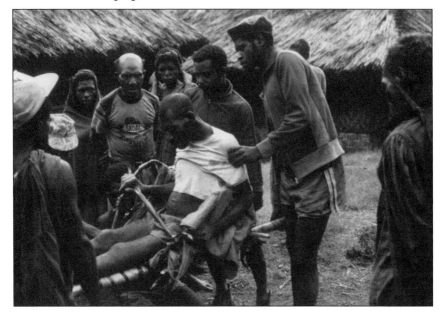

Births traditionally take place in the family's house, a familiar intimate environment, where the woman in labor will be assisted mainly by a woman who
has already given birth and is someone she knows well (see Chapter 3.3.). Hence
very few women prefer to give birth at the health center, which helps explain
why, in the Yupno region (according to the H.E.O.), there is a high infant mor-
tality rate (and an even higher number of cases not reported in the statistics).

Fresh supply of medicine. Very frequently, medicine runs out in Teptep,
and it can take three months until new supplies are flown in. The H.E.O. could
alleviate this problem with better stock-keeping and re-ordering in good time,
so motivation and responsibility are relevant in this case.

Communication problems and cultural barriers. Language problems are
linked both with "conservative" attitudes and the isolated location of many
villages. Very often, patients speak no Tok Pisin and also no Kâte,[30] so poor
communication increases the incidence of misunderstanding.

Jurenu, a man from Gua:

> If we could speak Tok Pisin, Kâte or English, that would be great, we
> could go to the health center and talk about the cause of our illness and
> get medicine. But we cannot do it, and we are the only ones to speak

our language. Therefore it is bad, if I go to the 'doktaboy' and speak in my language. How could the 'doktaboy' understand my words? That is why I take anybody, whoever can talk, take him with me and go to the health center.... It is an important reason, that we are the only ones to speak our language, which is why it is difficult for us to get medicine.

Praie, an old woman:

Sometimes, when we go to the house, where you get medicine [the out-patients' department], then we look, who could translate, and if no-body is there, we go out again. But sometimes we sit down, and they ask us, and we are like we are stupid, we do not understand a word, and the 'doktaboy' say to us: 'Do you not want to come with somebody who translates?' That is how they talk and they throw us out.

The younger (mostly male) Yupno have at least partly learned Tok Pisin in school or in town, though they speak it slowly and have a limited vocabulary; for them, Tok Pisin is and remains a foreign language. On the other hand, for the staff Tok Pisin is often the mother tongue (there has been a creolization, in the linguistic sense), so they speak it fluently, often quickly and with a great amount of Standard English in the vocabulary. The Tok Pisin-speaking Yupno often remain "speechless" when in the presence the coastal people's verbal skills; they only partially understand and often pretend that they cannot speak Tok Pisin. They are therefore unwilling to accompany patients from their village as translators. Were employees to talk more slowly in a simpler Tok Pisin and gauge from the reaction of their conversation partner whether they were un-derstood, it is likely that the Tok Pisin-speaking Yupno would be less inhibited about using their language skills. None of the employees working at Teptep dur-ing my research knew the Yupno language. Formerly, only Potin, a man from Kangulut who worked as an A.P.O. in Teptep, could talk to the patients. He was very popular, but after some disputes among the employees he was transferred.

Varenañ, a younger woman from Gua:

If I am ill, I am afraid of the 'doktaboy'. If I was to go there and they would talk to me, what should I answer? That is why I was somewhat scared. Once Roti [her "adoptive daughter"] got ill, and they said to us, we should go to the ward, I was afraid, but I went. At the time, Potin was there [the above-mentioned A.P.O.], and he translated, and I looked after Roti. She got well, and I came back [to the village].

Since the middle of 1987, a young man from Nian was employed at the Teptep Health Centre store and sometimes helped out as an interpreter. It would be an advantage if at least one A.P.O. (there are a few trained ones) from the Yupno region could work in Teptep. The politics resulting from the 'wantok' system led to a policy not to employ A.P.O. and teachers in their region of origin because of a potential role conflict and pressure from their relatives to give them preferential treatment. This policy brought a lot of problems to Teptep.

The details of the traditional concepts of illness among the Yupno to a large extent are, and remain, foreign to the health center employees. Quite isolated from the native population, they live in a sort of enclave with a different standard of living, language, and interests.[31] They experience Teptep as a hardship posting, for a variety of reasons. First, there is the isolation and the resulting concentration of social relations within the small group of their colleagues. There is also dissatisfaction about the lack of leisure activities available in Teptep (sports like badminton, football, and basketball). Most men frequent the social club, with its regular excessive beer-drinking, and many become involved in the drunken brawls that occur every fortnight when the wages are paid. For employees from the coast, the cold climate and the remote location of Teptep, which can only be reached by plane, lead to frustration and also to disputes among the employees themselves, which result in frequent changes in personnel. For all these reasons, it becomes difficult if not impossible for staff at the health center to attain the level of social contact, possible during a longer stay, which would allow them to gain the necessary insights into the cultural traditions of the population they are treating. This vicious circle of isolation, group conflict, frustration and high turnover of personnel is difficult to break, and so the Yupno remain "foreign" to the staff.

On the other hand, to the Yupno Teptep is "foreign" territory, where "foreigners" live and work (the 'kiap', a policeman, several teachers, a Japanese, a Swiss development worker, the employees[32] of the hospital); all are "outside" people, from other parts of Papua New Guinea or even farther away.

The Yupno point to a number of factors that impede their acceptance of biomedicine.

Modern medicine costs **money**, and although fees are low, old people, especially, have no money, since they are to a large extent excluded from modern economic life and from regular access to cash. Contrary to traditional therapies, payment in kind is not accepted at the Teptep Health Centre.

Centre employees often treat the local people **condescendingly**. Some people told me they had been insulted as "dirty," "backward," 'bus kanaka tru' ("real bush-kanaka") by medical personnel. The sanitary notions of the staff who orient themselves on Western standards certainly diverge. They live in houses with running water, contrary to the Yupno in whose concept the actually cold water of the Yupno River is "cold;" if they wash themselves in it, they therefore alter the "cool" ideal state—which is something nobody would do on purpose. The accusation of being backward is an expression of the conservatism of the Yupno, and results from the slightly frustrated basic attitude of the staff, who have been trained and employed to improve the state of health of the population, including the use of preventive measures such as education in hygiene, but they get little feedback and are therefore not strongly motivated to apply themselves to this large task.

Marone, an older woman from Gua:

> If I have a cold, then I do not go to the health center to get medicine. I feel ill and I stay here. The 'doktaboys' have a habit of talking a lot, and I am afraid, and that is why I do not go [there]. It is bad if I go and cannot express myself and the 'doktaboys' beat me; therefore, I do not go to get medicine. I did go once and they said to me: 'Sit down there, no, come and sit down here', this is how they shoved me around, from one corner to the other, and they gave me medicine, and I drank it and I threw it up and I went back to the village. This is what I am afraid of, too, and that is why I do not go to the health center. I stay here [in the village].

Susune (the mother of Mayu and grandmother of little Nstasiñge), a vigorous woman from Gua:

> I thought if I went to Teptep and they talk to me, should I answer in Tok Pisin or in 'tok ples' [Yupno] or what should I say? I thought a lot about this. I decided: I will just go. It doesn't matter if they talk to me or if they hit me, they will give me medicine. This is how I felt, and I went in [to the outpatients department], and I saw, they were all talking about something, but I did not understand about what, and I sat down and stayed seated. They gave me medicine, I drank it and then came down again to Gua. I do not know were they insulting me or did they say: 'Ah, this sort of woman does not even know Tok Pisin!', or did they say 'Why did this 'kanaka'-woman come here?' Did they talk about me like this or did they insult me? I do not know it.
>
> Once, I had *amek* ["swollen belly"], and therefore I went, and the nurse and the 'doktaboy' looked at me and said: 'This woman is pregnant.' They asked a lot: 'Is your husband alive, or has he died and another man gave you this belly?' This is how they talked to me. They talked like this again and again, and at that time I took Onerinke [a male relative from Uskokop who speaks Tok Pisin],

and we both went in [to the outpatients department]. And Onerinke said to them: 'Her husband, my *a* [mother's brother], lived in
Madang, and then he went to Buka and died there. They brought
him back here and we buried him.' This is what Onerinke said to
the 'doktaboy'. The 'doktaboy' answered: 'Other men have made her
pregnant, she is lying since she has a big belly. She is lying to you
and she came and got you and brought you here!' I stood up and
said: 'I, this wrinkled skin, I am old, how should I get pregnant?'
Something had gotten onto my skin, and the 'doktaboy' were lying.
And the relatives form Gua said to me: 'The deceased, your husband, had a *njɨgɨ* ["oppressing problem"], it went in [into you] and
it is now on your skin.'

This is how they talked, and I screamed and ran around. Some
thought: 'She is pregnant,' and others said: 'The *njɨgɨ* ["oppressing
problem"] of Mañnau gave her her belly, and that is why she
screams and carries this bad illness around.' I told this to Onerinke,
and the two of us went in again. They told me the same as before
when we had gone out. I was very angry, and I came out, and said:
'What kind of a belly do I have that they talk about it all the time!',
and I pulled up my blouse and let everybody know; they came together, I squeezed my breasts [which were not like a pregnant
woman's] and pointed to my swollen belly, we laughed about it for
a long time [about the "mistaken diagnosis" of the 'doktaboy'], and
I left them and came to Gua.

The Yupno find this condescending attitude of the employees insulting and
humiliating. They do not all react as self-confident and full of humor as
Susune, but avoid these accusations by refusing to visit the health center.
Sometimes a treatment demands admission to the health center as an inpatient; the patient has to spend the night in an **unfamiliar environment** and in
addition is dependent on a relative to look after him all the time and provide
him with firewood, water and food. More serious diseases may necessitate a
transfer to Madang, to the Modilon Hospital, a frightening prospect for many
(a majority) who have never left the Yupno region, do not speak Tok Pisin and
now have to endure this for the first time just when they are sick.

Ntsimantsiman, an old woman from Gua, reports her experience at Modilon Hospital:

When I was here and was splitting bamboo and making a fire, a
splinter broke off and shot into my eye [*ndel yamak*, "bamboo
splinter"], and they brought me to the Bameleñ "medicine-house"

[the aid post at Tapmañge], and the 'doktaboy' looked at it [the eye] and said: 'your eye is completely ruined, I cannot repair it here, you have to go to Teptep.' So they sent me down, I slept in Gua, and the next morning the wife of Faiu [her son] and Virin took me and dragged me to Teptep to the health center.

So I was there, and the 'doktaboy' looked at my eye and could not repair it there and the first 'doktaboy' said: 'you will go to Madang.' I was afraid and said: 'if I go, what would that help? I will soon die, leave me alone.' This is what I said and I stayed there for one day, I was scared to get into the plane and the 'doktaboy' thought I was sleeping in the ward, but I had run off and was running around and go to Bilewañ [a location near Teptep]. But my eye was almost totally dark [and I could only see very badly], and I walked around there, it was getting dark, and they brought me back to Teptep. I did not want to get into the plane, but the 'doktaboy' and the other men grabbed me very firmly and sat me in the plane.

I did not want to, but the men urged me into the plane and the plane started and flew off, it slowed down a bit and went down, and I was terribly scared and held on tight to my seat....I was much afraid and said to Nanjañne [a male relative who accompanied her]: 'Nanjañne, we are going to crash!'...This is what I said, and another small boy was also sitting [in the plane] and was very frightened and sang his *koñgap* melody [for fear]. We flew on and landed at Saidor, but I did not want to get out, I remained seated inside, and the pilot and Nanjañne opened the door and went out, but I didn't, I stayed seated inside. I sat inside, and they unloaded the 'kargo' from Teptep and loaded some 'kargo' from Saidor. This is how they did it, closed the door, the plane started, and we flew, flew and got to Madang airport. The plane left us at the airport, and I did not understand anything, I had never seen a car, and the houses were all different, too, and I was afraid and sat down.

Nanjañne sent a message to the hospital, and the car from the hospital came and came very close to me, and I jumped up with a start, and Nanjañne took my hand, they opened the door, I got into the car. I saw many cars coming, I was scared, that they would fight with each other and hurt me, and I was frightened and just sat there. The car took us and got to the hospital. I stayed at the entrance. They wrote down my name and sent us into a room, then

into another one, and sent us to bed. I slept, the next morning I
got medicine and an injection and I remained sitting in my bed,
and two of my children, Arenke and Namuñ, came to me, visited
me, and we sat there, at noon, I got medicine, and the two of them
took me and left me very close to a big road, I looked at the cars,
many cars came and went, I was just looking. This is how it went,
it was almost dark, and the two of them brought me to my bed and
went back to their house, and I and Nanjañne slept.

My eye was hurt, and I slept, and the 'dokta' very firmly said to
me: 'mama, get up and take your medicine,' this is how they said,
and I woke up, I sat up, and they gave me medicine, two young
men, and I did not know them. The two of them looked after me
well and I was fine, the two of them cared for me, this is how it
went, and then they had to work somewhere else, and the two of
them came in and said to me: 'we are sorry, Mama, this is now our
last task. Tomorrow, we will work somewhere else, then another
'dokta' will come and wake you up and you will wake up and he
will give you the medicine, and the two of us will go away!' This is
how the two of them talked, and Arenke translated it to me, and
the two of them went, and a white man came in, looked at my eye
and said: 'we will not take your eye out [operate on it]. It will stay
as it is. We give you medicine, and your eye will get well again,
and [then] we will send you back to your place.' This is what he
said to me, and I was no longer afraid and I was fine. I slept, woke
up, sat up high, and various big, fat men came in, and I was sitting there, and they all surrounded me closely and I got scared and
looked at their faces, and I was sitting there, and Arenke sat below
my bed. They stood themselves there, and many men looked at my
eye and they said to me: 'your eye is not all bad, it is a bit better,
and tomorrow you will go back to Teptep.' This is how they said, I
was just sitting there and listening, and Arenke said to me: 'tomorrow you will go to the village.' This is how he talked to me, I slept,
morning came, and I had not been walking around in town to
look at everything, I was just at the hospital and came back. They
sent me off and gave me a note with a message, and I came to the
airport, and the plane took me with it, and I came to Teptep, the
plane left me behind, and I left my netbag at the airfield and went
to the health center at Teptep, and the 'doktaboy' saw me and said
'good' and sent me home.

Some methods of treatment necessitate tests on **blood and feces.** Mostly, it is not explained to the patients why they are necessary since it is often assumed that they would not understand it anyway. According to traditional concepts, blood and stool are filled with *moñan* ("breath spirit"), so nobody would give them voluntarily; they would want to know the reason for such tests, out of fear of possible misuse at the hands of a sorcerer.[33] The Yupno have also repeatedly experienced **ill people dying** at the health center, a place they associate with death and many *koñwop*, "souls of dead persons" (see Mayu's story in Chapter 4.1.e.).

All the problems listed here hinder the acceptance of biomedicine among the Yupno. Still, despite language problems and cultural barriers, Yupno visit the Teptep Health Centre, even though older people and those not conversant in Tok Pisin hesitate to do so. If the population were asked (for example, in a questionnaire[34]) about their attitudes to Western medicine, this would very likely convey a false picture, since only a few Yupno would admit their fears. There is a wide gap between their own statements ("no problem, I willingly go") and their actual behavior once they fall ill.

The following report by Jowage, an old "heat extinguisher" from Gua, makes it clear that older Yupno, too, visit the health center in case of physical disorders and vigorously try to solve possible problems (such as difficulties of communication):

> I do not know Tok Pisin, that is why I tell [it] to my children, if I am ill and sometimes they go with me, and I get medicine, and sometimes Baldja [his daughter who attends school in Teptep] gives me a little letter, this I take along and give it to the 'doktaboy', and they look at it and give me medicine. A little while ago, we talked about the land [had land-litigations], at that time, everybody only thought about that and they were in the village. So I went on my own and came to the 'doktaboy' and asked them about medicine. They looked at me and were completely irritated [did not understand anything], and I left them and went up [to Uskokop]. I took Kawuek [a man from Uskokop] and Take, and we went back, went down, and Take explained my disorder [*kaldok*, "cough"], and they gave me medicine, some I drank, some I carried back [to Gua]. Yes, this is how I usually do it....I am not scared of injections, no, not at all, it helps my body. That is a big thing, I like them, and I go to the health center. Also, I am not afraid to take medicine, I saw other people who were afraid of it, but not I, I like to take it. Some people drink medicine and throw up and pull a face, but not I.

The reception of biomedicine by the Yupno is therefore marked by acceptance and refusal at the same time and is limited to the realm of drugs, the curative sector. Most of the preventive measures (which were presented in the excursus Chapter 4.1.a. "The Teptep Health Centre") aim beyond the needs of the population or do not meet them at all. Welsch's (1983, 1987) description of the appraisal of biomedicine among the Ningerum (Western Province) and the way they cope with it also applies to the Yupno:

> Ningerum people have not rejected modern medicines. They, like most Papua New Guineans, see aid posts as a valuable component of their health care system, though they are often accused of both ignorance and non-compliance. Such criticism generally stems from a fundamental misunderstanding between patient and health worker… By understanding how therapeutic knowledge and responsibilities are distributed in the community, health workers (and planners) could better serve their patients by anticipating non-compliance and averting it instead of being continually frustrated by it (Welsch 1987: 209).

It is mainly the younger people with school education who are most receptive to biomedicine, especially in the case of more recent sicknesses like malaria and venereal diseases for which traditionally there is no method of treatment, hence no concepts of causation, and in the case of physical disorders that per se are not called "illness." Modern pharmaceuticals increasingly replace the therapy offered by traditional "coolers" (*yawuro yawuro amɨn*). Since biomedicine cannot remove the cause of "real illness" and thereby cannot really affect the traditional concept of therapy, the Yupno welcome and quite rationally use it as a supporting and certainly helpful means that can supplement traditional therapy. As A. Strathern and P. Stewart (1999: 93) argue:

> Biomedical medicine and indigenous systems of medicine are often assumed to be in conflict with each other.… various contexts exist in which introduced and indigenous medical practices meet different requirements for the population in question. In this instance, then, the two systems are seen to be complementary rather than in conflict.

This observation is shared by other anthropologists, see Counts and Counts (1989: 292) for the Lusi, LiPuma (1989: 305) for the Maring.

Biomedicine is more readily refused by the older people. The main impeding factors are culturally defined: language problems, "feelings of unfamiliarity and inferiority," perceptions of the hospital as a place of "souls of dead persons" (*koñwop*), and the fear of giving away body substances like blood or stool, which are filled with *moñan* ("breath spirit").

The medical and technical infrastructure of the Teptep Health Centre (degree of education of the staff, technical and financial equipment of the hospital) is excellent compared to health stations in other provinces of Papua New Guinea or in most other "Third World" countries. If a greater acceptance of biomedicine among the Yupno were to be achieved, one that would not unduly disadvantage traditional medicine (since both systems are based on totally different concepts and their respective advantages are recognized by the Yupno) far more priority should be given to the predominantly social and cultural factors (differing concepts of illness, communication problems, prejudices, motivation of the medical personnel) as an intrinsic part of the training of medical staff, instead of, as so often happens, being preoccupied with issues of financing and technical and medical know-how. As long as the Yupno retain their concepts of illness, biomedicine is not likely to replace traditional medicine. As Aitken (1984: 48) has noted: "...the traditional understanding of and approach to sickness and curing is very different from that of scientific medicine. I believe that they are incompatible and, therefore, not capable of integration....In practice, the two systems are seen by people as different and used as alternatives, relevant to different health problems."

Medical pluralism enables the Yupno to receive medical care corresponding to their needs and to a modern public health plan.

2. Social Discord or the State of "Really Being Ill"

a) "Oppressing Problems": Concepts, Social and Temporal Setting

I

For the completeness and well-being of a human being, the maintenance of harmonious social relationships within the clan (*jalap*) and the partner clan (*ngapma*) is essential. If these social relationships are disrupted, or if they are burdened by a "heaviness" (*njɨgɨ*), a person or one of his or her relatives (as in little Nstasiñge's case) may fall ill because of an "oppressing problem" (*njɨgɨ*). To express it in Western terms, one gets sociosomatically sick. I would again emphasize that *njɨgɨ* means to be "heavy" in a physical and figurative sense; it connotes social tensions of any kind that settle "heavily" or "weightily" on a person, that "oppress" or stifle him or her and—if they manifest themselves as illness—torment, torture and hurt him or her. They result from conscious or subconscious offences or misdemeanors committed by one or several members of the kinship group, which then manifest themselves as illness. Since their ultimate origins are always social conflicts and tensions, they are, in the widest sense, a disorder of the social fabric, and of the ideal Yupno "cool" state.

The "oppressing problem" (*njɨgɨ*) may either directly affect the "problem causer" or make one of his relatives ill. From every intentional misdemeanor (such as theft, or an illicit sexual relation) something remains, called *nduara*. The term *nduara* derives from *nduat*, rest, something left over; the word appears in compounds like *mbut nduat*, "a piece of pork" or *ondeñ nduat*, "a small piece of leftover sweet potato."

From every action, something therefore remains, and this remainder in the case of a misdemeanor may develop into an illness-inducing problem (*njɨgɨ*) for the culprit or one of his relatives. In such a case, the people say: "*nduara abedak*," "he has gotten a remainder [of the misdemeanor]," or "*nak ngakdakon nduara pasat*," "I carry your remainder [of the misdemeanor]." *Nduara* is used as a term for a concrete, intentional misdemeanor, in the sense of an "offence" (like a theft or an intentionally incorrectly executed brideprice), but not for emotional states (like rage) or unspoken curses that remain confined to the level of thought.

Megau, a "big man" (*amdi*) from Gua, explains it like this:

> Let us suppose I shoot a pig of another man, kill it, cook the meat and eat it; the pig's owner did not see me. Therefore, I have stolen. So I kill it, carry it off, cut up the meat, cook it, eat it, and I do all this secretly. Good, I am here [go on living normally]. I am therefore here, but then [quite soon], then the pig's *nduara* [meaning: the remainder left over from his deed] will cause illness in me. My skin will get all loose.

> They [the others] look at me, my face looks like pig's fat, as if I had rubbed myself with it, all dirty, just like when we rub ourselves with fat, all greasy. So I am here. And my clan, my brothers and whatever relatives come and look at me and say: 'oh!' They look at me, they only see me on the outside, only my image [meaning: they cannot look at his thoughts], and they go away again and talk about it everywhere.

> 'Has this man killed somebody else's pig and eaten it and has the *nduara* caught him?' This is how they talk then and they tell one of my brother's or another relative: 'you can ask him, is it really true that he has killed another man's pig? Go and ask him and try to find it [out].' Well, and this brother or sister or father or father's brother or mother's brother will come and say: 'is it true that you have killed somebody else's pig, kept it a secret and cooked the meat?' I can then say: 'yes, really, I have killed a man's pig, cooked

the meat and, yes, I believe, this *nduara* has caught me.' Well, so I admit it, and my relative will tell me the following: 'very quickly you will pay back this man [a pig]!' Well, I give it back, if I have a [suitable] pig, I go there, tie it up and give it to this man, and my illness will be over.

Misdemeanor only becomes a *njɨgɨ* if it develops into illness. According to Yupno logic, our interpretation of the retrospective search for a scapegoat (somebody is ill, one looks for a cause and retrospectively assumes a misdemeanor, resolves it and the diseased gets well) is not correct. After all, something (*nduara*) remains of every previously committed offence, and is always "invisibly" there, even over a long temporal and spatial distance and, though not necessarily, lead to *njɨgɨ* and illness. Today, *nduara* is also used as the vernacular term for "sin" within the Christian context (in church and in the bible translations of the Summer Institute of Linguistics, SIL).

However, "oppressing problems" may also become active indirectly, when the person affected by a misdemeanor, the damaged party, reacts in an angry or insulted way, gets into a "hot" state and then unloads this "heat" onto either the person who has caused the "oppressing problem" or on his or her relatives. An angry, excited person is not only "hot" (*tepm*) and "different" (*tɨlagɨ*) but also "above," having "raised" himself over the others. People say to such an enraged person, as to a stubborn child, "*kwin wok ndɨma ki*," "you shall not go higher up!"

II

In everyday life, the outer social frame (for a male ego) of pathogenic social relations consists of the clan and the partner clan (*ngapma ngapma*), one's own clan (*jalap*, see Chapter 2.3., Figure 1, *nut*, I), father's sister and her children (*mami*, II), the kinship group of the mother (*pek*, III) and the wife's relatives (*mbasok*, IV).

Even though, as the Yupno repeatedly assured me, it is theoretically possible that unrelated persons may also cause each other to be ill by *njɨgɨ*, no such case became known to me, and if one considers that most of the socially risky transactions (like the brideprice transfer and return) always take place inside the clan and the partner clan of two groups (at the brideprice, therefore, the clan and partner clan of the husband and the clan and partner clan of the wife), hence within the kinship group, this seems unlikely. In addition, within the realm of the individual "signs" (*tauak*, see below, Chapter 5.2.d.) that denote certain groups of persons, only a limited term or "sign," that is, "sign for a woman" (*sak tauak*) exists that can also mean somebody outside the kinship group. To interpret it the other way around: in everyday life, the problem therefore does not pose itself. If one wants to injure a non-relative through illness or death, one would commission a *sɨt*-specialist or a *mawom*-specialist (see Chapter 5.4.) to do so.

The "hot" emotional states, which can only be explained by the social norms of the Yupno, are labeled differently; the Yupno distinguish among various forms (see below, Chapter 5.2.c.). They are the conditions of people who are not in a harmoniously "cool," integrated state and which can manifest themselves as illness (not only in oneself, but in others), but which are not inevitably illness causing. If they are regarded as a cause of illness (and not as a temporary disorder of an individual without consequences), they are called an "oppressing problem" (*njɨgi*). The misdemeanor, a public violation of the current social rules or a grave offence against the code of behavior, may also happen unknowingly; it can therefore be the result of an emotional outburst, an impulse or a cool calculation.

Possible reasons for *nduara* (the "remainder of a wrong act that lingers on") and for illness-causing, "hot" emotional states, which may both lead to an "oppressing problem," are: the killing of somebody else during a fight or by purposely caused illness and death (with a *sɨt-* or *mawom*-act), theft (like in Megau's preceding story of a theft of a pig), "wrong" sexual relations, lack of care for old relatives or parents, violations of prohibitions, incorrect brideprice transfers and others. The possibilities listed here that may lead to an "oppressing problem" are in no way complete but give a sketchy outline of possible offences. In every single case of illness caused by an "oppressing problem," possible reasons regarding the personal situation of the afflicted, the kinds of social relations therefore within the above-sketched frame are deliberated anew. Every "oppressing problem" is thus determined from a number of different factors and so, to a large extent, is defined by the ill person's biography.

The term "oppressing problem" (*njɨgɨ*) is used for all the illness-causing transactions taking place between people that are part of the social environment, but not for misdemeanors in the "non-social" domain, in the relations of a human being to the bush-spirit *sindok* or to his "strength-holder of the settlement" (*kokop kɨrat*).

An "oppressing problem" is not an unchangeable fact but may either grow stronger, "go up," or weaker, "go down." The more serious it is, the higher it is, hence the more it has distanced itself from the "cool" state of social harmony thought to be in the middle between the "high" upper position (*tepm*) and the "ice-cold" position down below (*mbaak*). If an "oppressing problem" (*njɨgɨ*) is assumed to be the cause of illness in a patient, its movement, which expresses itself in his state of illness through his physical condition and through "signs" (*tauak*, see below), is observed and commented on. If it intensifies, people talk of "*njɨgɨ ni wosak*," "his 'oppressing problem' goes up," "*njɨgɨ abani wosak*," "his 'oppressing problem' is (still) busy going up." If it moderates or goes down, they say "*njɨgɨ kale pisak*," "his 'oppressing problem' goes down," "*njɨgɨ kale yawurondak*, "his 'oppressing problem' has become (almost) cool." If it lingers on despite efforts at clarification, people say "*njɨgɨ tusokgen*," "his 'oppressing problem' is still there."

The "oppressing problems" may be caused by living human beings and by dead persons (also by persons deceased some generations ago, hence by "ghosts," *koñ*), so they are not temporarily fixed onto people actually living in the present time but relatively "independent of time." However, they rarely ever transcend the time remembered, that is the generally-known genealogy,[35] since their cause in no way reaches back to the "dawn of history."

This central concept of the "oppressing problems," which determines the Yupno way of coping with illness, is rather marginally touched upon in the Melanesian literature, with the exception of M. Strathern (1968), A. Strathern (1968, 1984, 1994) and Brandewie (1973), who present these concepts of pathogenic emotions among the Melpa in great detail. Most anthropologists tend to ascribe this phenomenon of "pathogenic emotions" to the realm of "ethnopsychology" rather than medical anthropology (see Schieffelin 1985 and the other contributions in White and Kirkpatrick 1985).

b) "Left-Overs"

If a Yupno falls ill through a *koñ*, a "ghost," people specify the problem by talking about a *bɨmjɨt*, an "oppressing illness-causing problem" for which a deceased person or his or her "ghost" is responsible. It is an "old oppressing problem" because the deceased, when still alive, either acted wrongly or, annoyed by others, was brought into a "hot" state in which he or she is still ensnared as a "ghost"[36] (see Chapter 4.1.c.).

Two examples of "old oppressing problems" (*bɨmjɨt*) caused by an annoyed "ghost" (*koñ*) may serve to emphasize what has been said. Both incidents occurred during my stay; and the descriptions below were compiled either from talks (Example 1) or long discussions (Example 2).

Example 1:

Koki, a younger man from Gua, was initially suffering from "swollen feet" (*kalañ baptok ak*). He is married to Mumbiañ, the daughter of the evangelist Oti, originally from Finschhafen, a respected, reputable man from Gua who has died in the meantime. Oti's wife died, he himself was growing old and feeble and lived in a household with his daughter, Mumbiañ, and Koki. His eyesight was failing, he could not walk anymore and could only sit in the house. Koki and his wife took little care of the old man and only very sporadically ensured that a fire was burning in the house. Often, they attended to their own business in the garden. Oti grew bitter about this, and repeatedly scolded Koki: 'why did you marry my child and don't look after me?' Around this time, Koki's complaints started. One day, when Oti was sitting in the house alone, he burned Koki's netbag by mistake. Koki was furious about it, so he took a stick and beat his old father-in-law, inflicting injuries on his belly with a burning *bumbum* reed. (In a different version, Oti inflicted the burns on himself, which, however, could only happen because he was left on his own.) Shortly afterwards, Oti died, and Koki's illness increased. Koki, his clan and a few leading men in the village talked about the possible causes of his illness in a meeting; Koki publicly admitted a series of (further) misdemeanors, but his condition did not improve. Thereupon he himself assumed that his illness was due to an "old oppressing problem" (*bɨmjɨt*), caused by Oti's "ghost" (*koñ*). In order to appease Oti's "ghost," Koki paid a pig to Oti's closest friends (since Oti, originating from Finschhafen, did not have any relatives in the village).[37]

Example 2:

Njano, a young woman, fell gravely ill. At the beginning of her illness, she complained of headaches (*mbisoñ tepm*) and therefore spent her day at home by the fire instead of working in the garden. In the afternoon, she dreamt of Popokop, the late mother of her father's half-brother (see Figure 3), who was cooking pork in a bamboo, some of which she gave Njano to eat. In the evening, she related her dream to her returning parents, then began to talk incoherently, to babble; her body movements slowed down and became uncoordinated, and people described her state as "heavily drunk" (*opmbal*). Her condition did not improve, and two days later the members of her clan (Tuwal II) met to discuss it, since they suspected an "old oppressing problem" (*bɨmjɨt*) emanating from Popokop (because of Njano's dream). In her lifetime, Popokop had been very angry about the following: for some time, there had been tensions between the clan Mambap and the Tuwal II clan (the clan of Popokop's husband Kirin; from this marriage came a son, Uñgwep, the half-brother of Quantsañne, Njano's

Figure 3: Njano's Relatives

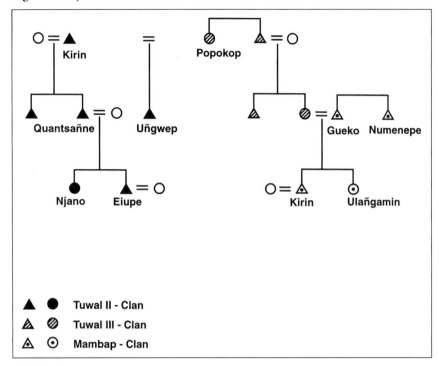

father). They insulted each other repeatedly, each clan called the other "the scum of the earth," stingy, unreliable, belligerent. The Mambap let the Tuwal II know that (in the case of a brideprice, for example) they would not even think of paying only as little as a pig to the Tuwal II since it could not be expected that they would get it back.

Popokop was very angry about these accusations against the clan into which she had married, and notified her son Uñgwep and his half-brother Quantsañne that they were never to help the Mambap with payments of pigs. Her anger was augmented by the fact that, at the confirmation of Gueko's daughter Ulañgamin (Popokop herself belongs to the group of the maternal kin group (*pek*) of this daughter), Gueko and Numenepe had killed pigs and promised Popokop a share, which she never received. Before her death, she proclaimed that after her death she would "stay with the Mambap clan" (meaning: ensure "old oppressing problems" there, to this concept of a "ghost" besieging a clan corresponds that after the death of a person a pig has to be paid to the maternal kin group of the deceased, a defensive measure to make the "ghost" (*koñ*) peacefully return to where he or his *amɨn-wop* ("shadow soul") originally come from. When Kirin (a Mambap), the son of a daughter of a mother's brother (MoBrDaSo) of Uñgwep, married, Quantsañne as an elder brother of Uñgwep wanted to help with the brideprice and kill a pig. But when he shot at the pig he only wounded it and it ran off. Day and night people were looking for the pig until Njano finally found it. People assumed that Popokop's "ghost" had invaded the pig and was now causing Njano to be ill (out of revenge on Quantsañne, who had not heeded his half-mother's ad-monitions). The matter was discussed, then some money was paid to Popokop's matrilateral kingroup (hence her *pek*), giving hope that her "ghost" was now appeased, thus solving the "old oppressing problem" (*bɨmjɨt*) and ending Njano's illness.[38]

Hence a "ghost" cannot, as the "old oppressing problems" (*bɨmjɨt*) of Oti and Pokopo show, suddenly become active and act retrospectively, since the reason for his annoyance and his "hot," "above" dwelling state happened while he was alive; in other words, he acts "chronologically." Following this princi-ple of chronological order, "oppressing problems" (*njɨgɨ*) stem from actions today by living persons yet manifest themselves much later, among grand-children or other descendants.

c) "Hot" Feelings

Certain emotions may lead to "oppressing problems." That these emotions, such as rage or hatred, originate at all has to do with disturbed social rela-tions. Conscious, controlled misdemeanors (as when certain persons author-ized to claim a share in the brideprice are deliberately overlooked, causing them to become angry, turn "hot," then unload this "heat" and cause illness) provide a reason for this conduct, exactly as in the case of previous disputes. Andrew Strathern (personal communication, see also Strathern (1994)), notes that the Melpa and Wiru possess a very similar concept:

> Yupno concepts are strikingly similar to those of the Highlanders with whom I have worked up until last year (1991), that is, the Hagen and Pangia people. Anger causes "heaviness" (Melpa <u>mbun</u>, Wiru <u>kenda</u>) and that in turn "sickness" (Melpa <u>kui</u>, Wiru <u>yene</u>), and major effort is expended on discussion, confession, reparation, in pursuit of end-ing a sickness condition. In Melpa, the focus is on "digging out the causes" (i.e. <u>pukl</u>, roots), and in Pangia it is on finding the <u>pine</u> (base

or basis); usually centered on exchange relations or past enmities, again as in Yupno.

Yupno people think of the potentially pathogenic, "hot" feelings (anger, rage, hatred, and so on) as localized either in the neck (*teak*) or belly (*mbɨt*). A similar division into two different kinds of "hatred" is also known by the Melpa. "One (kind of anger) comes up in the mouth…and is forgotten as soon as quarrelling is over. The other is anger which comes up in the heart… and is much more serious. This anger is deep-seated, established in the consciousness and intentions of a person, and is known as *popokl*" (M. Strathern 1968: 533).

With due caution,[39] it can be said that since thoughts and feelings are located in the belly, the emotional and mental states marked with "belly" (*mbɨt*) are longer lasting. The terms formed with "belly" (*mbɨt*) therefore more strongly emphasize the mental aspect, those states marked with "neck" (*teak*) can be interpreted as a short-lived version of the feeling located in the belly and signify a momentary state as well as the manifestation of this state. Somebody grows numb from anger or frustration ("something chokes me," "to be speechless from rage"), or the anger is vented verbally. *Mbɨt kaloñ*, "to be one belly," 'wanbel,' "to be unanimous" therefore also means a real, lasting unanimity, a relaxed basic attitude which is shared by all; *teak kaloñ*, "to be one neck," is a rather momentary agreement regarding a certain issue, a compromise reached in a dispute or after a discussion. In part, however, the terms are used synonymously.

The terms for "hot" states which can cause "oppressing problem" are:

- **teak tevan** ("different thoughts"). Description of the state and examples for the context of the term:

  somebody overlooks someone, is unfriendly, and shows his or her indifference.

  If a married man is often seen with another woman, his wife becomes "jealous" (*teak tevan*), has "strong negative thoughts" (see in the case of little Nstasiñge, the behavior of Kan).

  If someone has been robbed and knows the thief but does not (since the theft cannot be proved) take him to task, but over a long period of time is suspicious of him and angry at him, overlooks him, "cuts him dead" and does not answer his greeting.

  If someone runs off because he or she is angry, fed up with everything but does not openly talk about it and instead suppresses his or her rancor, so the anger stays in the belly.

Teak tevan ("with different thoughts") hence means the realm of feelings which we circumscribe with jealousy, suspicion, suppressed rancor, distrust.

- *Mbɨt tevan* ("to have strong thoughts") is used for someone who is stubborn, unwavering, and frantically and distrustfully continues to think the same. This term contains more the mental aspect; *mbɨt tevan* and *teak tevan*, however, are used in a similar way.

- *Teak ndapndap* ("repeatedly beaten, hurt thoughts"). Examples:

  an old man is married to a considerably younger woman, who leaves him and starts relationships with other men; the old man gets the feeling of being old, not being able to win against the younger men, and thus of losing, and being inadequate.

  Somebody watches someone else breaking something that belongs to the observer, but does not confront the offender and take him to task. Later, however, the observer talks about it with others, and one of the people present then conveys these comments back to the offender. In this way, the matter escalates.

Teak ndapndap ("repeatedly beaten, hurt thoughts") also means feelings and thoughts that are increasingly incited or stirred up, and the person in question again and again suffers further defeats, which continue to inflame his or her emotions. This term stresses the long drawn-out repetition and increase of this feeling.

- *Teak kandap* ("the throat is ablaze"). This state may end in an outburst of rage or in a brawl. Examples:

  the father of Tanowe (Mañnau, see the case of little Nstasiñge) was *teak kandap* when he declared he no longer belonged to his clan.

  Somebody wants to start a garden and pursues this aim single-mindedly, regardless of time or other considerations; when a person is possessed by something, like a thought or a project.

- *Mbɨt kandap* ("inner fire," "burning thoughts"). Examples:

  a continuous suspicion, somebody incessantly thinks of someone or of something bad.

  The rancor is covered up inside; on the outside, one is friendly towards the person in question, but inwardly one "curses" him or her.

The term is also used in the sense of jealousy, if, for example, a woman thinks that her husband has a relationship with somebody else but keeps her anger and her frustration to herself.

The term is also used in connection with work, *mbɨt kandap kot*, and means somebody who only thinks about doing business (making money), but neglects everything else. "Workaholic" would be the modern expression. *Teak kandap* ("the throat is ablaze") and *mbɨt kandap* ("inner fire") are often used in a similar sense, but *teak kandap* in addition often contains the verbal expression of this state as well.

- *Mbɨt njap* ("anger in the belly") means feelings like rage, indignation, fury, which one wants to get rid of and does so in public by yelling and starting a fight. Our terms "outburst of rage" and "venting of anger" approximate this concept. It may be used as a generic noun for "fight."

• *Mbɨt peak* ("increasing suspicion") means a state in which a suspicion increases, or "ripens." Example:

to turn it over in one's thoughts again and again ("you or who else"): who, for example, has stolen something or who is the one with whom one's wife is unfaithful?

Mbɨt peak ("increasing suspicion") means a suspicion or distrust which deepens, hence stresses the temporal factor ("to ripen") as well as the result, "to be formed, shaped."

• *Mbɨt opmbal* ("the thoughts are all topsy-turvy"). Examples:

term for somebody who does not know what he or she is doing, who attacks someone and hurts him or her or sets fire to a house.

The term is also used for somebody who is completely drunk.

As synonyms, the terms *nandak nandak opmbal* ("wrong knowledge," "turned-around thoughts") and *teak opmbal* ("the throat is wrong," "to babble," or "to say something wrong") are used. Two further terms are *nandak nandak yuki* ("to have bad thoughts," "to think badly of somebody") and *gen yuki* ("bad words," "insults" or "deceitful gossip").

A term belonging to a somewhat different domain (of reaction), *mbɨt pasil,* "my belly, my feelings got frightened," which can be translated with being afraid, being scared, to fear, mentioned here for the sake of completeness. "Oppressing problems" (*njɨgɨ*) cannot originate from this state but from the "misdemeanor" itself if somebody willingly frightens someone else.

The opposite terms, which signify positive states, thoughts or feelings, hence the end of a "hot" state that may have led to "oppressing problems" are:

- *teak kaloñ,* ("to be one throat," "to be unanimous");

- *mbɨt kaloñ* ("to be one belly," "to have shared thoughts," "to be unanimous");

- *mbɨt kuak* ("the belly is cold," in the sense of "something will get well"). This term is only used for illness caused by the bush-spirit *sindok* or by an "oppressing problem" (*njɨgɨ*) that one attempts to alleviate through an offering or a payment.

- *Ngɨlarɨ* ("to be good," "to be unanimous").

d) Diagnosis: "Signs" and Dreams

I

The basis of a therapy, that is of liberation from an "oppressing problem" (*njɨgɨ*), is thought to begin with the search for the cause[40] by attempting to clarify who, or which kin group, might have a reason to cause illness by unloading a "remainder of wrong conduct" (*nduara*) or a "hot" emotional state.

This search happens in various ways. The ill person, in line with the notion that illness is connected with places and persons, takes himself to various social environments (such as houses of his partner clan (*ngapma*), or of his matrilateral kin group (*pek*), and "tests" whether his condition improves or worsens (see the case of little Nstasiñge who was given to different people to hold, taken into several houses and to another place, Tapmañge, in order to find out the cause of possible "oppressing problems").

Very important in the search for causes are the "signs," *tauak.*[41] They comprise certain gestural or facial expressions of the ill person or of certain animals found close to him. Within the Yupno system of thought, these "signs" have a fixed meaning that is recognized and shared by all. Almost all the "signs" (with few exceptions) can in each case be assigned to a certain group of relatives; a part of them defines itself from the "hot-cool-cold"-concept which assigns "hot" or "cold" qualities to certain plants or substances, another part corresponds to the "right-left"-division (on the right, the strong, paternal side, the side which pulls the bowstring and shoots the arrow; on the left, the maternal side, the helping side which holds the bow), a part is based on the traditional rituals, for a further part, the original meaning could no longer be analyzed or had been lost. A (small) part points directly to other possible causes of illness outside the complex of "oppressing problems." All these "signs" (*tauak*) are also thought to be significant in dreams.

The individual "signs" are:

- *meññan tauak* ("signs of mother and father").

    If an ill person urinates in excess (*pɨsit pɨsit jok*), or his sickbed smells of urine, the cause of this illness points to his parents, because every child originates from the semen his father (*pɨsit niroñ*) entering the mother.

    If the penis or the scrotum of an afflicted man is swollen (*yawɨ nyɨvɨlɨ bapdak*) or the vulva of an ill woman is swollen (*kambul bapdak*).

Both signs belong to the domain of reproduction and sexuality. The cause of an "oppressing problem" may be that the mother slept with another man or that the father had sexual relations with another woman.

- *Nut tauak* ("sign of one's own clan"):

    many gestures made by an afflicted person with the right hand or on the right side of the body are assigned to his or her own clan. Right (see above) means the strong, paternal side.

    If the ill person often brushes his or her mouth with the right hand, this gesture is interpreted as "closing the mouth" (*ndol uroknok*); some member of the own clan has acted wrongly, kept the act a secret, and the *nduara*, the "remainder of the misdemeanor," has now affected the ill person.

    Other *nut tauak* are gestural movements at the head. Their origin lies within the complex of brideprice, if the sister of a man gets married, he as a classificatory or biological brother will get one or several pigs as payment and eat the snout, the eyes and the ears himself, but will pass the other pieces on.

    Such signs may be:

    if the afflicted "pulls his hairs" or pulls them out (*mbisoñ ndañgwan pilakndak*), "scratches his head" (*mbisoñ epmdaldak*), or if he "pulls at his nostrils" (*tɨmnɨ njagaldak*).

- *Tira tauak penyi patogo* ("rat sign of the elder and younger brothers"):

  a sign belonging to the realm of the various techniques for detecting *si t* is the small "red rat" (*tira goman*). If it runs around close to an ill person, this is taken as a "sign for a *sit*-act" (*sit tauak*, see below) or "sign of one's own clan" (*nut tauak*), but most frequently it signifies "causing to be ill on behalf of the elder and younger brothers," as *penyi patogo tauak*.

- *Ngapma tauak* ("sign of the partner clan"):

  if a small *njigngek* frog or a *ngolok* worm comes close to the afflicted person, the cause of the illness is looked for in a partner clan (*ngapma*) whose misdemeanor causes the patient to be ill or a member of which has already ordered the illness (*sit*).

  The *njigngek* frog and the *ngolok* worm are the "partner clan sign" for all the clans. At the time of the bullroarer (*obip san*), a level of initiation, the leaders of the initiation would take a *ngolok* worm and *njigngek* frog, and rubbed them and the *mbrombak* lizard (a *kokop kirat*, a "strength-holder of the settlement" of Gua) on the penis and vulva of different members of the partner clans (*ngapma ngapma*). They would then bespeak them and put all three together with the bullroarer *obip san* onto certain leaves. The *moñan* ("breath spirit") of the people in question allied itself with the *ngolok* worm. With this act, the fertility of the gardens was to be assured, drought avoided and the novices turned into healthy men and good warriors. There were always two partner clans to take part in this *obip san*-ritual, performing it as partner clans (*ngapma ngapma*), which is why the frog and the worm are interpreted as "signs of the partner clans" (*ngapma tauak*).

  If these small animals were to appear in dreams, they would be attributed with the same meaning.

- *Meñ tauak* ("sign of the mother"):

  if the ill person makes gestures on his or her left, "weaker" body side, this points to the mother.

- *Pek tauak* ("sign of the kin group of the mother"):

  if a child (or more rarely an adult) suffers from lasting and serious diarrhoea, this is interpreted as a "sign from the kinship group of the mother." The reason for this is too low a brideprice, which has caused the mother's relatives to feel themselves badly paid, so they unload their "hot" anger onto the patient and thus impede the growth of the child, as the "product" of the brideprice.

If a mother cannot breastfeed her child any more because she has run out of milk, for the same reason one also speaks of *pek tauak* (see the illness report of little Nstasiñge, Chapter 4.1.c. "oppressing problem" [5].)

- *Mbasok tauak* ("sign of the kin group of the woman"):

  if an ill man frequently opens his mouth wide as if wanting to call out, this points to the kin group of his wife, to which he and his relatives had paid the brideprice and which is now suspected of causing an "oppressing problem;" it must have thought the completed brideprice was too low, and thus became dissatisfied and annoyed. The sign is interpreted as a "call for payment." If such payment is later made, it is called *ngopmo* ("my covering," see Chapter 3.3.).

- *Koñ tauak* or *mbawo tauak* ("sign of the 'ghost' or of the ancestors"):

  if an ill person is excessively attacked by lice (*eyat*), this is held to be the "ghost sign;" the lice are an outward manifestation of the "ghost," which now "eats up" the patient.

Some of the following signs belong to the traditional religious domain, which today has to a large extent been given up, and so their underlying meaning could not be precisely analyzed.

If one dreams of the little *mbrombak* lizard and /or it enters a ill person's house, this points to a related ancestor who has assumed the form of a *mbrombak*, and people deliberate as to which clan the mother of this ancestor belonged (and from which he received his *amɨnwop*, "shadow soul"). If somebody from the patient's clan at the time killed this ancestor or one of his relatives through a *sɨt*-act, it therefore gave him cause for a "hot" feeling like anger or hatred. The *mbrombak* lizard is thought to be a "strength-holder of the settlement" (*kokop kɨrat*) for the Yupno and a "guardian" of the *mbema* (the traditional settlements).

The beetle *bɨmjɨtwal*, too, is held to be a *mbawo tauak* or *koñ tauak*, since its shape (head, neck, body) is similar to that of the bullroarer *obip san*, the voice of the "ghosts" (*koñ*).

The rat *kɨran*, which is also interpreted as a *mbawo tauak*, is an important indicator in the search of ordered illness (*sɨt*), held to be the main traditional cause of death. The rat *kɨran* thus indicates that this ancestor had been killed by *sɨt* and, filled with rancor about this, now ensures "oppressing problems."

- *Sak tauak* ("women's sign"):

  this "sign" points to an "oppressing problem," caused through an illicit sexual contact with a woman, which concerns the men and transcends the kinship system.

  If an ill man drinks a lot of water ("cold"), asks for sugar-cane ("cold" food, both things "one likes"), this points to an "oppressing problem" because of a woman (who is "cold" and with whom one would like to have a relationship); either the man in question has flirted too much with a young woman or started an affair with an already married woman. In this case he is considered to have engaged in improper sexual conduct. Frequently, the father or husband of this woman is already preparing to call in a *sɨt*-specialist, to perform pathogenic acts against the man concerned. Since illicit sexual relations are one of the main causes for inflicting an illness, this sign is also interpreted as *sɨt tauak* ("sign of a *sɨt*-act," see below).

  If a butterfly (*kabɨbɨt*) comes into the house of the patient and flies into the fire and burns, this also points to an "oppressing problem" to do with a woman, since the butterfly is the symbol of women.

  The *meñgak* frog is held to be "cold" since it lives near the water. If it hops around near the patient, this also points to a woman.

The following three signs do not point to an illness-inducing "oppressing problem" caused by a relative or a group but directly to the cause; for completeness' sake, however, they are listed as well.

- *Sindok tauak* ("sign of the (bush-spirit) *sindok*," see Chapter 5.3.):

  illness caused by the bush-spirit *sindok* can be detected from the condition of the patient's body. If the body or skin is very hot (*ngodɨm jusok*), or painful (*ngodɨm tepm tisok*), or if the patient suffers from burns (*kandap sañgamok*), this points to *sindok*-activities.

- *Sɨt tauak* ("sign of a *sɨt*-act," also *kalala* (no translation), see Chapter 5.4.):

    kalala means the condition of person who has been seriously ill for a long time and has grown very thin; his or her state is described as "sunken eyes and a white nose," and the assumed cause is a *sɨt*-act.

- *Mawom tauak* ("sign of a *mawom*-act," see Chapter 5.4.):

    if a patient suffers from shivering fits, violent headaches and pains in the joints and if his condition worsens over a very short time, this rapid course of his illness is assumed to be cause is *mawom*, a pathogenic or death-causing "technique."

II

As already explained in the case of little Nstasɨñge's illness (see Chapter 4.1.c., "oppressing problem" [6]), dreams (*dipmin*) of the ill person himself or his relatives and their interpretation provide information about the cause of an "oppressing problem." As with the Melpa: "attention is paid to dreams which kinsfolk have that may be interpreted in such a way as to point to the cause of a patient's sickness" (A. Strathern 1989a: 149); see also Strathern (1989b). Also, as M. Young (1989: 119–20) notes for the Goodenough Islanders: "Dream images and body 'pictures'…are material for interpretation by the curer, who is able to say with some authority where the patient's disturbed social relationship lies."

Dreams are a frequent topic of conversation among the Yupno, and their content is discussed most often among relatives. They are thought to be so relevant that, if a Yupno at night wakes up out of a dream, an experience of his *amɨnwop* ("shadow soul"), he may then awaken his relatives who are asleep in the same house and tell them the content of what he has dreamt. After a brief discussion, they all go back to sleep.

Part of the dreams are episodes of real or at least known, often stereotyped, acts, with certain "dream images" that are symbolic of certain things, and this connection is known to all Yupno, so their interpretations are unambiguous and relatively rigid. However, dreams may be interpreted differently according to the context, especially with those that point to the future, but less so for dreams in the context of illness, and for innovative dreams, containing elements unfamiliar to the culture. New social situations, new objects such as a plane, for example, are dreamt of and then interpreted within the thought system of the Yupno by ascribing to the foreign object certain qualities (for example, tinned fish is classified as "cold"). New dream images are also interpreted in the domain of "oppressing problems." If one dreams of a person

Survey 1: The "Signs"

kin group	tauak		
	animals:	plants, substances:	gestural and facial expression, physical signs:
meñnan (parents)			excessive urinating, swollen genitals
nut (own clan)			movements on the right body side, on the head
penyi patogo (brothers)	*tɨra goman* rat		
ngapma (partner clan)	*ngolok* worm, *njigngek* frog		
meñ (mother)			movements on the left side of the body
pek (maternal kin group)			diarrhoea, no breast-milk
mbasok (brideprice recipients)			to open the mouth wide
koñ or *mbawo* ("ghosts", ancestor)	*mbromak-*lizard, *bɨmjɨtwal* beetle, *kɨran* rat		
other agents			
sak (woman)	*kabɨbɨt* butterfly, *meñgak* frog	"cold" things, sugar-cane, water	
sindok (bush-spirit)			"hot" body, burns
sɨt (ordered illness-causation)			physical condition, sunken eyes, white nose
mawom (ordered illness-causation)			physical condition, rapid and serious course of illness

speaking Tok Pisin, for example, this points to an "oppressing problem" coming "from outside" and people ponder which of the dreamer's relatives goes to
school in Madang or elsewhere or works "outside."

If a person dreams that he receives betel nuts from other men but cannot
hold the betel nuts in his hand or that the men just put them down, this points
to his partner clan (*ngapma*). He then also dreams part of a *s*i*t*-act, where a
member of the partner clan has the task of going to the *s*i*t*-specialist to get
water or sugar-cane ("cold things") there and take them to the ill person, who
at this stage is sweating heavily (i.e. is "very hot"), in order for him to get well.
(See Jowage's story in Chapter 5.4.a.). Other dreams are interpreted with a
view to a specific case of illness.

An excerpt from an illness debate may serve as an example of one such
dream interpretation. It took place in the house of Quantsañne, a man from
the Tuwal II clan, at Mpagmbewoñok, "the "place of the originating lake" in
Gua on 27 July, 1987. His daughter Njano (see Figure 3 above) had fallen
gravely ill and her relatives suspected that she had caused the "oppressing
problem" herself (initially, an "oppressing problem," caused by the "ghost" of
her grandmother Popokop, had been suspected in Njano's case, see above).

A brief note is apropos here regarding the preceding events: her brother,
Eiupe, wanted to marry a woman from Nokopo. This marriage did not come
about since his kin group deemed this woman "unqualified," and so was reluc-
tant to raise the brideprice. In his absence (he was completing training as a
teacher on the coast), he was married against his will to a woman from Nian.
Njano, who had a very close relationship with her brother, opposed this marriage and said as much in a letter to him. Then Eiupe, of his own accord and
without a brideprice, married a woman from the coast. When, after some time,
he visited Gua with his new wife, his relatives were very annoyed because of this
break with tradition. Although they had bought a wife for him, he showed no
interest in her, and then, without their consent, had married another woman.
Because Njano had taken her brother's side and subsequently lived in a state of
constant tension with her relatives, she left the village with her brother and his
wife and went to live in Wandaboñ, where her brother had in the meantime
started working as a teacher. Some time later, Njano came back and fell ill.

> **Bribiañ** (the wife of Napone, a member of the Komin clan, which,
> together with the clans Ngandum and Kapbaga, forms the partner
> clan (*ngapma*) of Njano's clan Tuwal II, see Chapter 2.2.): I dreamt,
> and the two of us, Napone and I, talked about it. I dreamt, you
> here, this group [Njano's father Quantsañne as the representative of
> the clan Tuwal II, and Megau as the representative of the partner

clan Ngandum, with their families], you wanted to go to Tapen [place in the lower Yupno region] for good, and you put everything, bowls, pots and all that [in netbags] and carried it, and Megau's group, they gave us everything that stayed here [pigs etc.]. At that time, we saw Megau and his group, they went to Tetep-gowañ ["below Tetep," situated close to Teptep] and to Wangogokup [no translation], left it [this region] behind them and went around the hillside, and they were all gone. I tried to hold on to some of the little pigs that they had left for me, and they looked at me and were all upset. A small white pig which they had left here was completely mad and wanted to eat us. I did not hold on to it and did not tie it up, I let it go free, and I said: 'they have left us and are gone forever. What shall I do now, will the pigs understand my words and I, shall I tie them up?'

The pig I had set free tried to run away, and then it came again and was here again. Here, at this section of the path, we tied all [the pigs] together, and we went up to Gomevilka, where Beñgene has a garden. In former times, we had also made a garden there, and it was [a bit overgrown] still there, and there we tied all [the pigs] up. And in this place, I wanted to get sweet potatoes, and that is why I stood there.

And I turned around, looked around and, from Kunagatowa, the "place above the pandanus palm," there came a group of people. And a little girl, she had everything which belonged to her stuffed into a netbag, and she carried a digging-stick and a spade. She came and she went there, where Susune [the aforementioned mother of Mayu] ties up her pigs and where the small path goes up, she tried to climb up, but it was very hard for her, she made a big effort to climb. And I thought: 'that is Kamake's daughter, her name is Doke,' and she stayed down below and sang her *koñgap* melody.

But it was not Doke, it was Popokop [the late grandmother of Njano, see Figure 3]. She turned around and looked at me. She turned around, looked at me, carried her digging-stick and spade and went up [the mountain]. She followed the path which goes up, and I stood and watched, and her old husband together with his *wau* [younger namesake, Kirin and Napone], the two of them were also running around. Kirin was the first to go, Napone followed him. And I said to myself, 'Kirin cut this sugar-cane *kandat yaat* [*kandat yaat* is the only kind of sugar-cane thought to be "hot," hence a special sugar-cane] and tied it into a bundle and now he carries it and runs around together with Napone. The two of them tied the sugar-cane and carry it. They cut very many parts of this sugar-cane and tied them like a bundle and carry it.'

And Kirin was like before, healthy and without wounds, that is how he was. He came up. He came up, in plain sight, but he did not see me. I saw him, he came up, and he looked in the direction of Teptep, and he went. And Napone followed him, they both came up, they did not see me and did not say anything to me, they did not see me, they looked towards Teptep and followed the path to Mbɨvɨka, the "place of the broken-up ground," and they went.

And I stood there, I just stood there, and a small group came, a small group of children. I thought they were the children from Guap who came. All the children from Guap, Njano, Madevit, Bumbum. They all ran around and came down. They saw me, I was there, and they came down and said: 'owa' [grandmother], and I was pleased, was nice and said 'mbawo' [my grandchildren] to them and they all surrounded me and were pleased and I, I was happy with them. And on their skin, which they had washed well, they had rubbed fat or powder or such stuff [meaning: baby powder], they were all turned-out very well. And I was thinking: 'what is in my netbag that I could give to them?' And I thought about it and searched in my netbag. And I had some dried pandanus nuts I had filled into my netbag. I took them out and did not put them in a bowl and handed it to them, no, I gave them to them by hand.

And two stood a bit below me, in the direction of the valley, they stood there and ate. And one stood at my side, he took one [a pandanus nut] and put it in his mouth, I saw it. And what did he do? The skin of the pandanus nut hung [stuck] in his throat. What should I do to get the pandanus skin from his throat? And the boy was trying very hard to retch up the pandanus skin and his eyes were popping out. And I saw him and became frightened. I thought: 'what on earth am I to do to get out this skin? Why did I give it to him and he swallowed it and it stuck?' This is how I thought, and I grabbed him and turned him around, and I put my finger down his throat and tried to find the pandanus skin but I did not find it. He screamed and yelled and his eyes were popping out and he was already close to choking and it was very difficult for him. And I thought: 'what has he got in his throat, what is blocking his throat?' Because the pandanus skin did not stick in his throat, his throat was okay. And the pandanus skin had hidden in the cheek. The boy behaved as if the pandanus skin had wedged in his throat but he was only pretending and I was trying very hard and then I checked it and saw that the pandanus skin had hidden itself in his cheek. I took it out and the boy talked quite normally again and sat down.

The other half of the dream I did not see, I dreamt that far and you, Napone, you woke me up to start a fire and I did not dream on. And I said to him [Napone]: 'I was just dreaming, why did you wake me?' That is all.

Nanjañne [a man from the Kapbaga clan, a partner clan (*ngapma*) of Njano]: This dream is a dream about Quantsañne's parents [Kirin and his second wife Popokop who were angry about the unauthorized marriage of their grandson Eiupe], and hence I think this young girl [Njano] who is ill, is ill like the little white pig, this is how she behaves [stubbornly, aggressively]. This pandanus skin the boy has swallowed went into his throat and he cannot say anything, this shows the *njɨgɨ* ["oppressing problem"] of the two old people has grabbed her [Njano] and blocked her mouth.

Megau [a man from the Ngandum clan, also a partner clan (*ngapma*) of Njano]: Quantsañne and Paka, what do you think about this dream? Just talk and if we hear numerous different opinions, well, we will interpret them later.

Nanjañne: This pandanus skin which sticks in the mouth therefore shows…that the *njɨgɨ* ["oppressing problem"] has got a total hold on her [Njano] and it is very hard for her, you can see it.

Paka [a man from the Tuwal II clan, a *nut* (clan relative) of Njano]: This dream is not about this group of children, no. No, it is Njano, she is trapped, and the *njɨgɨ* ["oppressing problem"] has taken hold of her. The sign clearly points in this direction, can you see this, eh?

Everybody: Yes.

Quantsañne [Njano's father]: I have a thought and it goes as follows: this boy who has hung himself [almost choked] like in a trap, that is as you have just said. They [Njano and her brother] get up and leave us. I think, the pigs, pots, bowls, that they leave here for us…

Nanjañne: This sugar-cane which he [Kirin] carries around, that is like seed for all the food.

Quantsañne: It [the sugar-cane] does not point to something which comes from outside, the *kandat* sugar-cane is a sign that it [the "oppressing problem"] is situated in one's own clan. This sugar-cane is something "hot," it is a sign of a fight within the house group [the patrilineage, *jalap*]. This dream…points exactly to that. It does not point to anything else, really not.

Nanjañne: We are not little boys. This pandanus skin which she gave to the child from Guap and which stuck in his throat, that is something real. Njano has such difficulties breathing as if the pandanus skin were sticking in her throat, she is lying there as if the pandanus skin were sticking in her throat and we have a hard time with her. That is no pandanus skin, that is this *njɨgɨ* ["oppressing problem"] which constricts Njano's throat and she is having a hard time to get rid of it. This *njɨgɨ* here has choked her almost like that and it is difficult to throw it out.

Megau: Njano is ill but she did not think: 'I am ill and my mother and my father are here and look after me and I must not contradict them, I obey them and get well.' But just this Njano did not do. When she got ill, her parents wanted to talk to her but she was furious at them and beat her mother. And she said: 'my parents are not allowed to look after me, take me to another house!'

Bribiañ: This is what she said, and her tongue went into her throat, and she could not talk clearly anymore. She was furious at her parents, and her tongue went down, and her thinking became muddled.…I think, this is how she did it, and she alone is responsible for the *njɨgɨ* ["oppressing problem"].

The following dream images have been thus interpreted in this brief extract of the discussion:

- the behavior of the little white pig ("it was completely mad and wanted to eat us") was equated with Njano's aggressive, stubborn behavior.
- The pandanus skin which the little boy swallowed was interpreted as an "oppressing problem" by all the participants. First as one caused by the (late grandparents) Popokop and Kirin (interpretation by Nanjañne), then more vaguely as an "oppressing problem" which had taken hold of Njano (explanation by Paka) and, finally, as one for which she, Njano,

herself was responsible since she had rebelled against her parents (in the opinion of Megau and Bribiañ).

- The group Bribiañ saw leave the place in her dream was taken to be Njano, her brother and his wife, and about how they left Gua and went to Wandaboñ (interpretation by Quantsañne).
- "Special" ("hot") sugar-cane *kandat yaat*, which Kirin and his *wau* Napone had cut in great quantities, was interpreted by Quantsañne as something pointing to one's own patrilineage or the own clan respectively, hence again as evidence of an "oppressing problem" within the kin group.
- Not interpreted, since "more than clear" was the dream image of the appearing and turning away of Popokop, Njano's grandmother.

The interpretation of these various summed-up individual dream images can therefore serve as a clear indication of who is responsible for an "oppressing problem."

e) Therapy: The Release from the Burden

After the "signs" have reduced the group of persons causing "oppressing problems," the members of the clan as well as the partner clan (or depending on the "sign," the kin group of the mother, *pek*, or the brideprice recipients, *mbasok*) meet in a house in the afternoon or evening for a discussion, typically lasting several hours, and in the course of which all the participants describe their "remainder of a misdemeanor" *(nduara)* or the cause of "hot feelings" from their own point of view.[42] Often, several "oppressing problems" are brought up and the causal "oppressing problem" is determined through the interpretation of dreams. Once it has been pronounced, and if the participants in the discussion agree, are "unanimous" or "harmonious" about who, or which kin group, is in the end responsible for the "oppressing problem," the person in question will shortly afterwards appease and "cool down" the damaged party by the presentation of a pig or a certain amount of money. The patient, thus released from his "burden," should now get well again. If there is no improvement in the course of the illness, a new meeting is set during which other possible cases of misdemeanor are discussed. If after several discussions the patient still does not get better, therefore no "oppressing problem" can be unmistakably determined to be responsible for his condition, the relatives will assume a more serious cause and suspect that the illness is of the commissioned variety (*sit*, see below).

In the case of a *bimjit*, an "oppressing problem caused by a ghost," people who are more traditional in orientation, in addition to paying compensation to the ghost's maternal clan, will also ritually exorcize this angry "ghost." This ritual, *koñ mɨndak*, called "chasing away of the ghost" is performed usually by an older man well versed in the tradition, a *nandak nandak amɨn*, a "man with a lot of knowledge." For the competent performance of the "chasing away of the ghost" alone, however, he is not counted among the specialists in the complex of illness, but he is often at the same time a "cause-of-illness-detection specialist" (*pat amɨn*, see below) and a "causer of ordered illness" (*sɨt amɨn*, see below). There are slightly divergent variations within this ritual of "chasing away the ghost," depending on the clan.

A variant of the "chasing away of a ghost":

The performer collects various grasses and plants with thorns and barbs, breaks them and crushes them and puts them on leaves of the strong *zarak* plant. He kneads and presses some of the mud- or clay-like *wawɨt* soil into the shape of a thin dish, on which he places the *zarak* leaves. After these preparations, he goes to the former house of the deceased (previously, to his men's house) and lights a piece of bark-cloth. The stinking smoke attracts a black fly, a kind of blow-fly in which the angry *koñwop* ("soul of a dead person") is located. He catches it, puts it on the crushed thorny grasses, calls the name (of the owner) of the "ghost," puts the *zarak* leaves down, tightly encloses the bundle of leaves with the *wawɨt* soil, presses this parcel into a hollowed-out wild taro bulb, and again covers it completely with a thin layer of *wawɨt* soil. Together with the "victim" of the "ghost" (the patient) and his relatives, he then goes to a stream, and everybody starts to scream and yell: "you, you [name of the 'ghost'] have dwelled in the middle of this ill person, we have caught you, we will now throw you into the water and then you [your anger] are finished!" At the same time, the taro bulb is thrown into the brook and the "ghost" is eventually carried away down its place in the hereafter, the sea.

3. The Bush-Spirit *Sindok* or Breaking the Rules of the Topographical-Religious Environment

a) The Concept of *Sindok*, Its Dwellings and Prophylactic Measures

I

The *sindok* is a malevolent bush-spirit that is capable of causing burns and states of mental confusion. Although younger Yupno often called it by the Tok Pisin term, 'masalai', it does not belong to a rather diffusely conceived category of various "water-spirits" or "bush-spirits" but is looked upon by the

Yupno as a very concrete and real being. Morap, the creator figure of the Yupno, has called it into being.

The *sindok* bush-spirit is thought to be the mother of the marsupials. This is even more clearly formulated by the inhabitants of the villages like Devil and Meñan, which are situated very close to the bush, the actual hunting ground. From the explanations of the inhabitants of Gua, who live far away from the hunting grounds and thus very rarely hunt for marsupials, the image forms of a mischief-making figure that is half-human, half-animal. Among the very Christianized Yupno, it is sometimes also called Satan.[43]

The *sindok* bush-spirit is able to change its outer appearance. "Normally," it appears in the form of a tree kangaroo (as a *ndankwit*, a grey-black animal with a white belly, also called *nabada*). Thus in the small cult-object men's house (*tɨlagɨ yut*) in former times, *sindok kɨrat*, a marsupial bone, was kept as its bone and was used for *sɨt*-acts. Today, the *sindok kɨrat* are kept hidden in inaccessible and secret places (such as caves or hollowed tree-trunks) by the *sɨt*-specialists.

This bush-spirit may also take the form of a bird, a *ndagal*, which has many "hot" ginger roots (*maam goman*) growing at its dwelling, a *kawam* (Tok Pisin: 'tarangau', eagle or falcon), a white night bird with long talons, a *siñgeñ* (another bird of prey active during the day) or else a snake (*toñ amɨn*) or, more rarely, a lizard (*mbrombak*). These two latter forms of appearance depend on the "strength-holder of the settlement" (*kokop kɨrat*) of the clan in question. People who, for example, have a bird as the "strength-holder of the settlement" (such as members of the Ngupmevil clan at Devil) can see the *sindok* bush-spirit in the form of a bird, whereas the clans domiciled in Gua see it as a small *mbrombak* lizard. In stories told around the fire of an evening, the *sindok* bush-spirit often appears in human form as a man (*sindokwuli*) or as a woman (*sindoksak*) who seduces men. Children imagine the *sindok* bush-spirit to be a naked, savage man with talons and overgrown with lichen—a "wild man of the woods."

II

The *sindok* bush-spirit can be found in the bush or in generally inaccessible places (like rock-faces) which are attributed to it (*sindok kokop*). Such dwelling places are said to be steep mountainous regions that surround Gua village, as well as certain almost impassable parts of the Yupno gorge. However, the bush-spirit also lives where, in former times, a men's house (*mbema yut*) of two partner clans (*ngapma ngapma*) stood, and where the "strength-holder of the settlement" (*kokop kɨrat*) of this traditional settlement (*mbema*) was kept. Only members of these partner clans may stay there without danger; men from other clans would be punished with illness (burns, headaches, nausea and so on) by the angry *sindok*, because they lack permission to be in such a forbidden area. Because the *sindok* "normally" dwells outside the village region, it mainly becomes active during hunts (for its "children," the marsupials) and (more rarely) when a new garden is established in the bush.

To prevent the *sindok* bush-spirit being exposed to a possible hot annoyance, which might, for example, follow the making of a new garden or the construction of a new bush house within its area, people will place a bundle of white or whitish leaves and plants there, since these are thought to be very cold. This plant bundle is called *mbaak* ("very cold," "ice-cold;" see Chapter 3.2.), and is meant to make the bush-spirit cold and thereby inactive. The individual components of this *mbaak* bundle may vary depending on clan-specific knowledge and the availability of the plants. Typically, however, a *mbaak* bundle consists of the following components: the small flower *ndetkok*, "bird shit," the white ("cold") soil *kuak*, the light-green (to the Yupno: "white," "cold") leaves of the *joñwijok* and *nyaknkuak* trees, which are smeared with *kuak* soil. Also sometimes included are the white lichen *ilakilak*, the light-green plant *petmbat*, the banana variety *ngolda*, the plants *mbañgam*, *kwebekal*, *ngapmba*, the moss *boa* (all of them light-green, whitish or watery, "cold" plants) and *wuek*, an earth-worm; old money (for example, now-worthless coins such as Australian pennies or shillings) or *tiri* (Job's tears, which resemble the traditional shell-money *yimat*) and—as a more modern component—white ("cold") paper. The money or "money look-alikes" is meant to soothe the *sindok*. The idea of reciprocity that underpins Yupno social life also marks people's relationships with the anti-social *sindok* bush-spirit.

b) The *Sindok*'s Reactions and Their Consequences

Despite this ice-cold bundle (*mbaak*), which is intended as a prophylaxis against the *sindok*, the bush-spirit may become active and cause illness. Yet it does not harm people completely at random or without a reason. It controls and administers certain areas, animals (like marsupials) and plants that have been cultivated at certain places. These include the pandanus, which was brought to the Yupno by the *kunagat amin*, the "pandanus-man," from Yawan (the Yupno name for the Som-Orowa region). If a person, intentionally or not, behaves improperly in the realm for which the bush-spirit is responsible, the offender thus insults or angers the *sindok* bush-spirit, which then becomes "hot," and might inflict illness upon that person or a relative.

The *sindok* may become active in various ways, but most frequently it acts according to the following basic pattern: if a man goes hunting and shoots too many marsupials ("children" of the *sindok*), this annoys the *sindok*, which then punishes the hunter by putting him into a seemingly drunk state during the cooking and eating of the marsupials in the evening, through contact with his (charged, annoyed, "hot") *moñan* ("breath spirit"). The victim vomits, falls asleep, then rolls into the burning fire and is badly burnt. These burns are treated like normal burns with certain leaves (see Chapter 5.1.b.), but in addition a specialist, the *pieñ amɨn*, a "fumigator," is summoned to chase the *sindok* from the house of the patient, using certain formulae and the stinking smell of the smoldering bark cloth *pieñ*.

The following report, in which an old man tells about his mother's *sindok*-illness, also shows this typical basic pattern:

> At the time, we were living in the bush, at Mamal [a part of the bush above Gua], it was just at a time of fighting. And all the paternal relatives were still alive, everybody went to Mamal together, and there we remained, I was still very small. A *wau* [namesake] caught a tree kangaroo in a trap and gave it to me. We did not cook it, we just put it aside. We prepared everything to go to our *mbema* [traditional settlement] and we cooked a bit of food, and a part we put aside for all the men who were in the place. The recently-caught tree kangaroo was kept hidden. It was hanging in the sling and the *wau* gave it to me and I took *ndamba* [a kind of fern] and wrapped it and put it away in the netbag and we went up to Nikat. There I slept together with Njambe, and there we cooked it [Jowage, Kamda, Kamake and other men] and put part of it away in a netbag. And Njambe said to me: 'give this cooked piece there to your brothers and your mother.'
>
> And I went up and took the tree kangaroo with me, Njambe had gutted it and stripped off its fur. Its fur we gave to my mother, and Kamake and his father went away. And they had made a fire for my mother, and this *sindok* tree kangaroo burned my mother in the fire! It did not stop! And there I was up above, in a different house, I was in Kamda's house. There I was up there and I went down into the house where my mother was and I saw her. Njambe and his wife were sound asleep [in a different house]. And the *sindok* had grabbed my mother and thrown her into the fire. I saw it. What was I to do to get her out of the fire? It was not like it is now, I was a small boy and could not get her out. I pulled at her and pulled at her and I did not succeed, she was too heavy and she kept sliding more and more into the fire. And I gave up and called for Nawi and Derañge. The two of them were sleeping in the *mbema yut* [bachelors' house], they heard nothing, and I stopped calling and woke up

Njambe, and Njambe jumped up and pulled this woman to the edge of the fire. And she was lying at the fire's edge and out of the flame came a snake, long as a creeping vine, and wound itself past us to the door. And it was not afraid of us. I saw that.

And we [he and the men who had been notified in the meantime] banned the *sindok* [which had changed into the shape of the snake], made *pień* [smoked it out], and we said: '*morak mane kawam kuak tami!*' [Very freely translated: "*sindok*, you are now completely out in the cold and destroyed!"] Then we put the snake into a bamboo pipe and laid it down in the house, took *jońwijok* leaves, *petmbat*, *nyaknkuak* [an "ice-cold bundle" (*mbaak*)] and killed the snake and said again: '*morak mane kawam kuak!*' ["*sindok*, you are now completely out in the cold!"]

And half my mother's body had been burned. We tried everything possible [medicine against burns, *kandap arap*, see Chapter 5.1.b.], without success. We carried the mother around, into different houses, she stayed for a bit there, lived for a while in another house, stayed there, this is how it went, and after a time her wounds dried up. Later, she went to Gwamakkokop [Gobbayon in the Nankina valley] and died there.

The *pień*-ritual does not always succeed in banning the *sindok* bush-spirit, which may resort to other "tricks" to harm people—often over a longer period of time, as the following illness report about Esemi shows.

In Paiamba [an area near Uskokop village] Esemi and Añganeyu [two men from Uskokop] were once making a sweet potato garden, and found a *sindok kirat* [a bone of *the sindok*]…They picked it up, looked at it and simply threw it away. First, it [this bone, meaning: the *sindok*] hurt Añganeyu, burned him in the fire. And afterwards they all went, burned *pień* bark cloth and cut *umban* leaves and took *tiri* [necklaces of Job's tears] and put it down [there where the bone had been found] and left. This is how they did it, and Añganeyu got well. This is how it was.

Later he [Añganeyu] gave up the piece of bush he had cleared to make a garden and Esemi built a fence and he and his family planted sweet potatoes and cabbage. One day, they all went into their house, they wanted to sleep, and when they were all sitting in the house, they heard a woman from Mogatimin [an area near Uskokop], from that region, sing the *końgap* melody of Sipimi [a man from Uskokop], she sang it. And she also sang Esemi's *koñgap* melody. And Esemi was sitting there and heard her and said: 'I think they have stolen or are fighting or something like it, and that is why she is singing the *koñgap*.' And he was sitting there and listening and from the direction of Dalgowañ [an area near Uskokop] again two women were singing Esemi's *koñgap* melody. Esemi and his relatives heard them, but they remained seated, and the two women again sang the *koñgap* melody, and this is how it went, and Esemi and his relatives fell asleep.

The next morning, it was raining heavily, and it did not stop raining, and they slept on, and in the night Esemi dreamt that two women were talking about marrying him, Esemi. One said: 'I will marry him.' The other said: 'no, I will marry him.' This is how the two of them talked. He dreamt this, and then he woke up.

The next morning, it was still raining. They were all sitting in the house [the bachelors' house *mbema yut*] and they thought, a small boy, the child of Jim, Teñneka, or another small boy, the child of Takope, Soñok, had come and stood at the door and looked in and gone away again and they thought of the two small boys and asked: 'Soñok?' They were not sure which of the two it could be, and this small boy looked in and put his face against the door and went out. Teut [a relative of Esemi] and Gueko [Esemi's son] lay half-asleep on one side of the fireplace. And they called the name of the small boy, but he had left, and they stopped and thought, he had gone to the women's house [*sak yut*], and they stayed in the house. And they sat in the house, and from above, from the rack above the fire, something black fell down. Teut and Gueko and Teut's child Dabuñgen slept soundly on one side. Esemi felt this black thing fall onto his skin, and he thought: 'this just fell down like that.' He did not look at it but threw it off and went back to sleep. Then, again, some black particles fell onto Esemi's face. He wiped off these black bits of soot and turned around and looked up, and a tree kangaroo with a white belly [a *ndankwit*] was sitting up above, in the middle of the house, and was looking at Esemi.

Esemi woke up all the sleepers and said: 'just look at that!' Dabuñgen and his father Teut looked up and got scared and ran out of the house, Gueko also got up and went out, and only Esemi stayed in the house and said: 'hey, one of you should come and try to hold it [the animal], so we can take a closer look at it, if I alone try to catch it, it is not good.' And they said: 'normally it does not come into a house!' and they were afraid and went on standing outside. Esemi coaxed them to hold him since he wanted to climb up high into the roof. Thereupon Gueko went inside and got the tree-kangaroo. And he held it, and it did not show fear and did not bite him, no, it was completely tame.

He carried it outside and stuffed it into a netbag. They gave it tree tomatoes, and it ate a lot of them. And they gave it other food and put it away again into the netbag, and it slept underneath the house. They gave it sweet potatoes and fruit, and it ate well and lived with them, for quite some time. They got it out of the netbag and let it climb around in the house, and it slept in the house, ran around outside for a bit, came back into the house, slept, and it went on like this for a long time.

One day, Porenau [a man from Uskokop] took it, carried it to Bapsum [an area near Uskokop] and let it run around his garden, and it ate up everything. And this *sindok* [the tree kangaroo] hurt Koki, Porenau's brother, and burned his feet. They asked Esemi: 'why did you bring this tree-kangaroo? You, come now and do something [a *pieñ*-ritual] against the *sindok*, and the boy [Koki] will get well.' And Esemi did not do anything, he just did not do anything at all.

And one day Esemi's wife went mad [*wulawula*], and she went to Sandubo [an area near Uskokop] with Teñneka, Jim's child. Teñneka went with her and left her in Wakumne's pandanus garden. Teñneka went, to check on his traps. And I think, the *sindok* killed her in this place, and she died. Teñneka saw, she was dead, and he came back to the village, but he did not say anything, he was scared. And the old woman was lying there, rotting, and the men were running around, looking for her. And Teñneka saw all the men, how they were looking for her, but he did not say anything, he just watched. They were all running around to find her, they looked and looked and looked, and finally they found her bones. And the bones they buried.

The careless throwing away of the *sindok* bone (*sindok kɨrat*) found during the making of a new garden hence did not remain without consequences for Esemi. At first, the *sindok* bush-spirit lived as a peaceful tree kangaroo in his house, but then devoured everything in a garden and caused burns in another man. Esemi did not do anything, and as the next thing the bush-spirit induced in Esemi's wife a state of "mental disturbance," *wulawula* (mad, out of one's mind), in which she met her death. Either the afflicted becomes completely mentally deranged and disoriented, or suffers from fits, rants, and rages and may threaten other people, demolish houses, or shoot randomly with bow and arrow.[44] In such a state, the afflicted person is bound hand and foot and watched over by others until the seizure is over and he has calmed or "cooled" down again.

This illness is rare, and I was unable follow up a case of it. However, a coastal man living in Teptep, a 'didiman' (a Lutheran agricultural development planner), suffered such a seizure, and tore through Teptep station as if he was out of his mind, shot around himself with bow and arrow, and destroyed the furniture of his house and broke all the windows. He was eventually overpowered by other men and treated with sedatives at the health center. The inhabitants of Gua interpreted his behavior as a typical *wulawula* disturbance.

As therapy to end such an attack, a somewhat modified form of the ice-cold bundle (*mbaak*) is performed, the afore-mentioned cold plants are collected, crushed in a bamboo pipe and mixed with old peoples' urine (again, something very "cold"). The victim's skin is rubbed with it and thereby cooled down.

The *sindok* bush-spirit knows further methods to harm people. It can smuggle small stones (a small black stone, *tip pilɨn*, or a white stone, *tip kuakuaga*) or a small piece of bamboo into the human body. Nobody in Gua, however, knows anything definite about this, though it is supposed to be widespread in the villages of Kewieñ, Nokopo and Isan as well as in the Nankina region

As mentioned above, the *sindok* bush-spirit is also linked with the pandanus complex. The "pandanus-man" (*kunagat amɨn*) who brought pandanus to the Yupno was the child of the Uñdamon bird, the "strength-holder of the settlement" (*kokop kɨrat*) of some clans from Devil. He came in the shape of a bird (as the *ngamat* bird) to the Yupno region, stopped there and urinated. Out of his urine originated two small streams, and there he planted pandanus trees. Then he flew to a different place. The pandanus fruits from this region are "different," "forbidden" (*tɨlagɨ*), since the "pandanus-man" himself planted them, and the *sindok* bush-spirit, acting for the flown-away "pandanus-man" and his mother, the Uñdamon bird, may punish anyone who eats from these pandanus fruits.

Thus the activities of the *sindok* bush-spirit are many. Its most frequent action is to make people suffer burns (as in the case of Jowage's mother), which are mostly unambiguously recognized as *sindok tauak*, "signs of the *sindok*." Yet it can also do harm over a longer period of time, take on the form of animals (a tree kangaroo, in the case of Esemi) or also cause people to be ill through contact with plants like the pandanus fruit. In rare cases it causes mental disturbances. The major cause of its harmful behavior is a conscious or unconscious misdemeanor committed by people against its environmental domain: places where a men's' house once stood (hence places held to be *tɨlagɨ*, "different," "forbidden"), inaccessible places like the faces of cliffs or steep mountainous regions, and the bush area, as well as the animals living there (above all, tree kangaroos, but also certain birds, snakes and lizards) and trees such as the pandanus. In contrast to the inhabited village region and the cultivated garden land, for which the people are "responsible," the bush-spirit *sindok* rules over the "non-social," religiously marked, topographically conspicuous environment that is not controlled by humans.

4. The Sorcery Techniques *Sɨt* and *Mawom* and the Search for the Instigator

Very serious illnesses, which frequently end in death, are caused by men who specialize in two different ritual "techniques,"[45] *sɨt* and *mawom*, which are thought to cause the worst illness.

Y., an exceptionally clever "burner" (*sɨt amɨn*) and pragmatist, echoes the sentiments of many men when he discusses his attitude to the two alternatives, *mawom* and *sɨt*:

> There are two possibilities. You know the government has now prohibited killing somebody publicly. If I kill somebody in public, I am going to end up in prison. In order to end my hatred, there are only two ways: I commission a *mawom amɨn* or I take a little piece of left-over food from my enemy and give it to a *sɨt amɨn*. He will die, and my hatred is over. My friends ['wantok'] have thus solved my *njɨgɨ* [his "oppressing problem," meaning: his hatred for his enemy].

Both "techniques" have some things in common. Knowledge about *sɨt* and *mawom* acts is passed on in one's own clan (more rarely also between partner clans); the specialist chooses as an "apprentice" one of his (own) sons or the child of one of his brothers, a boy held to be discreet. The boy should be between twelve or seventeen years of age, ideally pubescent but "chaste," that is, very "hot."

The social setting in which the instigator and the victim find themselves varies greatly: *sɨt* and *mawom* may be ordered by family members among themselves, within the clan, the partner clan (*ngapma*), within the village or even against non-related people from other villages. Both kinds, however, are as a rule only applied in cases of conflicts with deep-seated causes (such as deaths in one' own family caused by *sɨt* or *mawom*, illicit sexual contacts, or repeated theft of pigs). Since a narrowing of the social space (to own clan or own family) mostly parallels an increase in social conflicts, most of the illness-causing *sɨt*- and *mawom*-acts happen within the clan or the partner clan.

Both *sɨt* and *mawom* are performed for a fee, and both kinds cause illness that may eventually kill people through the loss of their *amɨnwop* ("shadow soul"), but the concepts of action and effect on which they are based differ. The method of *sɨt*, more popular with the upper Yupno, is presented first.

a) *Sɨt*

I

Sɨt literally means: "I burn, heat, cook." The term, as already mentioned (see Chapter 4.1.e.), is the generic noun for "illness" in general, a condition therefore, which has a cause (*mevɨli toñ*). Furthermore, *sɨt* also means a certain cause of illness, called 'poisin' in Tok Pisin, which is described as "personal leavings and food remains sorcery" (Patterson 1974/75: 141) "parcel sorcery" (Knauft 1985: 110) or "leavings sorcery" (Strathern & Stewart 1999: 103). The Yupno themselves talk in the context of *sɨt* of *amɨn kasit*, "caused by the hand of a man," and thereby precisely express the central element (one that is different from the other causes of illness) of this cause: i.e. a "technique" employed by a specialist with the aim of making someone ill.

Sɨt is used in two ways: as a generic noun for "illness" and, to the Yupno, together with *mawom*, the worst and most threatening cause of illness. *Sɨt* is far more common in everyday life among the Yupno than *mawom*.

The precise manner of performing a *sɨt*-act varies from clan to clan and depends on individual and clan-specific knowledge. Even the paraphernalia differ from specialist to specialist, thus more modern substances may be used; for example, the red soil *mañot* instead of the more effective since "hotter" but difficult to obtain *kowa* paste. The ritual is therefore not at all rigidly fixed ceremonially but varies according to the knowledge of the specialist and the implements at hand. All the components applied, however, belong to the "hot-cool-cold"-system, and all the acts are anchored in the religious system. In other words, within the framework of the Yupno "hot-cool-cold" classification, which is strictly followed by all, and the shared system of belief, thought and knowledge, innumerable variations are possible.

Apropos *sɨt*, Patrol Officer Rylands (1945: Appendix) notes in his patrol report (1945) under the heading "NATIVE BELIEFS AND CUSTOMS IN THE URUWA AND YUPNA VALLEYS (HUON. DIST.):

SORCERY: Only the old men are supposed to know the rites and others pay them to cast spells [...] METHODS: Leavings of the victim's food are heated in a fire together with a stone. This can bring about most illnesses. The leaves of the KAWAL [probably 'kawawar', ginger] (an ornamental shrub) can be used instead of leavings and with equally good results, notwithstanding the fact that the victim has had no contact with the leaves. ANTIDOTES: If a man is sick and thinks a given individual has directed a spell against him; [sic] the sick man's brother or other male relatives go to the alleged sorcerer and demand the material with which the spell was worked, under threat of bodily violence. If the alleged sorcerer admits his part in the affair (and probably in any case if he thinks the sick man will recover) he hands over whatever materials he has on hand and the male relatives throw it into running water. If the sick man recovers, they then pay the sorcerer on the understanding that he will never work against that particular man again. My informants said that of course all these practices had stopped since the native Mission Teachers frowned on them (Rylands 1945:Appendix).

II

Knowledge about *sɨt*-acts is shared by most of the (older) Yupno men, and especially among the more tradition-oriented men, it is thought to be full of prestige and belongs to the general knowledge of a respected man. Nevertheless, nobody would call himself a "burner" or publicly admit to being one, since this would very quickly expose oneself to suspicion in a case of illness and could create enemies. Asked about this topic, many of the older men admitted knowing about *sɨt* and in part also being able to perform it, but at the same time insisted that they had never practiced it. But within the village and also with respect to other villages, people know who is a "burner" (*sɨt amɨn*) and who is not.

As with *mawom* (see below), the "burner" (*sɨt amɨn*) does not perform the act himself but supervises one or several unmarried, "hot" boys, for two reasons: every *sɨt*-act is dangerous for the performers, and the "burner" or the one or several of the boys[46] could be harmed if they make a "mistake" during the performance. The more important reason probably lies in the fact that a married man is no longer "hot" enough since he has progressively cooled down as a result of repeated sexual relations with his wife, whose "vital energy" (*tevan-tok*) and *moñan* ("breath spirit") are thought to be "cooler." For this reason, the "burners" formerly remained unmarried and mostly had their own small men's house (*mbema yut*, the same term as for the bachelors' house), where they kept the paraphernalia. This house in most cases stood in the village,[47] and in outward appearance did not differ at all from normal dwelling houses (*tedetedeyut*).

III

The basic pattern of a *sit*-act aimed at bringing about the death of a victim, and typical of the clan Y. in K. village, is as follows: the "burner" waits until he gets one or more parcels in which a particle[48] imbued with the future victim's *moñan* ("breath spirit") is contained. They are called *njaapndak*, "left-overs," people then say about the "burner" "*njaapndak awedak*," "he received left-overs." The "burner" takes these *njaapndak*-parcels into the men's house (his own clan's *mbema yut* or formerly the one owned together with the partner clan) and starts the preparations by looking for the leaves that are important for the performance. The collection of this ("hot") plant material is already dangerous since the heat may transfer to the specialist. As a counter-measure to ensure that these hot plants do not harm himself or one of his own relatives, the specialist lets a piece of bark cloth smolder. The smoldering of this bark cloth relates clearly to the activities of the *sindok* bush-spirit, since this act is meant to prevent it from doing harm. All hot leaves grow deep in the bush, the domain of the bush-spirit *sindok*, and are therefore potentially dangerous.

There are variations in the performance of the procedures that follow; here I present two of them. The first version was initially told to me by a man from Gua, during a long talk, and then was discussed and completed in subsequent conversations with him.

Version 1

After the completion of his preparations (collection of the "hot" plants), the "burner" chooses two or three boys from his own clan or the partner clan who have not yet had any sexual relations and hence still have a totally "hot," intact "vital energy" (*tevantok*). These boys are called *nap mbisap amin*, "knot-tier," since they tie the parcels (with the leaves).[49]

Special preparations are necessary for their task. The boys may not leave the men's house for a week; and they are fed special food (*luplup* bananas, taro, sweet potatoes). Their excrement and their urine are carefully filled into bamboo pipes in the men's house and stored, as they are "different," "forbidden," "taboo" (*tilagi*). Everything that formerly adhered to them, as, for example, the *moñan* ("breath spirit") of the women who cooked their food, has to be excreted. During the night before the actual performance, the *njaapndak* parcels are smoked over the fire on a rack and "heated up." Certain leaves are now mixed into the boys' food that make them vomit and act as if drunk; their physical condition has been once again fundamentally "made different" (*tɨlagɨ*) and they are now in a "hot" state.

The next morning, the boys, under the supervision of the "burner," put the *njaapndak* parcels in a row along the fireplace, on the other side of which a *sindok kɨrat* (a "bone of the *sindok* bush-spirit") and a *kokop kɨrat* (a "strength-holder of the settlement" of two partner clans or of the village) are placed. The direction of the rays of the sun and the wind are important in this: they both have to come from one direction, and in no case may the shadow of the boys fall onto the "bone of the bush-spirit" (*sindok kɨrat*) or the wind blow their breath in its direction and mix with the parcels, lest the *moñan* ("breath spirit") of the boys also be heated and destroyed. The boys now build a "nest" out of ("hot") *njogal* leaves for each parcel. The "burner" (*sɨt amɨn*) then calls the names of the one or several victims as well as of the instigator. The boys scatter a few crumbs of *kowa* (red, very "hot" crumbly paste) onto each parcel. Then for each parcel the tongue of a previously caught *kak amɨn* lizard is torn out with a *patndan* leaf and is then put on every parcel. The lizard is thought to be the substitute for the victim, and its tongue represents his or her *moñan* ("breath spirit"), which is in the parcel.

The boys now tie the parcels very carefully with the left ("colder") hand in order to avoid wrapping up any of their own *moñan* ("breath spirit"), which is more strongly present in their "hotter" right hand. Then the parcels are carefully carried by two boys, each with two sticks, to a little bush house *sɨt yut*, which had been erected beforehand, especially for this act, in a remote part of the bush belonging to the "burner's" clan. As a further precaution against unauthorized people, the path leading there is closed off.

The bush house *sɨt yut* is completely sealed off against the daylight, and is decorated with leaves that give the house "strength" (*tevantok*); these "heat" it and are supposed to make it "different" (*tɨlagɨ*). The leaves come from the following plants: *komndak maam* (a ginger species), *tapmat* (a thorny creeping vine species) and *mbomak*, the stinging nettle-like plants *kokopyaal*, *yaal* and from the *makum* tree (the leaves of which are thorny). In the house, a big fire is lit (traditionally with a fire-saw) using wood that burns well, from the *tekop kandap*, *ndalndal* and *tañgwin* trees. The ginger leaves (*komndak maam*) are put on the fire, then the parcels are placed on top, and the men close the door and leave the house. This phase is called "*meñ kalap mbɨsap*, "time of the origin of the flesh," meaning: the victim is to die and only his body (flesh) is to remain.

Inside the door, the "bone of the bush-spirit *sindok*," smeared with red ("hot") soil (*kowa* or *mañot*) and/or the ("hot") blood of a young girl, watches out, together with the "strength-holder of the settlement" (*kokop kɨrat*), so that the *moñan* ("breath spirit") of the one or several victims cannot escape. From the outside, everybody now listens to the *sindok* "devouring" the parcels, making the victims scream like tree kangaroos.

Some time after the burning of the *njaapndak* parcels, the "burner" gets the ash, carries it into the bush and rubs it between two trees with dry bark, which grow so close that they rub against each other in the wind. In versions provided by other men the moment of the victim's death remains uncertain, but in the one given by Y. from Gua death happens precisely when the ash is rubbed between the trees.

After completion of the *sɨt*-act, the "burner" and the "knottiers" have to cleanse themselves ritually, "cool down" and perform a *koñ mɨndak*,[50] a "prophylactic" ritual "chasing away of the ghost" to render harmless the certainly angry "souls of dead persons" (*koñwop*) of the victims. Without this "chasing away of the ghost," women and children are also exposed to the danger of getting an "oppressing problem" (*njɨgɨ*) through an angry *koñ* ("ghost") or of becoming ill through the *nduara*, the "left-over" of the *sɨt*-act.

First, all the participants go into the bush to hunt for marsupials, birds and/or wild pigs. The pigs' bristles and the feathers are cooked and wrapped in a leaf with which all the participants rub their skin. This is called *kawañ susoñ*, "to burn the smell." The "burner" now mixes and crushes the pig- or bird-blood with white soil (*kuak*) and ("cold") *petmbat, joñwijok* and *nyaknkuak* leaves in a bamboo-pipe; the resulting mixture has to be whitish in color. With a young banana shoot (of the "cold" *mbɨlañ*-variety) as a mortar, he again and again stirs the concoction and mixes *komndak maam*, the aforementioned ginger, in with it. With the banana shoot (beaten flat, like a spatula), the mixture is smeared onto the skin of all the participants. They all go to a river (Daldal or Yupno), where the "burner" takes a part of the *talbeñ* plant, a climbing vine which for this ritual has to grow on a rock. He stands next to this rock, close to the water, and pulls the plant off the rock; he then anoints all those present with the plant and afterwards throws it into the current. In addition, he says:

talbeñ	*koñi*	*talbeñ*	*dayañ*	*nyinda*		
plant name	ghost	plant name	as well	like you (pl.)		

kwinon	*ndima*	*awoñ*	*wo*	*teakkonni*	*abnjak*	
up above	no	come	go	into our throats	now	

pankuakeak		*kikañ*	*ndepno*	*mpagmbe*	*bamen*
to have cooled down		to go away	desert	water	big

tapmon	*kuañndo*	*mbɨtnyiren*	*kong.*
to the coast	go	like your feelings	see.

talbeñ plant, your 'ghosts' are like the *talbeñ* plant, you cannot settle on us [our skin], nor go into our throats. Now you leave, cooled down, you desert us for the ocean, you go to the coast, you will feel that you are there.

Hereafter, all the participants may go to their dwelling houses or into other houses without danger. The boys may first only eat *joñgat* bananas, and must remain tranquil and not start any fights, lest they immediately get into a hot state again. Two to three weeks later, the "burner" completes the sequence by killing some pigs, which he gives to the boys as his thank-you.

Version 2[51]

The "burner" sits next to the fire with a boy and prepares large, hard-to-tear leaves of the *kidiñ* tree as an outer cover for the *njaapndak*-parcels. Onto these he puts lilac-colored serrated *zarak* leaves, on top of them the smaller red ("hot") *mbok* leaves, then humid mushrooms (*yavɨt*) and fern of the *mbabuñ*-variety. On top of it he puts a paste from the sap and resin of the three "hot," special trees *sɨmbu*, *kulmak* and *ngoman*. The leaves of the ("hot") ginger *kokop kɨrat maam* are put over it. The *ndamba* fern is crushed separately, squashed and mixed with ash (or black soil) and the *mbok* and *zarak* leaves. The right elbow of the boy, the "knottier," is pressed into this mixture. The *njaapndak* parcel is laid on the prepared leaves, which are carefully rolled up and the tips of the leaves bent back. The boy then wraps the *njaapndak* parcels with two kinds of lianas: *ndaloñndaloñ* and *mambak*. He holds the parcel in the left, colder hand and wraps with the right, hotter hand. In the meantime, the "burner" breaks the stem of the *ndamba ɨsip* fern into pieces of about 10 cm while calling the names of the victims and instigators. With this, the *moñan* ("breath spirit") of the victims gets "broken." The parcels are stuffed into a bamboo pipe and smoked over the fire. Then the boy breaks the bamboo pipe with a special "black stone," *tɨp pɨlɨn,* and burns the remains. With this, the *sɨt*-act of this version concludes.

If a "burner" does not (as in version 1) want to kill his victim but only cause illness, he has various possibilities:

- if he does not burn the *njaapndak* parcel but envelops it with clay-like *wawɨt* soil, the victim will fall ill with *keaknok*, meaning to "continuously swallow what one has coughed up" (see Chapter 5.1.b).

- If, before all the preparations, he puts the parcel under a stone, the victim will first become (less seriously) ill, but can then be healed.
- If the "burner" does not burn the parcel but only smokes it or puts it on the ashes (see the following story), the victim will get seriously ill but will not die.

IV

Even though *sit* is the worst cause of illness for the Yupno, in no way is every *sit*-act deadly for the victim, as can be seen from the following reports. Most of the older men have survived several *sit*-attacks, though sometimes with complications.

Jowage, an old man from Gua, tells about his first *sit*-illness:

At the time, when Mapte [a man from the Ngangalbuk clan] wanted to marry Wolgañ, we were in Bapsin [a part of the bush above Gua]. And Asinu [a relative of J.] talked to me about his wife Jirat. [She had been raped by Timu]. The two of us [J. and Asinu] shot at Timu. And Guamda [a friend of Timu] got *njaapndak* [particles on which our *moñan* ("breath spirit") was adhering] of me and Asinu and gave it to the Teptep people.

Asinu had gone down [to the lower Yupno region] to get betel nuts. He followed the way of the betel nuts [the usual route] and shot into a *makum* tree [a tree with very big leaves into which the men often shoot arrows for testing], and a boy, Daop, found the arrow and came to the village and told the men about it. The men cut down this *makum* tree and took the arrow, and thus they also got the remains [the *njaapndak*] of the arrow [and thereby Asinu's *moñan* ("breath spirit")]. I do not know what they got from me, which part. Where was I at the time, and what did they get?

They took us [the *njaapndak* parcels with the *moñan*] and took us to Pitimka; in the middle of this piece of grassland there stands a tree. They built a house [*sit yut*] and made a huge fire. And they performed *sit* on us and cooked us [our *moñan*], but only in the ashes.

[At his time] a friend went to Nankina, and the men there said to him: 'your relative is dying now.' And Mian [a relative of J. from Nankina] came up [into the Yupno Valley] and made *kuak* [a "technique" to discover the culprit, see below], and *kuak* pointed to the way to Kangulut, but the men in Kangulut had already destroyed ["heated up"] this stuff [*njaapndak*]. Pisikaloñ, Dodek, Kaloñ, Yindapnaroñ [friends of J. from Teptep], this group was talking and came, to help me, and I got well. If they had not helped, I would already have died.

The two of us, Asinu and I, we almost died at the time. We both were very ill and slept in Kumamɨn. Asinu had made himself a bed from bark cloth, it was very hot, and he was sweating so much that the bark cloth got wet, he slept on it and I, it was the rainy season, I also made myself a bed out of a *ndavɨsal*-bark cloth, and I did not sleep, I sat there, and I was sweating, my sweat was running like water, and my *ndavɨsal* was completely wet. And I was very ill, I was only skin and bones, sweat was running from my nose, out of my back, from my armpits and it ran like water. And so the two of us were sitting there, and Jipa [another relative] was running around outside and was looking after us, and the two of us sweated so much, he became scared. And he said: 'you two are sweating so much. Where is there somebody running around to help you both?' [People fallen ill through *sɨt* sweat even more heavily when a member of the partner clan (*ngapma*) goes in search of "cold" sugarcane, which is provided by the *sɨt amɨn*. The partner clan member then gives this antidote for *sɨt* to the sick person (see Chapter 5.2.d.)]. This is what he said.

And Asinu slept, he slept like a lake. The bark cloth he was lying on was completely soaked. And my bed was also all wet. And so Jipa saw the two of us, became scared, the two of us were sitting there, and Yindapnaroñ came and had filled up a lot of betel nuts. He came to the door, and I pulled myself up and said: 'get some betel nuts!' Yindapnaroñ said: 'there are betel nuts!' He unpacked them all and put them down for the two of us. And Asinu and I, as we were close to death, got up and ate up these betel nuts. And at that time we got well. At that time, Yindapnaroñ first came to the two of us, and after him followed Kaloñ, and at that time the two of them helped us [meaning: got sugar cane from the *sɨt amɨn* and brought betel nuts], and now I am well.

Jowage reports on his second *sɨt*-illness:

[First, Jowage tells how he got into a fight with his father Kamda and Kamake, the latter's brother, over a brideprice. But the business seemed to have been settled, and everybody was living together in a hamlet.]

Kamda and Kamake were living in Kumamɨn. And so did I, I was together with them at that time. The two of them lived in their homestead and I in mine. One day, my wife Umbañne and my sister Sambañ carried sugar-cane up to Depok [an area near Gua], and I was on the way with my brothers, with Timu, Komda, Gunagbe, Take, Erana and Nayot. We were hunting for birds in the bush, and I parted with the boys in their homestead and came down, stood at my fence, and the two [women] brought sugar-cane to the pig fence, and I got a sugar-cane and ate it, I peeled off the hard outer skin, threw it away and ate the sugar, and the two of them sent me off, and I made fire in the house.

I was busy lighting the fire and sat down, when my sister Sambañ came back and said to me: 'I thought, your father, Kamda, wanted to smoke, but he broke a pandanus nut, put the skin into the 'tiktik' [reed grass], and he put it on fire and took the skin of the sugar-cane which you have eaten and thrown away, and he came down.' And furthermore she said: 'your two fathers [Kamda and Kamake] are doing something evil with you, they have got the skin of the sugar-cane, which you have eaten, I have seen it, and you have to keep your eye on the two of them, why are they running around?' This is how she spoke to me, and I watched Kamda and Kamake. The two of them had fetched the small piece of sugar-cane, and first they stayed around for a while.

Then Kamda left us and very quickly went down to Nankina and gave this little piece to the Nankina men and said: 'I watch, and you make sɨt.' This is how he spoke to Tsiñgoñgoñ and his brothers, and at that time they hence had me [the moñan ("breath spirit") adhering to the sugar-cane skin] and made sɨt with me. This is how it went, they put part of the little piece of sugar-cane from me against the trunk of a tree, it is called kisaran, and kept it there in a bamboo.

But the tree broke and smashed the bamboo [in which the little piece of sugarcane was stored]. They had therefore put the njaapndak from me at this tree and had gone to sleep, and in the morning they saw that the tree covered the njaapndak. They said: 'awa!' [roughly: "Goodness me!"] I had noticed that Kamda had slept in Nankina for two nights and had come up [to Gua], and I went around him [went out of his way] and went to Nankina and asked them: 'why did Kamda come down [to Nankina]?' This is how I asked, and Kuambe said: 'he brought down a *njaapndak* of a man, a little piece of sugar-cane skin. They touched the little piece and left it. They [Kamda and Kamake] cooked it in a piece of pandanus skin, and he [Kamda] brought it. We all touched this pandanus skin and the [other] little piece of sugar-cane skin and made *sɨt*, and the sugar-cane skin [one of the small pieces] is there!'

This is how they talked to me, and I brought the little piece of sugar-cane skin up here, and they had taken the pandanus skin [on which through its contact with the little piece of sugar-cane *moñan* from J. was adhering as well] and wanted to "burn" me [*sɨt*] and had put it [together with the sugar-cane piece] at the tree, but the tree had broken and was covering the bamboo.

Well, this is how it is, and always when trees fall over or when men cut down trees, they [the trees] want to kill me, and this [the little piece of sugar-cane and the pandanus skin under the fallen tree] does it and finds me out and follows me. Well, once a tree in Tapen broke and injured me and destroyed my voice, and I cannot talk well any more, and some other time, in Kamkwam, a branch broke off and also injured me. And always when trees are cut down, I stay away. [He points to a tree standing far away] If you cut down this tree and I stand here, it will hit me, and it will fall up here and hurt me.[52]

Partially completed but actually failed *sɨt*-acts may over a long period of time also result in consequences for the person concerned that could hardly be interpreted as "accidents."

V

Generalizing at a more abstract level, we may note for a *sɨt*-act that, if someone wants to make somebody ill or kill a person whom he feels is an enemy through *sɨt*, he has to obtain something with which the person concerned has been in contact. This object, called *njaapndak*, was part of him (hair, saliva, etc.) or had been touched by him (e.g., left-over food), and is therefore impregnated with his *moñan* substance ("breath spirit"). It is wrapped in leaves, put into a bamboo pipe or—as in the story above—stored in a pandanus skin; the *moñan* ("breath spirit") thereby transfers also to the wrapping enveloping the *njaapndak*. With this, part of his *moñan* ("breath spirit") has been taken from the victim. The "burner" (*sɨt amɨn*) and his helpers heat the particle through "hot" materials (certain leaves, red soil, etc.), and in analogy the *moñan* ("breath spirit") remaining on the victim and not

taken away is also heated; the victim's illness commences, and he or she develops a fever. Although the leaves covering the *njaapndak* are also very hard
to tear, for safety's sake the *njaapndak* parcel is sometimes additionally covered with the clay-like *wawɨt* soil and sealed off; "packaged" like this, the stolen
moñan ("breath spirit") cannot return to its owner. The victim gets worse,
and his *amɨnwop* ("shadow soul") slowly gets ready to leave him and follow
the stolen *moñan* ("breath spirit").

It could not be discovered when this point of time had arrived and whether
it could be fixed at all. The Yupno did not regard such deliberation and questioning by anthropologists about exact points of time as very important. A
few informants insisted that the *amɨnwop* ("shadow soul") would leave the ill
victim and follow the stolen *moñan* ("breath spirit"), so it had to remain uncertain how it connects itself to this *moñan*-particle. Most informants thought
that the *amɨnwop* ("shadow soul") only leaves the victim at the time of death.
Soon afterwards (in most cases immediately, but some days may also pass),
the "burner" and the boys light an especially big, hot fire, then the "burner"
calls out the name or names of the one or several victims, and the boys burn
the *moñan* ("breath spirit"). This "hottest" and most dangerous part of the
act, the killing of the victim (who may not, however, die immediately), is
watched over by the "bones of the bush-spirit *sindok*" and the "strength-holder
of the settlement" (*kokop kɨrat*), which have been previously heated and
brought into a "different state;" depending on the tradition, further "hot" objects may be added. After the *moñan* ("breath spirit"), which is in the *njaapndak* parcel, has been burnt, the remaining *moñan* still on the victim is over-
heated and also burnt, thus destroying the part that forms his personality.
Without *moñan* ("breath spirit"), the *amɨnwop* ("shadow soul") now also
leaves the human body, and the victim dies. The *amɨnwop* ("shadow soul")
becomes a *koñwop* ("soul of a dead person"), which wanders around "heated
up" and angry about the death of its owner. It may become dangerous to the
participants of the *sɨt*-act, settling on them or their relatives as an "oppressing problem" (*bɨmjɨt*) caused by a "ghost" and cause illness, so it must to be
prophylactically rendered harmless and scared away with the help of the ritual of the "chasing away of a ghost."

It is essential for the treatment of an illness caused by *sɨt* to find out who
has stolen the *moñan* ("breath spirit") contained in the *njaapndak* parcel and
heated it. The manifold "techniques" used to identify the "burner" or instigator are presented below (see Chapter 5.4.c.). If the *sɨt amɨn* is thereby identified, a *ngapma,* a member of the victim's partner clan, will go and demand
from him a piece of sugar-cane (something very "cold"), which the patient
then eats and thus may recover.

The *sɨt-*"technique" practiced by the Yupno may be taken as a "classic" example of 'poison' in Papua New Guinea, if one follows Patterson's (1974/75: 141–42) typical description of this act. It corresponds to many ethnological descriptions of 'poison' where the "heating" or "burning" of particles a person has touched is repeatedly stressed as the central aspect; see, for example, Jones (1980: 225–35), Bowden (1987: 187), Schmitz (1959: 39–40).

b) *Mawom*

The story of the Kiri *amɨn*

[This myth was told by a man from Kwembun, a village in the lower Yupno Valley.]

One day, a man was clearing a piece of bush, because he wanted to make a yam garden. He planted the yams, and some time later he wanted to tie it up, so he took a bamboo shoot and went to the garden. He had already planted the yams, but he wanted to tie up the shoots. Thus he went up, and he saw that a *njɨmuk* [a kind of liana] was growing out of the bamboo shoot. He wanted to tear it out, but no, he pulled and pulled and still pulling it went into the bush.

He thus went into the bush, and the other men went looking for him, and his wife also went looking for him. They looked and looked, without success, and finally they came to the village, and his wife said to them: 'he wanted to go to the garden, where did he go? I went looking for him, without success, and now I have come.' They told all the relatives and acquaintances in the various villages about his disappearance and asked where he was, and many times they looked for him, but they did not find him.

One day, a man came into the bush, and he saw a tree whose fruit was being eaten by many marsupials; again and again, a small piece of fruit fell down. He took a treefruit already bitten into, went to his house and prepared everything, to observe the marsupials. He went back, observed the marsupials, sat there, his eyes closed, and he went to sleep.

The [disappeared] man had decorated himself sumptuously with *mañot* and *noñgum* [red and black earth pigments] and all the paraphernalia for *sɨt* and *mawom* and pigs and hunting [paraphernalia to make the state of pigs or the hunting grounds "different," to "heat up" or make "ice-cold"], everything he got ready, put it ready on a branch, then took a treefruit and threw it at the sleeping man, who was sitting under the tree. He got scared, looked at it and held it, and this fruit was smeared with *mañot* and *noñgum* [earth pigments]. And he went back to sleep again, and the man in the tree again threw down a treefruit. The man below looked at it, turned it, looked at it from all sides. And the man who had formerly run away sat above on a branch. The one below spotted him and told his relatives about it, and they all came, started a fire at the trunk of the tree, cut off all the leaves of the tree, observed the man in the tree, waited around the fire, and it became night; late at night they built a ladder, and they burned a small piece of *mbowañ* [barkcloth belt], which he [the man on the tree] had sometime before thrown away, they made *pieñ* [smoked the piece of bark cloth], and the ladder became longer and longer, reached this man, and he climbed down on it. They brought him to the village. And this man showed them the following: this ginger [*maam*] is for pigs, that one there for yams, this here for *sɨt*, that there for *mawom*. Thus he taught them all and gave it to them, this is for this and that is for that, thus he instructed everybody, and then he died, and they buried him. This is how it [*mawom*] started, the man brought it and gave it to the people, and they make *mawom*.

Mawom, called 'sanguma' (or 'sangguma') in Tok Pisin and referred to in the literature as "assault sorcery" (Glick 1973: 183–84; see also Patterson 1974/75: 143–44),[53] is widespread in Melanesia. In the Yupno region it is confined to the people of the lower areas,[54] but is highly feared by the inhabitants of the upper half of the valley. The whole *mawom*-complex originated on the coast. Danger of *mawom* is suspected (among the upper Yupno[55]) if, for example, strange, unknown men are seen in the village. Word quickly gets around and no inhabitant of Gua will then leave his house on his own. In former times, the Yupno living close to the coast practiced only *mawom* and those living at the upper course of the Yupno River only *sɨt*. Today, knowledge about these two "techniques" may be bought at a very high price, but in fact this very rarely happens.

Mawom is ordered only in the case of conflicts which—as with *sɨt*—have deep-seated causes, and only then a *mawom amɨn* (a man who has the mastery over *mawom* and practices it, a "*mawom*-specialist") will accept the commission. The causes are most often deaths in one's own family caused by *sɨt*- or *mawom*-techniques and for which revenge is sought. Somebody commissions the "*mawom*-specialist," tells him the victim's name, describes his or her appearance and habits in case he does not know the victim and pays him a fee.

Like *sɨt*, *mawom*, too, may only be performed by young, "hot" men. Before a boy performs *mawom* himself, his skills are put to the test. For this initiation, the "*mawom*-specialist" in most cases chooses two to three boys. First they eat the liver of a marsupial—like good hunting dogs—in order to develop the skill to find "meat" quickly. Corresponding to this concept, the *mawom*-novices are called *pañan kalap amɨn*, "hunting-dog men." They are instructed in the correct ways to behave: it is forbidden to eat or drink on the way to or during the *mawom*-performance, to urinate or to defecate, since they (or their adhering *moñan* ["breath spirit"]) could easily be identified through these carriers of contact (left-over food, urine, feces), or to talk to people they meet en route. After this, they have to perform *mawom* on a mentally handicapped person (somebody who is *kadɨm*, mad). If this person does not die, the boy is unsuited for *mawom*; if he or she dies, the initiation is thought to be completed and the boy may now perform this act, though under the supervision of an experienced *mawom*-specialist. A *mawom* team consists of the *mawom*-specialist who supervises the act,[56] and two to three boys.

Once a "commission" for *mawom* has been given, the experienced specialist starts the preparations. First, he looks for *ndamba kuak* plants whose leaves have sharp thorns. Only the inner, rotting, stinking part of the plant is used, so dried outer leaves are removed. Then he collects leaves of the "hot" *mawom* ginger (*mawom maam*). Both plants are only used for the preparation, to make the skin of the boys, the "hunting-dog people," hot and different. In the bush, in a hidden place, he and the boys construct a small *mawom*-house (*mawom yut*), build a rack over the fireplace, and then on top of it put the collected plants together with a *sindok kɨrat*[57] (a "bone of the *sindok* bush-spirit") as well as a bow and arrow (the same that is used to shoot pigs). In this house, the young men who perform *mawom* sleep two to three nights, then they first have to (as with *sɨt* also) excrete all the previous food, cooked by women, and prepare themselves ritually. Again and again they rub their hands in the soot over the rack under which a fire burns and pull on their fingers. This makes their hands flexible for the later act. This preparatory phase is called *moñan milgañ*, "to prepare the breath spirit." Its effect is to remove everything the men had previously been in contact with, hence all the "contact carriers."

After this preparatory ritual, the participants camouflage their bodies with the black earth pigment *noñgum*, pack the "bone of the bush-spirit *sindok*" into a netbag and start out for the victim, carrying this bag and a small piece of wood, *kodok bop* (no translation), which is used again and again for every *mawom*-act and otherwise is kept in the *mbema yut*, the men's house.[58] The aim is to encounter the intended victim while he/she is alone. If the search is unsuccessful, the victim's child may be targeted as a substitute (which, however, is rare). There are cases where the *mawom*-victim is forewarned by a friend or relative, and then will never walk about alone. The victim cannot recognize the *mawom*-men since they camouflage themselves; they may dress up, for example, as a woman with a grass skirt, netbag and a large bundle of *bumbum* reeds on the head, or, should people approach, pretend to be a pair of lovers and run off, driven away by the people. Sometime later, they will try again to catch their victim alone. Once the *mawom*-group has reached its victim, one of the boys sticks the *kodok bop* piece of wood into his mouth, and thus prevents the surprised victim from screaming. Another one draws the arrow, the tip of which has to touch the "bone of the bush-spirit *sindok*" in the netbag, and shoots it at the victim, who is hit. The arrow is removed from his or her body but, because of the "bone of the bush-spirit *sindok*," it never leaves a visible wound. One of the boys scatters a bit of soil in the direction of the victim, calls his or her name and fixes the day on which the victim is to die. The victim goes home but is unable to tell what has happened.

There are varying statements: sometimes the *mawom*-men leave behind a "sign" (*tauak*) of their deed. If a young man or a child was the victim, they cut down a planted tree or a banana shrub, something which has been planted by a man; if the victim was a young woman, they cut down a young bamboo, as the sign for an old man or an old woman, they cut some grasses growing at the spot or on the way. As a "sign," a branch of the *mbɨtkuak* tree may also be broken off in such a way that the whitish side underneath the leaves points up.

After the completion of the *mawom*-act, the *mawom*-men return to their house in the bush. Unlike *sɨt*, no ritual to "chase away a ghost" (*koñ mɨndak*) is performed. The men first sleep two to three days in the *mawom*-house, kill a marsupial, pig or chicken and rub themselves, the "bone of the bush-spirit *sindok*" and the used bow and arrow with the burnt fur, the singed-off pig's bristles or the burnt feathers, and thus return from their "hot" to a "cool" state. Only then can contact with family, wife and children be resumed. The "bone of the bush-spirit *sindok*" is returned to its storage-place, and is admonished to remain there and not follow the *mawom*-men, who promise to come to it again with a new commission.

Very shortly thereafter, the victim will fall seriously ill (since his or her *amɨnwop*, "shadow soul," already prepares itself to leave the injured body[59]) and suffers from shivering fits, headaches and pains in the joints. Not long before the fixed date of death, he or she falls into a state as if drunk and then perhaps tells of his or her *mawom*-experience. If a man well versed in the signs of illness (*tauak*) diagnoses *mawom* as the true cause of illness in good time, only the eating of a coconut picked in a special way may help the patient; it has to be cut when ripe from the coconut tree and cannot be taken from the ground. It cleanses the part of the body where the *mawom*-arrow hit and where (internally) blood may be clotted. The victim vomits this "impurity" and may then recover. "Endangered" men, the people who themselves harm other people, practice *sit* or other "techniques," therefore generally keep a small piece of coconut hidden in their house for such an emergency. The meaning of the coconut is unknown to the upper Yupno, but this is not surprising since the whole *mawom*-complex originally came from the coast.

To identify the instigator, people look for bodily signs (fast, serious course of illness, *mawom tauak*) and wait for other "signs" that may point to the reason why somebody has commissioned a *mawom*-act against the victim. These are interpreted in the usual way: if, for example, the patient calls out for sugarcane or water, hence makes a sign pointing to a woman (*sak tauak*), people are quickly led to consider whether the ill person might have had illicit sexual relations with a married woman, in which case her husband might be the instigator. If this does not lead to the clarification of the cause, the same techniques for finding out are used as in *sit*, the *aminwop* ("shadow soul") of the afflicted or the "soul of the dead person" (*koñwop*), of the deceased, unmask the instigator (see below).

While the effectiveness of *sit*, the conscious altering of substantial parts of a human being, is based on the concept of the human being ("breath spirit," "vital energy," "shadow soul," "soul of a dead person" and "ghost") and on the "hot-cool-cold" system of the Yupno, that of the *mawom* appears to be atypical. No substances had been taken from the victim and nor is he or she "heated up;" instead, he or she is attacked perfidiously and injured, but the injury remains invisible, and the victim has been manipulated towards speechlessness without the use of the "typical" "ice-cold objects" (for the "ice-cold" arrangement, *mbaak*, of various substances, see Chapter 5.3.a.). The victim is in the end going to die of the loss of his or her *aminwop* ("shadow soul"), which leaves the human body through the injury, but every death is defined by the transformation of the *aminwop* ("shadow soul") connected with the human being into the unconnected "soul of a dead person" (*koñwop*) and its later change into a "ghost" (*koñ*). This explanation of the *mawom*-death remains very superficial because the upper Yupno have only relatively recently built the whole *mawom*-realm into their concept of etiology.

c) Identification: The Search for the Instigator

Since the classification of illness is made according to the assumed cause of the illness, each diagnosis and therapy concentrates on the search for this cause. Hence the central questions are: who has misbehaved? And, especially in the case of *sɨt* and *mawom*: who has, out of personal revenge, made somebody ill?

As already explained, "oppressing problems" (*njɨgɨ*) and "oppressing problems caused by a ghost" (*bɨmjɨt*) are first "localized" with the help of "signs" (*tauak*) from the afflicted person and the interpretations of dreams, and then resolved in group discussions lasting many nights. Disorders caused by the bush-spirit *sindok* are first treated like "normal" disorders (burns, and so on), and the bush-spirit is "made cold" and chased off with the help of the "smoking ritual" (*pieñ*). For illnesses where a *sɨt*- or *mawom*-act is the suspected cause (either because the afflicted makes typical *mawom*- "signs" or *sɨt*- "signs" or because the illness does not end despite exhaustive discussions of all the "oppressing problems," in which case one has to assume the worst), the Yupno have several divinatory techniques. They are all aimed at finding out who has stolen the *moñan* ("breath spirit") of the ill person or has "burned" it (like with *sɨt*), or who has given orders to injure a person and thereby chased away his or her *amɨnwop* ("shadow soul") from its owner (as in *mawom*). While with *sɨt* the instigator as well as the "burner" (who are often identical) are looked for, in *mawom* the search is only for the instigator. He alone is responsible for the illness, and the *mawom amɨn*, as the executor of the order, does not attract any rancor.

These various techniques or methods for which only a limited[60] generic noun, *pat*, exists, are executed by various specialists, the *pat amɨn*, "trap-men," who, with few exceptions (see below), are men. "Trap-man" (*pat amɨn*) is the generic noun for the individual specialists who, depending on the method used, are specifically named. Some techniques are used only in case of actual illnesses to find out who is responsible, some only when the victim has died and people look for the culprit; some methods are only applied in case of illness, others also in case of a theft. The knowledge of a method is passed on from the father to one of his sons. Rarely does a man know more than one technique or a complex of methods. Important for successful performance, however, are not only the components used but the "charging" accompanying sentences or formulae. Thus, for example, several men of different clans may use the same technique but every one of them has his own accompanying formulae. Without these formulae, which are carefully kept secret from others, the technique has no effect.

I

A specialist among the "trap-men" (*pat amɨn*) is the *tɨra amɨn*, the "rat man," whose technique is called *tɨra pat*, "rat trap." It is only performed in the case of a death and normally comprises three steps. For a start, the "rat man" and some people who help him, build several rat-traps (gravity- or hatch-traps)[61] during daylight. They are put down next to each other or underneath each other, in the bush or close to the settlement. Every trap is assigned to a clan or its partner clan (or a village). For example, the trap standing on the extreme right of a row "represents" the Talon clan (and its partner clan Mambap or, for example, the village of Uskokop), the one next to it represents the Ngangalbuk clan (or, for example, the village of Kangulut), and so on. Later in the afternoon, shortly before dusk, the specialist blows on these traps with a small bamboo pipe, *amɨn ndañgwan*, called "human hair." Beforehand, some of the deceased's hairs (on which were still adhering residues of his *moñan* ["breath spirit"]) were stuck into this bamboo pipe, along with several grasses and leaves. When it is dark, the specialist and his helpers check the traps: if a rat has been caught in a trap, then the clan or place this trap "represents" is responsible for the deceased's death. It is here that the culprit must be looked for. To confirm the first result, the specialist may cook this rat in the fire and afterwards cut it open: if its blood (after the cooking) is still liquid and runs out, this is further proof pointing to the social environment (clan or village) of the culprit previously marked by the trap.

For further proof, that is, for a second verification, the additional method employed is also called "rat trap" (*tɨra amɨn*). On the cemetery (formerly in the place where the dead were buried), the "rat man" catches a rat and stuffs it alive into a bamboo pipe. A bundle of leaves serves as the plug of the bamboo pipe, into which some of the deceased's hairs have been rolled and which has been pierced by a sharpened bone of a marsupial in such a way that it points at the rat like a thorn. Its upper part has been smeared with red earth pigment *mañot*, the lower part with black earth pigment *noñgum*. Hiding it in a netbag and accompanied by some men, the "rat man" carries this bamboo pipe around everywhere, from village to village. If these men find themselves on a path which leads directly to a certain village, or if they are getting to a village sector and suddenly hear the rat's tail beating against the bamboo, they open the pipe: if the bone has pierced the rat's head, penetrated its eyes, forehead or cheeks, and if the rat is dead, the culprit is to be looked for in this village or a sector thereof (formerly: in this men's house, *mbema*).

In the third verification, the suspicion is further checked with the help of a different technique, *tɨra susoñ*, "cooking the rats." In the bush, men and women startle rats (of the kinds *tɨra goman*, *kɨran* or *siwan*) and catch and kill them. The "rat man" and a helper burn off their fur and disembowel them. Now the "rat man" blows into the anus of each rat with a small thin bamboo pipe, "human hair" (*amɨn ndañgwan*, see above) in which there are hairs of the deceased. The rats are tied into *umban* leaves and individually cooked, each in a bamboo pipe. Each rat "represents" (as with the individual traps) a clan and its partner clan or a village. Each of the two men secretly decides this for himself, so it is a kind of double check. After some time, the rats are taken out of the fire again and carried to the cemetery (or the former place of the burials), where they remain for some time. Later, the rats are taken into the house again and cut into two pieces:[62] if no blood remains in the rat, the clan and his partner clan or the place it represented are innocent. If, on the other hand, the rat is not done and blood streams out of its cut-up body, this is a further and now final confirmation of the knowledge gained from the two other rat experiments about the group or the village of the culprit.

Normally, as it was repeatedly explained to me, in order to definitely mark the culprit, the "rat man" applies his method in the sequence presented here (1. rat trap, 2. living rat with the bone, 3. cooking of the rats in the bamboo). But since the methods are clan specific and correspondingly individually marked and can be handled flexibly, one or the other step may be left out or the order reversed.

Another specialist, the *mbut mɨndak amɨn*, the "pig cutter," also acts only in the case of a death. In the house of the deceased, the "pig cutter" gets banana bast ready and wraps individual pieces around the legs and/or the arms of the deceased, thereby assigning the wrappings to certain villages or men's houses (*mbema*) or clans and partner clans (for example, he defines the first three ligations on the left leg (starting at the foot) as the village of Kangulut, the next three as the village of Meñan, and so on). The deceased is thus bound into sections as, for example, with the pigs that are killed and cut into pieces for a brideprice before their meat is cooked in the earth-oven or in bamboo pipes.

After some hours, the specialist checks the ligatures: if the "soul of a dead person" (*koñwop*) of the deceased has "eaten" the skin and the string, thus if the bast string is missing in certain places, then the culprit is to be looked for there, within this kin group or in this place. The "pig cutter" may also fix the ligatures without attributing them to kin groups or settlements, and the result is then interpreted according to "signs" (*tauak*). If, for example, the ligature on the left leg or arm is missing, the person responsible for the death is to be found in the maternal kin group of the victim, or if the markings on the right half of the body are gone, the culprit belongs to the one's own clan. A different method, no longer practiced today, was known to the *ɨlok amɨn*, the "reed grass man;" it was also only practiced in the case of a death.[63]

The most respected specialist is the *kumbu amɨn*, a kind of "medium," a man who in dreams or in a kind of trance identifies those who are responsible for a case of death. In many ways, he corresponds to the *tawak amine* among the Wantoat as reported by Schmitz (1960b: 163–68).[64] A "medium" inherits his skills from his father (also a *kumbu amɨn*). As a boy (still unmarried, "hot"), he is initiated at a *kumbu* tree[65] (probably the traditional tree for burials) by some experienced men. I could not get any information about the process of the initiation, but the novice seems to get things to eat from the complex of the *sindok* bush-spirit (maybe grated parts of a "bone of the bush-spirit *sindok*," plants belonging to its domain) and thereby has formed or strengthened his skills as a medium.

If a medium is now to identify the person responsible for a death, he will first sleep some time at the foot of the *kumbu* tree. A pendant *pɨdɨm* liana was fixed to this tree, which is thought to be the "ghost"-liana, and touches the boy, who has smoke from the "human hairs" bamboo-pipe (see above) blown over him by various men. The parts of the deceased (hairs, etc.) imbued with *moñan* ("breath spirit") and various kinds of ginger are mixed and given to the boy to eat while he is closely watched. The boy falls asleep or into a trance, and he becomes like drunk. In the meantime, the "soul of a dead person" (*koñwop*), of the deceased, climbs down the liana and enters the boy. The boy starts to say incomprehensible things. He is asked (since he now as a "medium" has the "soul of a dead person," of the deceased, inside him): "who has killed you?," and the boy states the place and the name[66] of the performer (of the *sɨt*- or *mawom*-man or of the instigator) and sings the latter's *koñgap* melody. He is now as if beside himself, rages all about, and has to be tied down lest he otherwise immediately run up to the culprit and kill him. After a while, he quietens down. He is taken to a house with a big fire, then emerges from his trance-like state and becomes normal again.

He keeps his special skills as a "medium" all his life. If, for example, he is sitting in a house and a man enters who has just had illicit sexual relations with a woman, the delinquent's *moñan* and *amɨnwop* ("breath spirit" and "shadow soul") go into the *kumbu amɨn*, who then proclaims the misdeed. *Kumbu amɨn*[67] are also specialists in the interpretation of dreams, and themselves often dream very meaningful dreams.

II

Two specialists who are sought out in cases of illness (hence not in cases of death) to identify the "burner" (*sɨt amɨn*) or the instigator of *mawom* are the *komup amɨn* and the *kuak amɨn*, who are the most numerous practitioners today. A *kuak amɨn*, "white man," may apply two different techniques:

1. Out of the afflicted person's urine and the white earth pigment *kuak* he mixes a paste with which he rubs the patient. Then he bespeaks his instrument, a kind of dog dummy,[68] *pat kɨrat*, called "trap bone" and rubs

some of the paste onto it. The "trap bone" remains in the patient's house, but the *moñan* ("breath spirit") of the patient (now transferred as urine in the paste to the "trap bone") goes outside, lures the *amɨnwop* ("shadow soul") with it, and it in turn (analogous to a sniffing dog) looks for the culprit and leaves white marks like small stains on the stones or light-green (Yupno: "white") leaves which lead to the house or the village of the culprit and which the "white man" (*kuak amɨn*) follows.

2. The other procedure goes as follows: the "white man" cooks white soil *kuak* (maybe red soil *mañot*, this may vary individually), *komup* (red sap of a pandanus kind, 'marita') and certain grasses in a bamboo and adds a small piece of *njaapndak*, "left-over food" of the afflicted, i.e. a particle imbued with his *moñan* ("breath spirit"), mixes everything well and stirs it into a paste. He cuts banana leaves and with them closes the house door of the patient from the inside. Then the ailing person has to sit up and is rubbed with this paste with the help of a little stick. Afterwards, the specialist throws the little stick in the direction of the banana leaves, it penetrates them, goes outside and leaves red marks on stones and trees. At first—according to this notion—it goes straight away to the ill person's men's house to strengthen its "vital energy" (*tevantok*), then it would have formerly gone to the traditional *mbema*-settlement but now goes to the village of the culprit. The "white man" and some relatives simply have to follow these red marks. If the culprit, the "burner," is found, he will give the relatives a piece of ("cold") sugarcane for the "heated" patient to carry away, and then the patient can get well. If a instigator of *mawom* is responsible for the illness, the "white man" and the relatives will at first not publicly announce his identity but, rather, retreat discreetly. Once the time and the occasion have arrived, one of the patient's relatives will take revenge by giving an order to a "burner."

The *komup amɨn*, the "red man," also knows two variants of the procedure, *komup pat* or *komup erap*.

1. *Komup erap*, "bowl with the red liquid": first, the "red man" gets his instrument ready, the "bowl with the red liquid." It consists of half of a hollowed-out coconut which is filled with red pandanus juice, into which he puts a small bean, *mbasip*. The coconut bowl is suspended in a net made of *mbep* bark cloth, with a bundle fastened to the top of it consisting of a small piece of the victim's carriers of contact (hairs, saliva), hairs from the nose of a good hunting dog, and two kinds of

ginger, wrapped in leaves. The bundle is decorated with fragrant flowers and grasses, the same that which are used as ornaments at the *koñgap* dance: they are meant to lure the *amɨnwop* ("shadow soul") of the
culprit, to flatter it so that it shows itself (on the culprit). The "red
man" now breaks off a leaf of the *pɨpnameñ* plant, calls the name of
his partner clan (*ngapma*), which is supposed to help him in this act,
and bespeaks the leaf. Afterwards, he walks around with his *komup
erap*-instrument and again and again very carefully hurls it around in
a horizontal circular movement so the red sap does not splash over.
Should the little bean *mbasip* fall out, this is taken as a sign that the
culprit lives at his place or in the direction in which it fell.

2. *Komup pat*, "trap with the red liquid":[69] the instrument *komup pat* con-
    sists of the lower part of a piece of *teet* bamboo pipe, which the "red
    man" fills with red pandanus juice very carefully (so the bamboo pipe
    does not get smeared inside). The lower part is wrapped with *mbalgerk*
    banana bast. The upper part consists of *sukuak* leaves, *njakngak* leaves,
    mamnaknak grass, *manjit* and *pɨpnjaap* grasses, into which red *mañot*
    earth pigment, feathers of the *ndakal* bird as well as some of the pa-
    tient's hairs have been wrapped and which is tied up with *mbalgerk*.
    Into this plug, the specialist sticks a *teet* bamboo stick, to which a white
    bird-feather has been tied. After the pipe or the red pandanus juice is
    bespoken, the "red man" takes a *popmdeñ* leaf and gives it "vital en-
    ergy" (*tevantok*), that is, "charges" it and beats on it. It breaks, and the
    parts are tied to the bamboo pipe. During this, the "red man" bespeaks
    the plants *teetgoman, dimdim, ndamba* and *ndauña ndamba*, which the
    Yupno himself has planted and which therefore are "hot," "different,"
    "extraordinary":

teet	*goman*	*dimdim*	*poñbat*	*bamañsulek*	*ndamba*
bamboo	red	kind of reed	stalk	break, bend over	fern

pagat	*ndauña ndamba*	*pagat*	*bamañgsulek*	*keki!*
root	kind of fern	root	to break, bend over	go!

Break this red bowstring [which is made of *teet* bamboo], and break
this *dimdim* stalk and the roots of the *ndamba* and *ndauña ndamba*
plant and go!

Now the "red man" puts the bamboo pipe into a netbag and goes on his way
with the other men. The *moñan* ("breath spirit") contained in the hairs of
the afflicted person has lured his *amɨnwop* ("shadow soul"), which,

encouraged by the plants whose names are invoked to overcome all the obstacles, then marks the way with red signs (red leaves, red flowers, small reddish stones) for the men to follow. Arriving at a garden house, in a village or at a fork in the road, they check whether the bird feather is colored red, indicating that the culprit is to be found here.

The various procedures of the two specialists, "white man" and "red man," are based on the same principle, involving the activation of a small piece of the *moñan* ("breath spirit") of an afflicted person (contained in the urine in the case of the "trap bone," through skin contact in the case of the other procedure of the "white man," in the hairs for the methods of the "red man"). It is meant to lure the patient's *aminwop* ("shadow soul") so it can unmask the culprit. It either leaves signs (white or red marks) that the specialists have only to follow, or it points out the direction where the culprit is to be found.

All the "trap men" (*pat amin*) are paid a fee; the price for a commission to a "red man" (*komup amin*), for example, amounts to one pig or 50-70 Kina. Most older "trap men" also possess skills in *sit* and in the methods (*pat*) of discovering, and can therefore bring illness and death as well as identify the culprit.

5. Key Points in the Yupno Medical System

From this systematic survey, in which various causes of illness have been presented, it is possible to summarize salient characteristics of the medical system that determine the way the Yupno cope with illness in everyday life and search for explanations.

1. In case of an "altered behavior," a "harmless bodily disorder" is first (normally) assumed. It is not held to be ill, is accepted without investigation into the cause and first treated with home remedies (diet, rest, massage); hence patients themselves (or the family as the largest possible reference group) try to eliminate the disorder. If this has no effect and the disorder continues to be present or gets worse, then

    a) a "cooler" is consulted, who, for a fee, applies his therapy with herb remedies and ablutions whose effect is based on the "hot-cool-cold" concept, to "cool" the "heated" person. Under this generic noun of "cooler" there are different specialists; thus the therapy managing group now consists of the afflicted, the family and the specialist. This domain of the "cooler" has recently increasingly been taken over by

b) biomedicine. It is available at the aid posts as well as at the Teptep Health Centre. Thus modern pharmaceuticals more and more replace traditional phytotherapy and ablutions, and the therapy managing group then consists of the patient, the family and a representative of biomedicine.

2. If traditional phytotherapy or biomedicine does not help, people suspect a *njɨgɨ*, an "problem." The focus of the therapy shifts from the roppressingemoval of the "bodily disorders" that accompany this *njɨgɨ* to the cause of the *njɨgɨ*; the patient is now deemed to be really ill (*sɨt asak*, "he is ill"). An "oppressing problem" is always based on social tensions or breaches of norms, which bring illness such as *nduara* ("left-over" of a deed) or dangerous "hot" emotional states in persons still living and already dead, hence in "ghosts." Since this "oppressing problem" is always connected with a group of persons and ceases to concern only the individual, the search for its cause includes observing the "signs" (*tauak*) of the patient, interpreting dreams and attempting to localize the group of persons causing the illness. In collective discussions among all the participants, the "oppressing problem" is more precisely defined and pronounced, and compensation is finally paid to the angry, "hot" group. The family afflicted by an "oppressing problem" is therefore the smallest group, since their social network may extend across the clan, the partner clan, and the matrilateral relatives to the group of the in-laws, to encompass the entire kin group as the largest entity.

3. If, despite these illness debates, no improvement results, or if the patient shows a typical "bush-spirit sign" (*sindok tauak*) such as burns or in rare cases complete mental disturbance manifested in raving madness, the bush-spirit *sindok* is held to be the agent. The ill person or one of his relatives has violated the borders of the *sindok* domain, either by hunting for too many marsupials or the "wrong" kinds, dwelling at tabooed places that are reserved for the *sindok*, or eating forbidden food (as certain pandanus fruits) ruled over by the *sindok*. The bush-spirit *sindok*, once angry and therefore "heated," now reacts and passes on its anger (as "heat") by causing illness. As a therapy, the *sindok* is "smoked away" by the "smoker" (*pieñ amɨn*) and pacified with small gifts. An individual, his or her clan and the *sindok* bush-spirit itself form the social background of a *sindok*-illness. In order to avoid certain confrontations with the bush-spirit, (as, for example, during

the making of a new garden), it is prophylactically "put out in the cold" with an "ice-cold arrangement" (*mbaak*) and thereby inactivated.

4.   If the ill person gets worse and if "oppressing problems" (*njɨgɨ*) or the bush-spirit *sindok* have been excluded as the cause, or if he or she exhibits clear "signs," the two "techniques" *sɨt* or *mawom* are assumed to be the cause. *Sɨt*, the cause more frequent among the upper Yupno, is performed by a specialist on commission. A small piece of *moñan* ("breath spirit") is stolen from the victim and "heated," which by analogy results in a "heating up" (falling ill) of the victim. If the victim is to die, this *moñan*-particle is actually burnt and without *moñan* ("breath spirit") the *amɨnwop* ("shadow soul") will also leave its owner. In the end, the victim dies of the loss of self. With the help of various techniques, an identification of the person who has stolen the *moñan* ("breath spirit") from the victim is eventually possible: the victim can thus get well again. The specialist who has heated his *moñan*-particle, the "burner" (*sɨt amɨ n*), now has to give to the afflicted something "cold" (like sugar-cane). The one who hurts and the one who heals are thus identical.

Mawom, the other extremely serious cause of illness, is also performed at someone's request. The unsuspecting victim is assaulted, injured and in no time will fall gravely ill. If the victim in good time eats a certain coconut and if the instigator can be found out, recovery is possible. Both causes, *sɨt* and *mawom*, like the "oppressing problems," arise from social tensions, fights, discords or breaches of norm and moral code, all of them a threat to the social fabric. The social space, encompassing relations between victim, instigator and specialist, may be quite small or may transcend the kinship system.

It is significant, that at the level of diverse individual concepts of causation (hence within the culturally defined "framework" shared by all), the Yupno cope with illness in a highly variable way. Individual variation is expressed in the interpretation of the illness, which in turn depends on the range of a person's knowledge. The narratives of various people about their experiences with illness show clearly how in each case people deliberate anew on the cause; and this is always to be found (with the exception of the "bush-spirit"-concept) within a network of social relationship that is constructed and experienced differently by every individual. On the other hand, the search for a cause— for example, with the help of a debate—is a collective attempt.

Survey 2: Simplified Representation of the Yupno Medical System

generic noun	*sɨt* (illness)				
special term	no, individual bodily disorders are named	"oppressing problems" (*njɨgɨ, bɨmjɨt*)	*sindok* "bush-spirit"	*sɨt*	*mawom*
degree of illness	increasing threat ⟶				
cause	natural (climate, overexertion)	social tensions, misdemeanor (in the social sector)	misdemeanor (in the religious sector)	private fights, hate, discord	
agent	"normal" bodily reaction	misdemeanor leads to *nduara*, transfer of "hot" feelings	*sindok* unloads "hot" anger	*moñan* stolen, heated or burnt, injury, loss of *amɨnwop*	
diagnosis	subjective feeling of the person in question	1. *tauak* ("signs"), 2. dreams, which make misdemeanor public	burns, *sindok* "signs"	*sɨt*-"signs," *mawom*- "signs," to find the cause by *pat* techniques	
therapy	massage, diet, rest (lay sector), "cooler" with phytotherapy and ablutions, biomedicine with pharmaceutical drugs	debate: making public the problem, compensation, i.e. "cooling," chasing away of the "ghost"	"smoking out" (*pieñ*) by the specialist	identification of the "burner or instigator, "cold" food from the "burner," coconut prophylaxis	

prophylaxis	no		holding onto norms, con-form behavior in the group	*mbaak*, i.e. prophylactic "putting out in the cold"	interpersonal re-lationships with-out conflict
social frame	individual, maybe family	own kin		individual, own clan and *sindok*	open, transcend-ing kin group
therapy managing group	individual (family) and "cooler," repre-sentative of biomedicine	own kin		ill person and "smoker" (*pieñ amɨn*)	ill person and "trap man" (*pat amɨn*)

Chapter 6

Conclusion

I

I began this book about the medical system of the Yupno with the conviction that concepts about disease and illness and treatment practices constitute a central complex of ideas for all peoples. After all, disease, illness and health are fundamentally connected with life—its origin, quality, maintenance and cessation. While disease belongs to the realm of the biomedical model, illness refers to the perceptions and experiences of the patient and his or her social group, which are culturally determined. Disease and illness may coincide, but this is not inevitable, and both are different ways of looking at the reality of "sickness."

The evaluation of what a given people or community thinks is "ill" or "healthy," and the opinions and attitudes of its members regarding these two states of being are both culture-specific and closely connected with their world view. Any adequate assessment must thus take account of the way people perceive their environment and structure it, the characteristics of the social, moral and religious system, values, and ideas about person, self, body-mind and emotions.

To provide an emic representation of the Yupno medical system, while at the same time considering the biomedical point of view as the other major avenue for the interpretation of "sickness," I decided on interdisciplinary cooperation with physicians. The resulting division of labor was clear: while the physicians biomedically investigated the "disease" complexes and state of health of the Yupno, I focused on and attempted to grasp the cultural complex of attitudes and behaviors concerning "illness" from the perspective of the Yupno actors. My specific aim was not to be the kind of anthropologist for whom "biomedicine serves as 'the reality through the lens of which the rest of the world's cultural versions are seen, compared and judged'" (Singer 1989: 1195, quoting Hahn and Gaines 1985: 4).

The centerpiece of my study is the case study of the little boy Nstasiñge, around which my objective has been to provide a synthesis of the two contrasting but intimately interconnected perspectives: Yupno conceptualizations of illness and data derived from the biomedical perspective. Thus the conjunction of these two points of view around a single case facilitates both the demonstration and evaluation of these differing modes of interpretation.

II

Fundamentally, "illness" (*sɨt*, literally: I burn, heat, cook) for the Yupno means to be in an extraordinary, "different," "dwelling above," "hot" state. The corresponding opposite term is *sɨtni mi*, "I am not ill." The concept of the human being is basic for the understanding of illness. Several parts belong to a "complete" human being: next to his or her body, a "vital energy" (*tevantok*), which is relatively "impersonal" and supra-individual, as well as the aspects *moñan* ("breath spirit") and *wopm* ("shadow soul"), which are decisive for the personality of an individual. Whereas the *moñan* ("breath spirit") dissolves at death, the *wopm* ("shadow soul") becomes a *koñwop* ("soul of a dead person") and over the course of time an anonymous *koñ* ("ghost"). Of equal importance beside these dimensions of the human body and soul are the *koñgap* melody possessed by every individual, together with his social relationships and their quality.

The state of "illness" that translates as "being hot" forms the extreme point of a continuum, which encompasses the concepts "hot" (*tepm*), "cool" (*yawuro*) and "ice-cold" (*mbaak*). The "ideal state" of a human being is the "cool," balanced, socially integrated, "dwelling in the middle" position; the "hot" state, on the contrary, is exceptional, undesired, and dangerous. Thus every therapy aims at "cooling down" the "heated up" (patient) to bring him or her back to the "cool" ideal state. The third state, "ice-cold," is, like "hot," an undesired state since the person concerned has moved away from the "ideal" middle position, although he or she is not thought of as ill and is therefore unimportant apropos concepts of illness. All three states can be changed. Both the initial position and the desired result are decisive. As a rule, complex knowledge about the manipulation of these states is vested in the men, and the principle of contact is fundamental. With "hot" objects, somebody who is in the ideal, "cool" position may be "heated," that is, made ill. Similarly, through contact with "cold" substances somebody who is "heated," i.e. in an ill state, may be "cooled" down to the ideal measure, and thus healed. The target of the manipulation is the "vital energy" (*tevantok*) of a human being. In a healthy, socially integrated human being it is "cool."

If it is now brought together with "hot" or "cold" objects that act as an agent, the "heat" or "cold" transfers onto it, and as a consequence the human being either gets ill or gets well.

In simplified terms, the basic pattern of how the Yupno cope with illness and determine the diagnosis and the therapy is as follows: they initially assume a "harmless disturbance of well-being" (which is not held to be "illness") and then turn to the investigation of the cause, following the principle of "trial and error" and working up to the most serious illness. The (bodily) "disorders" (symptoms) do not necessarily have to change for this, as the same "disorder" may be traced back to varying causes.

The Yupno have a system of four levels of illness (if one combines the two worst causes of illness, *sɨt* and *mawom*), and can accordingly choose among different curative options. This pattern follows what Romanucci Schwartz (1969) has described as a "hierarchy of resorts."

The first large group of "states," the "lowest level," is formed by the "natural disorders" that cause somebody to be "hot" but not yet "ill." These "disorders" are recognized and named but little importance is accorded them.

This first level—and it alone—can be correlated with the symptoms of biomedicine. From the Yupno point of view, these are fairly banal bodily disorders, not "illnesses," which gain another dimension only if indigenous therapies show no effect or there is no cure. From a biomedical perspective, however, these symptoms and diagnoses may already indicate a serious disease.

Illness begins only when suspicions are voiced that such "disorders" originate from a cause, and the diagnostic aim then consists of divining this cause. Hence the decisive question is not what someone is ill of (to be deduced from possible bodily disorders) but why someone is ill, and this question leads to the next level, where the "real illness" begins. This second level is subsumed under the generic noun *njɨgɨ*, as the consequence of an "oppressing problem." Serious "oppressing problems" are caused by a conscious or unconscious misdemeanor of one or several relatives. They can act directly upon the person afflicted with "guilt," hence on the one responsible for the misdemeanor, or also become active indirectly when the injured person reacts angrily, gets into a "hot" emotional state and unloads this "heat" on the culprit or a member of his or her kin group in a pathogenic way.

Not only the living but also the already deceased or their "ghosts" (*koñ*) can, if they have died angry or full of hate, transfer their "hot" anger and cause somebody to be ill. Such "oppressing problems" are diagnosed with the help of "signs" *(tauak)* indicated in the patient's behavior and through dreams. Therapy consists of an open discussion about this misdemeanor, the attempt to reach consensus among all the participants (in other words: the establishment of social harmony) as well as an ensuing payment of compensation, which is meant to soothe the "heated maniac" and cool him or her down. If an enraged "ghost" is responsible for the illness, it can be chased away with a special ritual. Ackerknecht (1971) repeatedly stressed this aspect of illness as the most important social sanction which may well befall every member of a kin group as well as the one who has misbehaved. It is certainly a central element in the Yupno medical system, as indicated by the long duration of discussions about "oppressing problems" and misdemeanors.

The bush-spirit *sindok* (third level) may also cause illness. It is thought to be the "mother" of the tree kangaroos and opossums, and reacts in the case of violations within its domain of responsibility, the non-social environment (bush, mountain forest, cliffs, and so on), by causing burns or states of mental disturbance. Its pathogenic acts become manifest in special signs attributed to it, so it is chased away by a specialist and/or calmed with gifts and cooled, or even rendered "ice-cold" and inactive.

The most serious illness, the fourth level, is caused by two "techniques," *sɨt* and *mawom*. *Sɨt*, the generic noun for illness, in this context is also the name of a certain procedure for which a specialist commissioned by someone else steals a small particle of "breath spirit " (*moñan*) from the victim and heats it, which by analogy results in the illness ("heating up") of the victim. If the victim is meant to die, this particle of "breath spirit" is actually burnt and without it the "shadow soul" (*amɨnwop*) will also leave the victim: in the end, the victim dies of the loss of the self. However, if the wrongdoer who has stolen this little piece of *moñan* from the victim and "heated" it is identified early enough, the patient may recover, but the "thief" has to give something "cold" to the victim to "cool" him. *Mawom*, the other serious cause of illness, is also performed on commission, but only by the people of the lower Yupno region (the practice is known to the upper Yupno, who fear it greatly). The unsuspecting victim is assaulted by *mawom*-men and injured and will very quickly get seriously ill. Should the instigator be identified in good time and if the patient eats a coconut picked in a certain way, he or she may survive. The category under the generic noun "oppressing problem" as well as the other two levels, illness caused by the bush-spirit *sindok* as well as illnesses caused by the "magic techniques" *sɨt* and *mawom* resist any comparison with biomedicine since they have no clearly defined biomedical correspondences but can only be distinguished by a rather generally conceived course of illness which is looked upon as increasingly threatening.

All four levels are marked by a pervasive principle of organization: the "hot-cool-cold"-concept. This "hot-cool-cold" continuum comprises all the circumstances imaginable, but it is still difficult to determine its beginning. Even though somebody afflicted by a "harmless disorder" is "hot" since the therapies of the "heat-extinguisher" are aimed at a "cooling down" as well. On this first level, however, the physical "cooling down" is still in the forefront. "To be hot" in its more comprehensive meaning starts on the second level, when someone is "really ill." The "heat" increases continuously up to the most threatening level of illness, *sɨt*, "I burn." Thus all the therapies aim at "cooling" the "hot," "dwelling above," i.e. ill human being, to bring him or her back to the "cool" ideal state. At the level of the "natural disorders," the "coolers" ("soothers," "heat-extinguishers," "restorers") approach this task with "natural" means (plants, water, and so on). The plant therapy as practiced by the Yupno practitioners for these bodily disorders has many parallels in other ethnic groups in Papua New Guinea

For "oppressing problems," the causes first have to be clarified in the group and then the "angry" ("hot") instigator cooled down through payment of compensation; in a similar way, action is taken against the bush-spirit *sindok*. Even the worst states of illness, caused by the "techniques" *sɨt* and *mawom*, can only be alleviated through "cooling," the application of something "cold." Comparison with another study of Yupno classifications shows that this "hot-cool-cold" concept is not only an important category in the realm of "illness" but that almost all the phenomena of the environment are also classified according to this model (see Wassmann and Dasen 1994b).

III

This pattern of coping with illness also becomes manifest in the interpretation of little Nstasiñge's illness, which has been reconstructed from the report of the child's mother, the proceedings of a protracted debate, and from talks with informants. To begin with, the mother, Mayu, told how she noticed the first—bodily—changes in her then seven months old son, Nstasiñge. He was screaming incessantly, his skin was hot, his eyes were red, and nothing could calm him down. When all the home remedies had no effect, she took the child to the nearby small health center at Teptep to get treatment for these bodily disorders. There, she was put off till the next day. She went back to the village and began to think about all the possible causes for her child's behavior; in other words, she was now interpreting his behavior as "ill" (*sɨt*). She started out with one "oppressing problem" (*njɨgɨ*) and thereby the social space expanded beyond the family circle: the illness became a social event. She excepted herself as an illness-causing person: "I had not walked far away with him." Her remark must be understood as defensive, a justification directed towards her husband Tanowe's clan and partner clan. Because they had raised her bride price, they had a vested interest in the welfare of the child and expected Mayu as a mother to take good care of the baby, the product of the "purchase" and therefore a new clan member. A mother who removes herself from the control of the village runs risks the anger of the bush-spirit *sindok*, and is in danger from *mawom* attacks. Mayu first accused her husband Tanowe of being responsible for her child's illness, but then, she and her husband were both accused by those who had contributed significantly to her bride price; out of jealousy, a woman accused Mayu's mother of being guilty of her grandson's illness and a neighbor was severe in his blaming of Mayu, the little boy's mother. To clarify the causes, the relatives (the baby's patriclan), in some cases living in other villages, were invited to the village for a discussion. At the same time, the child was given to different persons to hold and carried into various houses to see how the child would react to the various persons and places (if he would stop screaming, for example, which would be a "sign" that this person or this house—meaning this kin group—was not responsible for his "oppressing problem"). Two possible causes were talked about in this first discussion:

- A "ghost" and/or its living son from the more distant matrilineage might possibly be angry because they did not receive the part of Mayu's bride price to which, owing to extraordinary circumstance, they had a claim and so were now making the child ill. This suspicion was substantiated by the fact that the child hardly drank any milk anymore—a "sign" pointing to the matrilineage.
- The other "oppressing problem" was found in the patrilineage. Tanowe, the baby's father, ignored the orders of his own now-deceased father, whose "ghost" was unloading his "hot" anger onto Tanowe's child. This assumption was confirmed by various people's dreams, in which they had seen the deceased man cutting down bamboo in exactly the same spot where he once had planted it—a sign pointing to the patrilineage.

Since it could not be clearly defined which "ghost" was responsible for the illness, the participants in the discussion, the therapy managing group at this stage of the illness, combined both "ghosts," performed a ritual to chase them away, gave the child a new name originating from another clan, and transferred a small sum they collected to the account of the Teptep church district. Yet the child continued to be ill, and this led to the scheduling of a new debate. There were no "signs" pointing to other causes and thus this discussion ran along quite vaguely on the subject whether, possibly generations ago, a member of the mother's clan might have killed a member of the father's clan with the *sit*-technique or vice versa, and was now angry that two members of the formerly hostile clans had married. Again, a sum of collected money was paid into the account of the church district. The child did not get better, and the mother moved in with relatives in another village for one week. At a third meeting, two further possible causes of illness were discussed:

- a woman who for some time had been jealous of the (maternal) grand-mother of the child had come into Mayu's house, then shouted out and beat about with a stick. As a result, the "shadow soul" (*wopm*) of the baby became so scared that it left the baby.
- As a further cause, there was discussion of Mayu's bride price return, which had not been performed correctly according to tradition. Tanowe, the child's father, had fetched the half of the bride price to be returned in his wife Mayu's village of origin, but had not handed it over to some of his patriline relatives because he had fallen out with them; instead, he sold it and used the money he received on himself. The participants in the discussion could not agree whether Tanowe's misconduct or the anger of the people who had been left empty-handed had now caused the child to be ill.

When all the misdemeanors had been proclaimed, the jealous woman publicly regretted her behavior and called out to the baby's "shadow soul" to return to its place in the child. She called the little boy's name and sang his *koñgap* melody. Subsequently, she put around the child's neck a one Kina coin, which all those present had touched, and the mother, Mayu, gave him drinking water that had been consecrated by the evangelist. The child did not get well, and the mother now assumed one of the worst causes of illness, *mawom*. Yet her fears were not shared by her relatives—or at least not followed up. She again visited the health center with her child, and from there was transferred to the Modilon Hospital in Madang. For the first time in an unfamiliar environment, alone and with no knowledge of Tok Pisin, she there had to decide whether she wanted to return to the village with her child or wait to see if the child would get well. This decision was in part influenced by her fear of a potential condemnation from the relatives in case of the child's death.

The same sickness episode as seen from the point of view of biomedicine, reconstructed from conversations with personnel of the Teptep Health Centre and from the interpretation of the clinical record of the Modilon Hospital by the physician Sandra Staub, is as follows: the little boy Nstasiñge was taken to the Teptep Health Centre by his mother on February 3, 1987 for the first time. He was then seven months old and weighed 7 kg. The boy showed signs of a cerebral inflammation, which pointed to meningitis. For further clarification, a lumbar puncture was made. The results confirmed the diagnosis of a bacterial or tubercular meningitis. Therefore, a two-week therapy with the antibiotic Chloramphenicol was administered. A second lumbar puncture after this period of time showed that the spinal fluid was clear. The child was discharged from the health center.

More than two months later, on 13 April 1987 (and after all the traditional means, such as the public admission and the "cooling down" of possible "oppressing problems" were completed), the mother again consulted the Teptep Health Centre. The Health Extension Officer in charge described the child's state as follows: without fever, but with stiffness of neck, back, feet and hands, staring eyes, loss of weight, and signs of malnutrition. As he himself was unable to make a precise diagnosis of the child's disease — he supposed that "he has a big problem in his head," — the HEO treated him for eleven days with Phenobarbital (to stop the spasms) before having him transferred to the Modilon Hospital in Madang. On 24 April, 1987, the introductory examination there showed: loss of weight (the child only weighed 5,5kg), skin affected with scabies, ulcers, rumors on both lungs, decreased turgor of the skin, sunken fontanels. Based on these results, the following was diagnosed: brain-damage at status after meningitis, possible meningo-encephalitis, suspected tuberculosis as well as pneumonia. As an initial therapy, the following drugs were prescribed: the broad-spectrum antibiotic Chloramphenicol, the tranquilizer Phenobarbital which was meant to suppress the child's spasms, Pyrantel, a highly effective antihelminthic, the drying of the ulcers and the treatment of the scabies as well as physiotherapy. Following a blood test on the same day, Amodiaquine, an anti-malaria drug, was prescribed. The child was also vaccinated during the first week of his stay at Modilon Hospital. They vaccinated him against diphtheria, tetanus, whooping-cough, polio, tuberculosis and measles. The frequently repeated blood tests pointed to an inflammation yet did not result in any distinct finding. The almost daily performed lumbar punctures at the beginning of the therapy also produced little result. All too often, they proved to be traumatic. The few successful lumbar punctures produced normal results, no agens could be detected. For weeks, the child's condition hardly changed. He put on weight only very slowly but the symptoms of the stiffness as well as the frequent high temperature continued. The notes in the clinical report read again and again: "neck still stiff," "fever," "feeding o.k.," "condition much the same." On May 8, he was transferred from the "A-Ward," the ward of the acutely ill, to the "B-Ward," the ward of the convalescents, which Mayu mentions: "we were sent to a different ward." On May 26, tuberculosis therapy was begun. During the following four weeks, there were still no real changes in his condition. The child continued to have peaks of temperature, he also continued to be restless, and he gained barely any weight. He was then transferred to the "C-Ward," where there were no daily rounds. In mid-July, after a three months' stay at the hospital, an improvement in his condition was diagnosed for the first time. The child was now without a fever and had no further spasms, had lost the stiffness of neck and ate and drank well. On July 31, 1987, the child was discharged and flew back to Teptep with his mother.

Two points are notable in the biomedical treatment:

1. The child received a large number of highly effective medications, in part administered at the one time, without his disease even being exactly identified. Treatment thus proceeded according to the "trial and error" principle. In addition, numerous lumbar punctures were performed (according to the patient's report, ten alone at Modilon Hospital), and in five cases vessels were injured.
2. The child's condition was repeatedly reduced to four criteria: stiffness of the neck, fever, level of appetite and nutritional status, and state of excitation.

After these four criteria had been successfully treated from the biomedical point of view, the child's therapy was ended and he was discharged as healed. However, when I again saw the child, in 1988, on my third visit to the village, he was more than two years old and was clearly both mentally and physically handicapped.

In the case of little Nstasiñge, where both kinds of treatment, the traditional and the biomedical, had failed, this was interpreted in different ways: according to the statements of relatives and friends of the child's family, there had been too many "oppressing problems," both between the child's father and mother and within the kin group. Consequently, the situation had been too heavily charged with conflicts, and these "oppressing problems" had never really been solved. Although various such problems were discussed and identified, it still remains open which one was responsible for the child's illness. Since, the initial cause could never be identified, the illness could not be removed.

From the biomedical point of view, the child's admission to the Teptep Health Centre probably came too late. The delay in the start of the antibiotics therapy may well have been crucial for the course of the disease. The further sickness episode shows that the child, who weighed only 5.5 kg, was immoderately "filled up" with drugs of many different kinds, and that he received several vaccinations and had to endure many critical treatments and examinations (such as the many lumbar punctures) which can easily cause permanent damage if not carried out correctly. A modern Western medical diagnostic process was equally unable to identify the precise cause of the disease, i.e. the decisive agent was not detected. The child was discharged as cured from the Western point of view, that is, in a stable condition that could not be further improved.

IV

For the Yupno, "illness" (*sɨt*) begins after people other than the afflicted individual become involved. "Illness" is never a private, personal misfortune but an event in which several persons enmeshed in a network of relationships participate, which is of concern to the group involved, and for which there is a cause. "Illness" always means a disturbance of the ideally "cool" median state of a human being as of the social group; the ill person is "hot" (*tepm*) and has risen above this middle, is "above" (*kwin*). All therapies aim to "cool" afflicted persons down and bring about their social re-integration via the restoration of equilibrium.

Social discord, tensions and conflicts in the group are worked out and solved by diagnoses and treatment of "illness," which is held to be closely implicated with actual or alleged breaches of norms (such as theft, adultery or murder). To the Yupno, illness is therefore always a breach of culturally-defined norms:

a) in the realm of the social relationships, of the social environment: "oppressing problems," *njɨgɨ*, originate; in case of more serious conflicts, the order for *sɨt* and *mawom*, the elimination of the opponent through illness and death, may be issued;

b) in the realm of the "environment," in the relationship of a human being to the surrounding (non-social) space: it is structured by culturally-religiously determined concepts and norms, and the bush-spirit *sindok* is believed to pay close attention to their maintenance. Those who trespass in "illness-causing places" or engage in "wrong" behavior towards certain animals (especially tree kangaroos, "children" of the *sindok*) or those parts of the landscape founded by mythological beings and under the surveillance of the *sindok* may suffer illness as a consequence.

V

The research for this study was conceived and conducted as interdisciplinary. The rationale should by now be quite evident: as an anthropologist and non-physician, hence without an already internalized system of biomedical concepts, I found it easier to concentrate wholly on the Yupno point of view of "illness." My objective, especially in the data-gathering stages, was to avoid becoming strongly involved with the biomedical associations, to minimize any tendencies to try to force data into Western categories. The perspectives of the Yupno with regard to little Nstasiñge's illness have made it clear how greatly the realm of illness as conceptualized by them differs from Western biomedical perspectives, and how strongly their attitudes and behaviors are contextualized within an indigenous anthropology that pervades everyday life and intimately affects both individual and group conduct.

On the other hand, by investigating the same case of sickness from the biomedical point of view as well (based on the analysis of the laboratory results, and medical evaluation by the physician Sandra Staub of the medication and treatment administered to the little boy), the other major aspect of the sickness was foregrounded: "disease," as opposed to Yupno views of "illness."

The famous anthropological pioneer fieldworker, Rivers (1924) very early on concerned himself with the "inner logic" of traditional medical systems. He was aware that traditional medicine (or in today's terms: a traditional medical system) was a set of social, interdependent practices that by no means represented simply a potpourri of unconnected and meaningless customs; rather, they were determined and linked by ideas concerning the cause of illness. The conclusions that Rivers deduced regarding the rationality and logic of indigenous medical activities are totally applicable to Yupno concepts of illness.

The subdivision of a medical system into the various aspects or causes of illness and the anthropological discourse about it, in which these phenomena are analyzed cross-culturally, certainly contribute to a better and deeper understanding. One thing they cannot do, however, is explain the inner, culture-specific logic of a medical system in terms of which the members of a given culture cope with illness in everyday life. The aim of the present study has been to present a detailed example of this cultural logic in action. For the Yupno, illness, far from being a biological accident affecting the body, is very closely bound up with the structures and dynamics of social relations. It can be explained adequately only in terms of the underlying systems of belief, knowledge and thought that determine and structure their behavior, both interpersonal and in relation to the physical environment.

Chapter 7

Epilogue: Years Later

After the more extended field research between 1986 and 1988, when the material here presented originated, I visited the Yupno region and the village of Gua twice more, for shorter stays, but on both occasions my research agenda was focused on topics other than medical anthropology. The first visit, in August and September 1992, was directed towards issues of change, development, business, the role of 'kastom,' and the emic dimensions of disability. I lived in Gua village and rarely visited Teptep. The second visit, in August and September 2000, was for five weeks, which I again spent in Gua.

Illustration 12: Years after (2000): Zaka, Faiu and Sibik (from left to right) looking at the German book about their society

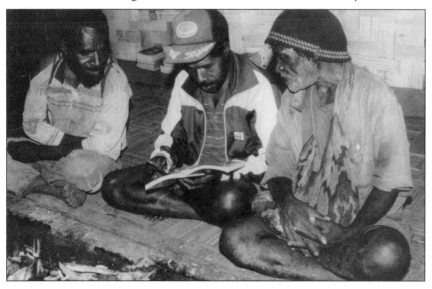

During my time there, I was preoccupied with the collection and enlargement of life histories, and the documentation of the many changes that were occurring among the Yupno.

Changes in 1992

The little boy Nstasiñge died in 1990. His parents Mayu and Tanowe are again living together in Madang and no longer want to go back to the village. Sauno and many of the older people, too, had died.

Gua village has also undergone some changes, and Western impact has increased: 'bisnis' (business) and 'senis' (change) are topics much discussed by the young people (see Keck 1993b.). Only very rarely can a Yupno be seen in traditional clothing.

The small 'tok ples' school has been closed down. The village store is today managed by Paul, one of Megau's sons. In 1989, a young evangelist from Finschhafen was assigned to the village and since then pressure from the Neuendettelsau Lutheran mission has increased. Church services are held regularly, traditional burial customs have been prohibited, and many of the old people have been baptised. The new "Oti and Saunu Memorial Church,"[1] a brightly coloured, solid wooden construction with a corrugated iron roof, has been erected at the location of the old church and was inaugurated in 1991. As a further innovation, today every village sector has a water-pipe with several taps.

Some of the young people have founded the first village "string band" called Makatu (Makatu is put together from abbreviations of three clans, Mambap, Ngangdum (Ka) and Tuwal, to which the band-members belong). Marijuana has recently reached the Yupno region and is secretly cultivated by the adolescents, but is sold only rarely or in small quantities because of the strict prohibition. The migration of the young people to the towns of Lae and Madang has significantly increased; many young people from Gua are today living in Madang; at the market, they are selling vegetables, tobacco and fruit (oranges), which arrive via airplane from Teptep. In Madang itself, they frequently grow peanuts for sale or are without employment.

Ginson Saunu, the son of the evangelist Sauno, was elected as representative of the Sapmanga District to the Morobe Provincial Government as the first ever Yupno, in 1989. He is a strong advocate for the construction of a road from Wantoat via Teptep to Saidor, and initiated the building of a Cultural Centre and a 'haus turis' in Teptep. In the summer of 1992, as independent candidate of the Kabwum-District, he won a seat in the House of Assembly, the national government in Port Moresby. Upon his first return to the village after winning the election in August 1992, he was celebrated and given benediction by the pastor of Teptep. The disputed borderline between Madang and Morobe Province was also settled. After years of discussion and confusion, Teptep station and the villages of Uskokop, Taeñ, Windiluk, Kwembun and Wandaboñ now belong to Madang Province, while the other upper Yupno villages (and therefore Gua as well) are part of Morobe Province.

The staff situation at the Teptep Health Centre has also changed: all five of the A.P.O. employed there today now come from the Yupno area.

Changes in 2000

Mayu, the mother of the small boy Nsatsiñge, is again living in Gua, and now has five children. Tanowe, the father, lives in Nadzap (Lae), supporting himself through casual work.

One of the most obvious changes in the village of Gua are the many new buildings, almost all in the traditional style as *tedetedetyut*; some are above Gua 1 in Gualbok and adjacent plots. A kind of hamlet or small settlement, consisting of several houses, has been built close to the road to Kangulut. Many of the young people who had migrated to the cities of Madang and Lae at the beginning of the 1990s have returned to the village, quite disillusioned about the possibilities of living and earning money in the cities as well as about the social climate, and are living in these new houses with their families. The income of those few who hold governmental or church positions in Teptep supports the whole lineage, and is used especially for paying the school fees for their children. This is a major and oft-discussed concern for the Yupno parents, who have only limited ways of generating a cash-income in the region. Smaller clans and their partner clan help each other, as a main co-operative task these days, to raise the necessary school fees.

The vegetable project still exists, but there are many difficulties in transporting the vegetables rapidly to their destinations, Madang and Lae. Transport problems (reliability, and high air fares) also apply for the other products planted or raised to generate an income: tobacco, coffee, and chickens.

The hotly debated road connection to Teptep via Wantoat or via the Rai Coast and Saidor still does not exist, although politicians continue to make plans. For the people in Gua with whom I spoke, however, the expected negative effects, such as 'raskals' entering the region, or the fear of women being taken away by outside men without paying a brideprice, outweigh the positive ones.

In 2000, both Provincial Governments, Madang and Morobe, have their representatives and offices in Teptep. The administrative border runs right through the Upper Yupno region, with the villages of Uskokop and Taeñ belonging to Madang Province, the other villages to Morobe. The population sees this competitive situation with regard to services as an advantage.

The changes the Yupno society underwent over the last 20 years are not unique, but can be compared to many other Papua New Guinea peoples' experience. Michael French Smith (2002), in his most recent book *Village on the Edge: Changing Times in Papua New Guinea* describes the transition of the local world of Kragur village on Kairiru Island. Among the many topics he raises are money, the increasing individualism and the changing of social relationships—a concern the Yupno discuss frequently, since they now have urgent need of cash for school fees, church collections, clothes, food from the store and traveling. The younger and middle-aged Yupno are especially sceptical about their and their children's future.

Wuli, a younger Yupno man who possesses a lot of traditional knowledge and who frequently reflects and discusses the pros and cons of 'kastom' and 'misin' (mission), is himself very much concerned about the future, and he should be given the last word:[2]

> I think like this: Our country is falling apart, and our government does not provide good services or bring development in our region, not really. And many of us have great worries about finding money and paying school fees, and our everyday life isn't too good. Why? The way our government is changing our country, and money and its way are becoming more important, but we can't see how we will get anything of this. What way will we have to get money? And take care of our families? And we all here, we all only know and understand little about the work of the 'haus sik', or the 'kiap' or the 'wok didiman' or whatever little work is around, and we find it hard, and our situation is not good, and we are having many children, and later we have worries about that too.

And, a bit resigned, he adds: "Now we are just here waiting."

Presentation of the Informants

I would like to make particular mention of the people of Gua who in some many ways made my time with them so enjoyable and productive. They gave me considerable help with everyday problems (housing, food, water, firewood), displayed wonderful patience during long talks, and readily cooperated with all my many demands on their time. Above all, their attitude towards me was warm and reassuring, and for all these things I am extremely grateful. *Mbit kuak tok madep si.* Those with whom I had the closest contact and to whom I owe most are briefly introduced here as representatives of all the others.

Faiu (Illustration 13), 33 years old in 1987, from the Kapbaga clan, was the first and until the end of fieldwork also my closest co-worker. He had completed training in Finschhafen to become a Lutheran pastor, and at the time of my stay was awaiting a posting on the coast. Faiu is married and has three children. As one of the best Tok Pisin speakers of the village, he had also been trained to translate concepts, and so was a big help with all the linguistic problems in addition to acting as my interpreter in many interviews. A reliable person who is full of humor, Faiu, with his diplomatic, considerate ways, was an indispensable advisor and mediator with all the other villagers in the case of disputes, and for me he arranged many additional visits and contacts. Even though he himself knew little about the traditional religious system, in the discussions with old men he nevertheless approached these questions totally undogmatically. Through the investigation of this complex of topics, he told me, his level of interest in the own tradition was raised. In the years following my initial field research, he worked as pastor in different upper Yupno villages (in the year 2000, he lived in Isan), but he still maintained close connections to Gua village.

Sibik (Illustration 14), about 40 years old in 1987, from the Talon clan; I got to know him better only during the second half of my stay. As a young man, he had worked as a cowboy in the Markham Valley and thus picked up some Tok Pisin. He was not easily ruffled and almost always in good spirits, so I enjoyed his frequent visits; towards the end of my stay Sibik would come on a daily basis. He helped in at least two respects: he, his wife Akñwal and

Illustration 13: Faiu

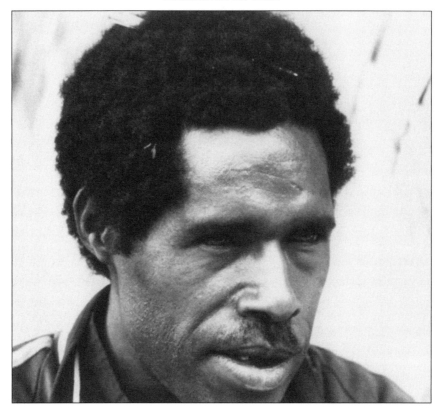

his five children reliably solved most of the everyday problems of logistics; also, he had great expertise in the interpretation of "signs" (*tauak*), and knowledge of people's ability to cause illness and to divine causes of illness. Most of my genealogical information I also owe to him. His pragmatic manner and calm were usually sufficient to soothe my bouts of irritation about the totally different notion of time held by the Yupno. He reacted with unlimited patience to any expressed difficulties on my part in interpreting the Yupno world. When we met in 2000, he did not seem to have changed at all, and immediately slipped again in the role of generously providing whatever help I needed.

Jowage (Illustration 15), about 65 years old, belonging to the Talon clan, an especially vigorous, energetic but also sensitive man who, as a "cooler," gave me much information regarding bodily disorders and the traditional possibilities of curing them. Apart from a brief stay in prison at Saidor, he had never left the Yupno and Nankina regions and so did not speak Tok Pisin, so

Illustration 14: Sibik

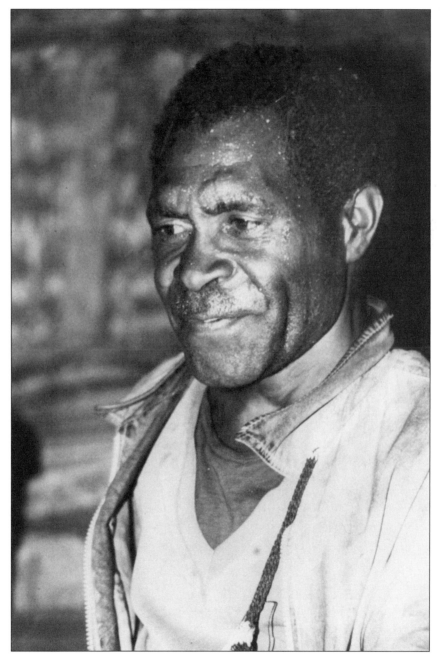

Illustration 15: Jowage

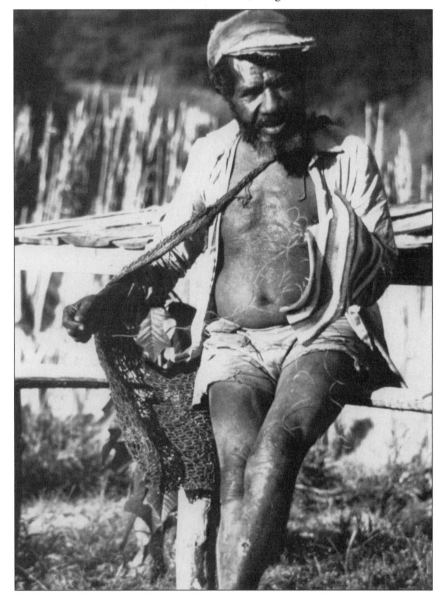

my conversations with him were conducted with interpreters. He is thought
to be one of the best mythologists and among the men most fully versed in
the traditions in the village. I was much touched by his impressive, long life

history which he told me over several hours, again and again breaking into tears when speaking about deceased relatives. One of his notable features was that he was extremely eloquent and could hardly contain his verbosity—a characteristic to which the villagers usually reacted with amusement but sometimes became impatient or annoyed. Jowage spent many days as a visitor in my house, all the while making (he was almost the only man in the village still doing so) small close-meshed men's string-bags, and was both very curious about and critical of my cooking ("pigs' food," he remarked on one occasion). His wife died in 1988, an event that sapped his spirit and seemed to age him; subsequently, he seldom spent the night in his house, where he lived alone, but often went to stay with relatives in the neighboring village of Uskokop. Jowage died in the early 1990s.

Zaka (Illustration 16), in his twenties, from the Talon clan. Zaka had gone to the mission school in Tapen and in 1987 was, at that time, the only young man living in the village who had attended high school in Madang up to Grade 10. He was an excellent Tok Pisin speaker, and to him I owe almost the complete translation of little Nstasiñge's illness report. He frequently also was an uncomplicated, caring companion on my many strenuous walks around the Yupno area. He could perhaps be regarded as an example of the "lost generation" of adolescents in the village: after finishing school, he could not find work and for a short while was at a loose end in Madang and Lae. He then married Rose, a woman from Nankina who had grown up in town, brought her back with him to Gua, and tried without success to get a training job as an A.P.O. Their first, prematurely born child died few days after the birth. Shortly before the termination of the second pregnancy, his wife moved back to her relatives in Madang and vowed never to return to Gua. In 1988, Zaka opened a small store in Gua, which he soon gave up, then later worked at Wasu in coffee processing, and hung around for a few troublesome years in Madang before he found work in the Yupno-Sepmanga region as an assistant in the election campaign being mounted by the then Provincial Government member, Ginson Saunu. He now (in 2000) has five children with Rose, and prefers life in the village over town. He was elected as 'komiti' and as magistrate at the village court, where he is responsible for mediating in conflicts arising in Gua and Kangulut villages.

Megau (Illustration 17), a man of about 50 years from the Ngandum clan, the former 'hedman' of the village. He is married to Metareñ, a very practical, energetic and hospitable woman and has children who are almost grown up. As a young man, he worked as a houseboy in an Australian household in Lae. In the beginning, he was very reticent, pensive and quiet since he mistakenly thought he did not know enough Tok Pisin for a conversation. His statements were well thought out, and my talks with him were intense and complex. After

Illustration 16: Zaka

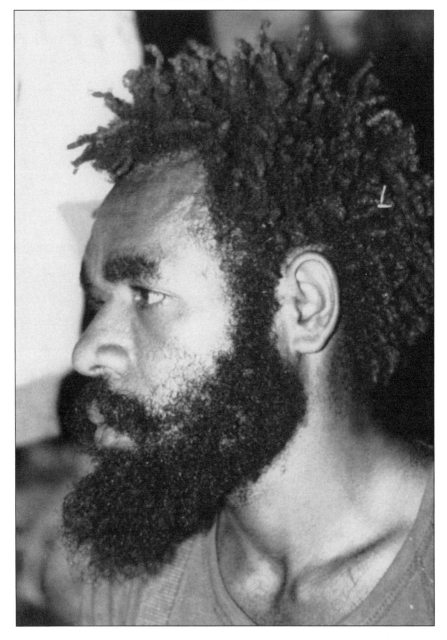

Illustration 17: Megau

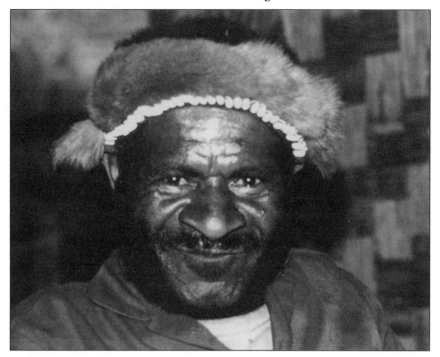

a few months, a very cordial relationship developed between us. Aside from much valuable information, I am especially grateful to Megau for his role in as a negotiator in connection with my purchasing of certain artifacts for museum collections in Berlin, Basel and Port Moresby, especially the large *nsaguo* wheels of feathers. By 2000, he had many grandchildren and was living a less active life, having built a small house for himself, in which he loves to chat with other elderly men. He had planted a lot of tobacco as a cash crop, which he was planning to sell in Madang, and this activity kept him very busy. His wife, Metareñ, was spending a lot of her time with the grandchildren.

Danda (Illustration 18), a quiet man of about 60 years from the neighboring village of Kangulut. I am indebted to Megau, because it was through his efforts that I managed to gain the confidence of his rather solitary relative, Danda, as an informant, who would accept only Megau as his translator in the case of secret material. Danda was a mine of mythological information and possessed a comprehensive knowledge about techniques to divine causes and to make people ill. An excellent flautist, he was a lone wolf who frequently

Illustration 18: Danda

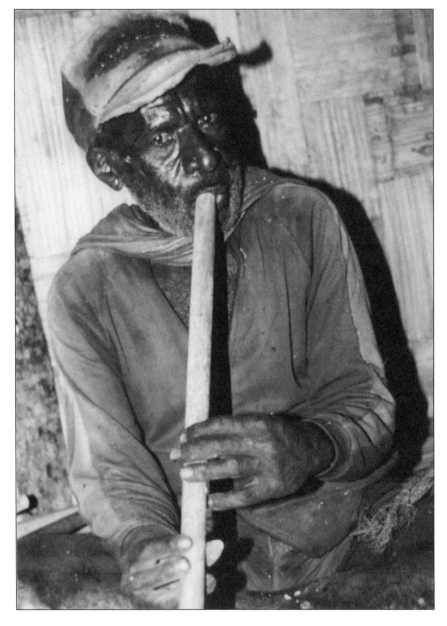

Illustration 19: Varenañ with a neighbor's newborn baby

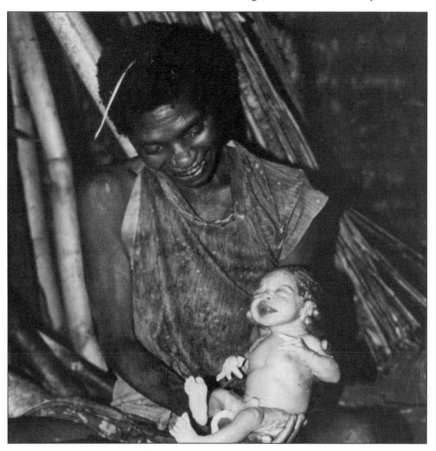

went off on trips into the bush or into neighboring valleys to gather materials for his magical practices. Danda died in the early 1990s.

Varenañ (Illustration 19), a woman approximately 30 years old, was originally from Nian and was married to the clearly older Motamba. Varenañ was my close neighbor, and because of the similarity in our names we were in a *wau-*, a namesake-relationship. Varenañ visited me daily (often several times), helped me with a lot of things and was my best friend in the village. Her cheerfulness and cordiality were contagious. Even though she did not speak Tok Pisin and I did not work with her a lot, I learnt a great deal from her: many important Yupno words and expressions concerning women's everyday life and their various skills, such as making net-bags, and much more. She, her

Illustration 20: Motamba with a child from his kinship group

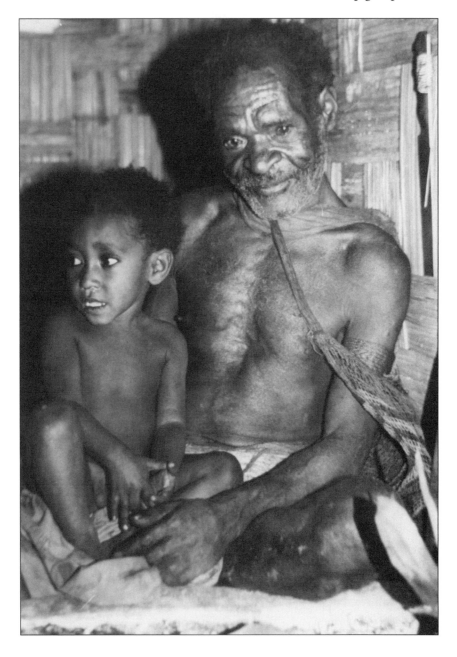

husband Motamba, her ten year old son Uñgwep and little daughter Roti were among my closest friends in Gua. In 2000, Roti was married to Nian, Uñgwep was living near Kabwum and, after the death of Motamba, Varenañ was remarried to one of Motamba's relatives and had moved to him to Devil village.

Motamba (Illustration 20), aged about 50, was a man of the Tuwal II clan and husband of Varenañ (above). As a younger man, Motamba had lived in the Wantoat valley for some time and maintained close links with people there. His first wife died years before, as well as the daughter from his first marriage who had given birth to his granddaughter Roti. From his second wife, Varenañ, he has a son, Uñgwep. He seemed older than he actually was; he preferred to stay close to his house, where, movingly and with great patience, he took care of the infants of his relatives. He was a gentle, quiet guest who shortly before dusk every day would visit me, and after skillfully lighting a fire he sat sipping tea while he awaited the return of his wife from the garden and his son from the community school in Teptep. Motamba died in 1993.

Botanical Classifications

(by Robert Kiapranis, Botanist, and Verena Keck)

The botanical classifications of the following plants were made by the botanist Robert Kiapranis of the Ecological Institute in Wau (Morobe Province), who came to Gua for several days to carry out this work. A scientific classification of all the plants was not possible (of the total of 242 to be classified, only 147, or approximately 60%, could be ascribed), for the following reasons:

- some of the plants used in the causation and cure of illness grow in the bush at a distance of two or more days by foot from Gua, others in lower-lying regions, and from there are brought to the Yupno region in a dried state; during the short visit of the botanist, they could not be collected.
- Some of the samples collected by the Yupno were not complete enough for classification (e.g. blossoms or bark were missing) or in a bad (withered) state.
- Some plants which the Yupno call by different names, hence classify differently and clearly distinguish, are exactly the same according to the botanical classification.
- Conversely, the Yupno give the same name to plant samples that are clearly distinguished according to botanical classification.
- Within the individual "major groups" like bamboo, cordyline, fern, sugar-cane, bananas, which are to be found in many different varieties, no further distinction could be made under field conditions.

The abbreviations signify: sp. = species, fam. = family. The plants in the alphabetical order of their Yupno names:

amɨn sisap   (*amɨn*: man, *sisap*: no translation), botanically unclassified, a kind of grass *amɨn tekok* (*amɨn*: man, *tekok* from *teet kok* from *teet*: kind of bamboo, *kok*: excrements, *tekok*: also name of the fire-saw), Compositae fam., a kind of grass

apmbɨlapmbɨl (*apmbɨlapmbɨl*: no translation), botanically unclassified

arap silup (*arap*: a kind of reed, 'kunai', *silup*: blossom), botanically unclassified kind of tree

boa (*boa*: no translation), botanically unclassified, a kind of moss

bumat (*bumat*: no translation), Dendrocnide sp., Urticaceae fam.

dimdim (*dimdim*: to grow thick; a kind of reed that grows very straight and thick and has a firm stalk), Mischanthus floridulus (Labill.) Warb., Graminae fam.

elin (*elin*: no translation), botanically unclassified, grasses with small barbs that prick people

ɨlaklɨlak (*ɨlaklɨlak*: to sway [in the wind], also called *ngodan kuak* [*ngodan*: moss, *kuak*: white]), Lichen sp., a tree lichen

ɨlok (*ɨlok*: name for a kind of gras, 'tiktik'), botanically unclassified

joñgat (*joñgat*, from *joñ*: gras, *gat*: to hang down; this plant grows only in grassland areas), Musa sp., Musaceae fam., a kind of banana

joñwijok (*joñwijok*, from *joñ*: grass, *wijok*: stem, stalk), Buddleja asiatica Lour, Loganiaceae fam., a mythologically important tree with light green (*Yupno*: "white"), "cold" leaves

kalañ kuak (*kalañ*: foot, *kuak*: white, "cold"), Zingiber officinale L., Zingiberaceae fam., a kind of ginger

kalit sewak (*kalit* = *karit*: cabbage, *sewak*: long, hence wild, "sprouted" cabbage with thorns), botanically unclassified

kalo (*kalo*: mould, the tree has whitish "hairs" on the trunk), Laportae decumana, Urticacea fam.

kamam kuok (*kamam*: new, raw, *kuok*: to originate, shoot), botanically unclassified

kandap arap (*kandap*: tree, wood, fire, *arap*: to glimmer, to burn down; a kind of tree whose wood does not burn fiercely, but only glimmers), Blumea lacera, Compositae fam.

kandap pokat (*kandap*: tree, wood, fire, *pokat*: flat), botanically unclassified *kandat yaat*   (*kandat* = *kindat*: name of area on the Yupno River, also: to collect, *yaat*: name for sugar-cane), Saccharum officiarum, Graminae fam., a very white sugar-cane

kauak   (*kauak*: no translation), Desmodium rapandium (Vahl) DC., Leguminosae fam.

kɨdɨñ   (*kɨdɨñ*: griddle, basis of the construction of a fireplace in the house, "base," name of a kind of tree), Macaranga triloba, Euphorbiaceae fam.

kokmbɨsap   (*kokmbɨsap*, from *kok*: excrements, *mbɨsap*: knot, time), Cordyline sp., Liliaceae fam.

kokop amɨn kamam   (*kokok*: place, settlement, *amɨn*: man, *kamam*: new, e.g. newly introduced by the mission, hence something newly planted in a place populated by the people), Bides piles, Compositae fam., a fragrant flower

kokopkɨrat maam   (*kokopkɨrat* from *kokop*: place, settlement, *kɨrat*: bone, meaning: "strength-holder of the settlement," *maam*: name for ginger), Zingiber officinale, Zingiberaceae fam.

kokopyaal   (*kokopyaal*, from *kokop*: place, settlement, *yaal*: stinging nettle, 'salat'), Dendrocnide sp., Urticaceae fam.

komndak maam   (*komndak* shortened from *ko* = *koñ*: "ghost," *mndak* = *mɨndak*: to cut, to chase away, to remove, *maam*: generic noun for ginger), botanically unclassified

komupkomup   (*komupkomup*, from *komup*: 'marita', a certain kind of pandanus from which the red liquid *komup* is gained; the blossom and fruit of *komupkomup* resemble that of the *komup* plant), Rubus rosifolius J.E. Smith sp., Rosaceae fam. or Rubus fraxinifolius Poir.sp., Rosaceae fam., a plant with thorns. *Komupkomup* is one of those cases where the Yupno give the same name to two botanically different plants, and hence do not classify differently.

kua   (*kua*: to grow, to originate), Vaccinium fissiflorum Sleum, Ericaceae fam.

kulbɨt   (*kulbɨt* from *kul*: no translation, *bɨt* = *mbit*: belly, thoughts, feelings), Ficus sp., Moraceae fam.

kulmak   (*kulmak*, from *kul*: to plant, *mak*: downwards), Dacrydium nidulium, Podocarpaceae fam., the tree is thought to be the "house" of the creator deity Morap *kumbu* (*kumbu*, from *kum* = *koñ*: "dead spirit," *mbu* = *mbɨt*: belly, thoughts, feelings, name of a tree through which the "souls of a dead person," the ghosts, talk to a "medium"), botanically unclassified

kunagat (*kunagat*: name of a kind of pandanus), Pandanus sp., Pandanaceae fam.

kunagat pɨsɨt (*kunagat*: name of a kind of pandanus, *pɨsɨt*: liquid, urine), botanically unclassified, a liana growing on the trunk of the pandanus tree

kwawɨl (*kwawɨl*: no translation), botanically unclassified, edible kind of vegetable, similar to spinach

kwebekal (*kwebekal*, from *kwebe*: Kewieñ name for pandanus, *kal*: to strengthen), Pilea sp., Urticaceae fam. or Begonia sp., a "cold" plant growing close to the water. *Kwebekal* is another case where the Yupno give the same name to two botanically different plants

luplup (*luplup*: saliva), Musa sp., Musaceae fam.

makum (*makum*: to flicker, the wood of this tree burns excellently in a dry state), Osmoxylon sp., Araliaceae fam., it has a thorny trunk and thorny leaves

mamba (*mamba*: no translation), Begonia sp., Begoniaceae fam.

mambak (*mambak*: no translation), Ficus augusta Corner, Moraceae fam.

mamnaknak (*mamnaknak*, from *mam* from *mambil*: chin, jaw, *naknak*: down [also the little hairs on grasses], botanically unclassified

maam goman (*maam*: generic noun for ginger, *goman*: red), Zingiber officinale L., Zingibearceae fam.

maam si (*maam*: generic noun for ginger, *si*: good, very, real), Zingiber officinale L., Zingibearceae fam.

manañgan (*manañgan*: no translation), Begonia taffaensisi aff., Begoniaceae fam.

manjit (*manjit*: a term from the Nankina language, to hang up, to strangle, trap), Crassocephalum sp., Compositae fam.

mawom maam (*mawom*: name for a certain "technique," 'sangguma,' kind of sorcery, *maam*: generic noun for ginger), botanically unclassified

mbabuñ	(*mbabuñ* = *mbebuñ*: to whirl), Cyathea sp., Cyatheaceae fam.
mbañgam	(*mbañgam*, from *mbañ*: to receive, to get, *gam*: cool), Oenanthe javanica DC., Umbelliferae fam., a "cold" plant growing near the water
mbasip	(*mbasip*: no translation); a kind of bean, botanically unclassified
mbep	(*mbep*, term from Uskokop for to make, to hem, to fabricate, a planted tree whose bark is used for bark cloth), Laportae sp., Urticaceae fam.
mbiagoman	(*mbiagoman*, from *mbia* = *mbiap*: no translation, *goman*: red), Acalypha sp., Euphorbiaceae fam.
mbiap	(*mbiap*: no translation), Acalypha insulana L., Euphorbiaceae fam.
mbiawandat	(*mbiawandat*, from *mbia*: a kind of bird, *wandat*: to fetch, meaning: the bird eats this plant), Cyrtandra sp., Gesneriaceae fam.
mbilañ	(*mbilañ*: to put up a mark), Musa sp., Musaceae fam.
mbitkuak	(*mbitkuak*, from *mbit*: belly, thoughts, emotions, feeling, *kuak*: white, "cold"), Leukosyke sp., Urticaceae fam., a tree with leaves which are white on the lower side
mbok	(*mbok*: fragile), Plectranthus sp., Labiatea fam., a cultivated plant with red leaves
mbomak	(*mbomak*, from *mbom*: red clay, *ak*: to fall down, meaning: the plant grows where the red clay crumbles down), Plectranthus sp., Labiatae fam.
mbutndañgwan	(*mbutndañgwan*, from *mbut*: pig, *ndañgwan*: hair, hence pig's bristle), Eleusine indica, Graminae fam.
mewe	(*mewe*: a kind of mushroom), botanically unclassified
miañmiañ	(*miañmiañ*, from *mian* = *meñ*: mother), botanically unclassified
ndalndal	(*ndalndal*, from *ndal* = *dal*: to rub, to twirl, to whirl around), botanically unclassified
nalok goman	(*nalok*: generic noun for banana, *goman*: red), Musa sp., Musaceae fam.
ndaloñndaloñ	(*ndaloñndaloñ*: to trickle down; name for falling pieces of wood and bark which fall down from the trees when the tree

	kangaroos climb around at night), Dennstaedtia nouguineensis, Dennstaedtia fam., thorny growth
ndamba	(*ndamba*: name for a fern-like plant), Sphenomeris chinensis, Lindaea fam.
ndamba isip	(*ndamba*: name of a fern-like plant, *isip*: sour, burning), botanically unclassified, a plant growing near the water
ndamba kuak	(*ndamba*: name of a fern-like plant, *kuak*: white, "cold"), Nephrolepsis cordifolia, Oleandraceae fam.
ndankwit kasit	(*ndankwit*: a kind of marsupial, *kasit*: hand, the leaves look like the paw of a marsupial), Ranunculus psedolowii Hj. Eichl., Ranunculaceae fam.
ndauña ndamba	(*ndauña*: to come first, *ndamba*: name of a fern-like plant), Cyathea sp., Cyatheaceae fam.
ndavieñ	(*ndavieñ*: no translation), Cucurbita maxima, Curcubitacea fam.
ndavɨsal	(*ndavɨsal*: no translation), botanically unclassified, the bark of this tree which grows on the coast is beaten into bark cloth
ndetkok	(*ndetkok*, from *ndet*: name of a small bird, *kok*: excrement, the flower grows in bird excrement), Ameyema finisterrae (Warb.), -Danser, Loranthaceae fam.
ngagngak	(*ngagngak*, from *ngak*: to stick, something which sticks well), Bulbuphylum cf. bolanum Schltz, Orchidaceae fam.
ngambum	(*ngambum*, from *ngam* = *gam*: cool, *bum*: ripe), Musa sp., Musaceae fam.
ngapmba	(*ngapmba*: no translation), botanically unclassified, a kind of *kwebekal*
ngasu	(*ngasu*: to hang up), Syzygium clafilorum (Roxb) - Cowan & Cowan, Mytraceae fam.
ngavɨ	(*ngavɨ*: name of an insect that dwells on the stem of this kind of bamboo in large numbers), Bambusa sp., Graminae fam.
ngodan	(*ngodan*: no translation), Lichen sp.
ngodɨm tiraptok	(*ngodɨm*: body, *tiraptok*: to get right), Astilbe papuana Schl., Saxifagraceae fam.
ngolda	(*ngolda*: no translation), Musa sp., Musaceae fam., a "cold" kind of banana said to have been washed up by the Yupno River, and important in religion

ngoman	(*ngoman*: red), botanically unclassified, big tree in the bush
ngwawan	(*ngwawan*: no translation), botanically unclassified, the bark of this tree is used by the "coolers," it tastes like nutmeg
njakngak	(*njakngak*: to smack one's lips, to bite), Pteris wallichiana sp., Pteris fam.
njɨmuk	(*njɨmuk*: name for the process when one gets something out with the fingernails), Orchid sp., Orchidaceae fam., a cultivated plant
njogal	(*njogal*: glowing fire), Alpina lephrochlamys K.Sch. et faut., Zingiberaceae fam.
numbun	(*numbun*: no translation), Acorus calamus L., Araceae fam., a "cold" plant growing near the water
nyaknkuak	(*nyaknkuak*, from *nyak*: to see, appearance, *nkuak* = *kuak*: white, hence of white appearance), botanically unclassified, a fern-like plant
nyingwalmelbi	(*nyingwalmelbi*, from *nyingwal*: a kind of bird, *melbi*: yams), Hebanaria tricoglossa Ranzr., Orchidaceae fam.
obip	(*obip*: no translation), Areca sp., Palmea fam., a tree
paña	(*paña*: to pick, meaning: the leaves are tiny, they can never all be picked), Solanum inodiflorum Jacq., Solanaceae fam.
patndan	(*patndan*: to bend something, to fold it and then wrap it up), Leukosyke sp., Urticaceae fam.
petam	(*petam*: no translation), Adiatum sp., Adiantum fam.
petmbat	(*petmbat*: no translation), Crinium asiatica sp., Amaryllidaceae fam.
pɨdɨm	(*pɨdɨm*: no translation), botanically unclassified
pɨpnameñ	(*pɨpnameñ*, from *pɨp*: chicken, *nameñ*: neck, meaning: red skin fold of the rooster which the flower resembles), Iresine herbstii, Amaranthaceae fam.
pɨpnjaap	(*pɨpnjaap*, from *pɨp*: chicken, *njaap*: food, eating), Vicia sativa sp., Leguminosae fam.
pobalok	(*pobalok*: no translation), Hydrochotyle javanica Thumb, Umbelliferae fam.
popmdeñ	(*popmdeñ*, from *pop*: to blow, *mdeñ* = *ndeñ*: onomatopoetical: to crack (if one hits the plant), Desmodium rapandum (Vahl) DC., Leguminosae fam.

rap silup	(*rap*: a kind of tree, *silup*: blossom), botanically unclassified
simbu	(*simbu*: black), botanically unclassified
sukuak	(*sukuak*, from *su*: no translation, *kuak*: white, "cold"), Blumea lacera, Compositae fam.
talbeñ	(*talbeñ*: no translation), botanically unclassified
tañgwin	(*tañgwin*, from *tañ = tam*: leaf, *gwin*: dry), Dodonea viscosa, Sapindaceae fam.
tapmat	(*tapmat*, from *tap = tepm*: hot, fast, pain, *mat*: fast), Rubus moluccana L., Rosaceae fam.
teet	(*teet*: good), Bambusa sp., Graminae fam.
teetgoman	(*teetgoman*, from *teet*: good, *goman*: red), Bambusa sp., Graminae fam.
tekok kandap	(*tekok* whereby *teet kok* from *teet*: good, *kok*: excrement, name for the fire-saw, *kandap*: wood, fire, a kind of tree which burns especially well), botanically unclassified
timni kadim	(*timni kadim*, from *timni*: nose, *kadim*: mad, firm), Musa sp., Musaceae fam.
umban	(*umban*: no translation, name for different kinds of 'tanget'), Cordyline sp., Liliaceae fam.
umban bap	(*umban*: no translation, name for different kinds of 'tanget', *bap*: big), Cordyline sp., Liliaceae fam.
woral	(*woral*: to curl upwards), botanically unclassified, a kind of reed-like grass
wuok	(*wuok*: brain, the plant's strong odor emanates from the inner part of the blossom), botanically unclassified
yaal	(*yaal*: all is said herewith, end of speech), Dendrocnide sp., Urticacea fam., a kind of stinging nettle
yaat	(*yaat*: open, name for sugar-cane), Saccharum officinarum, Graminae fam.
yaat si	(*yaat*: open, name for sugar-cane, *si*: good, very, real), Saccharum officinarum, Graminae fam.
yabam	(*yabam*: oily), Piptrus sp., Urticaceae fam.
yavit	(*yavit*: a kind of mushroom), botanically unclassified
zarak	(*zarak*: a Kâte name), plant with lilac-colored, serrated leaves, botanically unclassified

Glossary

Yupno Words

a: term for MoBr

aljoko pok, aljoko from *aljok*: axilla, *pok*: to come down, "swollen armpit"

amek: term for "swollen belly"

amɨn: human being, man

amɨn amdi, amɨn: man, *amdi* shortened from *amɨnti*, whereby *amɨn*: man, *ti*: very, true, good, "real man"

amɨn kamam, amɨn: man, *kaman*: new, also raw, "new man," term for newly wed man

amɨn kasit, amɨn: man, *kasit*: hand, caused by "the hand of man"

amɨn komakmbe, amɨn: man, *komakmbe* from *ko*: to go, *makmbe*: to be totally over, to be finished, "dead person"

amɨn koñwak, amɨn: man, *koñwak* from *koñ*: "ghost," *wak*: no translation, "recently died person"

amɨn monji, amɨn: man, *monji*: child, "little man"

amɨn ndañgwan, amɨn: man, *ndañgwan*: hair, "human hair"

amɨn ngop, amɨn: man, *ngop*: skin, wrapping, "human wrapping," payment for a dead person

amɨn pilañ, amɨn: man, *pilañ*: from *pi* or *pe*: big, and *ilañ*: to descend, slope, "old man"

amɨnwop, from *amɨn*: man, *wop = wopm*: image, shadow, "soul," "shadow of man," "shadow soul"

añgumgumañ from *añ*: to do, *gumgum*: to soothe

aññok from *añ*: to do, *nok*: food, nutrition, "to prepare food [and give it away]," brideprice

arokarok, from *arok*: to rub against something, scratch, also a place the pigs rub against, a stone, tree-trunk etc.), term for an itchy skin disease, "scabies" *awɨda sañnamok, awɨda* from *awɨ*: lime, *da*: suffixed particle, *sañnamok*: it burned me, "lime has burned me," meaning: "burn in the mouth"

Bapiayutyoma, from *bapiayut, bapia*: paper, *yut*: house, hence school; *yoma*: fence, hence area inside a fence, "school-fence"

bɨmjɨt, from *bɨm*: term for a fallen down, rotting tree, metaphor for a deceased person, *jɨt* heavy, an "oppressing problem" caused by a "ghost" or dead person

bɨmjɨtwal, from *bɨmjɨt*: stinking, rotten, *jɨt*: heavy, term for a fallen over, rotting tree where this beetle lives, *wal*: no translation, a kind of beetle

bumbum: term for reed-like stalks, used as torch

bumum: no translation, baskets for keeping the pandanus nuts

Daldal from *daldal*: "to swirl around" (a stick between two hands), "to twirl"

dipmin: dream

Eka, *eka* from *et*: sliding ground, *ka*: many, "landslide"

Ekatuwal, from *et*: sliding ground, *ka*: many, *tuwal*: keel, spit of land, "sliding spit of land"

eyat: lice

gen yuki, gen: speech, talk, language, *yuki*: bad, "gossip," "rumors," "bad words," "insults"

Gowañon, from *gowañ*: below, *on*: locative, "below"

Gowañowa from *gowañ*: below, *owa*: above, "above from below"

Guagowañ from *gua = guam*: centipede, here: place of the Gua-*mbema*, *gowañ*: below, "below Gua-*mbema*"

Gualbok, *gual*: no translation, *bok*: kind of 'pitpit'

guam: centipede

guammbema from guam: centipede; *mbema* from *mbe*: name of a tree that was traditionally of religious importance, and *ma*: fenced-in section around a center, hence "fenced-in section around the *mbe* tree." *Mbema* also means men's house; it used to always stand inside the fenced-in section near the *mbe* tree

ɨlok amɨn, ɨlok: name of a reed-like grass, *bumbum*, 'tiktik', *amɨn*: man, "reed grass man"

jalap: entry, entrance in a fence, an opening, term for kin group

Jogakluk from *jogak*: a sort of tree, *luk*: tree crown, branches, "place of the *jogak* tree crowns"

kaandap yukidak, kaandap: leg, *yuki*: bad, grave, *dak*: to be, "bad leg"

kaandapno komokndok, kaandap: leg, *no*: my, *komokndok*: to have died, "my gone to sleep leg"

kabɨbɨ: kind of butterfly

kak amɨn, *kak* = *kok*: to go up, to climb, *amɨn*: man, hence "the climber" (the lizard only lives on high trees and in pandanus trees)

kalañ baptok ak, *kalañ*: leg, foot, *baptok* from *bap*: big, *tok*: to exist, *ak*: he makes, "swollen feet"

kalañe kadɨmtok, *kalañe* from *kalañ*: foot, *kadɨm*: firm, mad, *tok*: to exist, "totally numb foot"

kalañno komokndok, *kalañ*: foot, *no*: my, *komokndok*: to have died, "my gone to sleep foot"

kalapno ko, *kalapno* from *kalap*: meat, *no*: my, *ko*: go!, meaning: "in the name of my ancestors, go!"

kaldok: "cough"

kalsɨt nywok, *kalsɨt*: loin, *ny*: no translation, *wok*: to come up, "swollen loin"

kamam kuok amɨn, from *kamam*: new, raw, *kuok*: to originate, a (plant) shoot, *amɨn*: man, "restorer"

kambul bapdak, *kambul*: vulva, *bapdak*, from *bap*: big, *dak*: to be, "swollen vulva"

Kamkwam from *kamkwam*: fast, "place where everything grows fast"

kandap: tree, wood, fire

kandap arap amɨn, from *kandap arap*: a kind of tree the wood of which burns very quickly, from *kandap*: wood, fire, *arap*: to burn out, to die out, *amɨn*: man, "somebody, who quickly extinguishes the fire or the heat," "fire extinguisher"

kandap sɨt, *kandap*: wood, also fire, *sɨt*: I burn, heat, cook, "I made a fire"

kandapda sañgamok, *kandap*: fire, wood, *sañgamok*: to burn, "burns"

Kaparɨkandom, from *kaparɨ*: variety of sweet potato, *ka*: many, *ndom*: hill, mountain, "hill of the *kaparɨ* sweet potatoes"

Kapbaga from *kap*: name of the leaf serving as a base for carrying burdens on the head, *baga*: hill, mountain, here: crown of the head, "[people with the] head-covering"

kasɨro wanpelak, *kasɨro* = *kasɨt*: hand, arm, *wanpelak*: to break, "hand- or arm-fracture"

kasok: recipients of the brideprice

kawam: kind of bird, 'tarangau'

kawañ susoñ, *kawañ*: smell, *susoñ*: to cook, to burn, "to burn the smell"

keaknok from *keak*: something that comes from below, cough, *nok*: food, to swallow, hence "to continuously swallow what one coughs up [phlegm]"

kɨnam kɨrat, *kɨnam*: bamboo, *kɨrat*: bones, "bamboo pipe"

kɨran: kind of rat

kɨrarogen, *kɨraro* from *kɨrat*: bone, *gen*: only that, "only skin and bones," "very skinny" *kɨrat*: bones

ko: go!

kokɨlɨt, from *kok*: excrement, *ɨlɨt*: to drip, to trickle, to run, "diarrhoea"

Kokndekmon from *kok*: excrement, *ndek*: no translation, *mon*: mountain, "toilet mountain"

kokop kɨrat, kokop: settlement, place, *kɨrat*: bones, "strength-holder of the settlement"

Komin, from *komin*: kind of tree, "[people from the] *komin* tree"

komup amɨn, komup: the red sap of a pandanus kind, 'marita,' *amɨn*: man: "red man"

komup erap, komup: the red sap of a pandanus kind, 'marita,' *erap*: bowl, basin, "bowl with the red liquid"

komup pat, komup: the red sap of a pandanus kind, 'marita,' *pat*: trap, "trap with the red liquid"

koñ: "ghost"

koñ mɨndak, koñ: "ghost," *mɨndak*: to cut, to chase away, to remove, "expulsion of the ghost"

koñ tauak, koñ: "ghost," *tauak*: "sign"; "sign of the ghost"

koñgap from koñ: "ghost," *gap* = *kaap*: melody, "personal melody," "dance feast," 'singsing'

koñwop, from koñ: "ghost," *wop* = *wopm*: image, shadow, "soul of a dead person"

kosum kalɨmdak, kosum: ear, *kalɨmdak*: to be closed, to be blocked, "blocked ear"

kosum mi, kosum: ear, *mi*: not existing, "deaf"

kosum tawa, kosum: ear, *tawa*: pus, "festering ear"

kowa: "hot" red soil

kuak: white, white soil

kuak amɨn, kuak: white, *amɨn*: man, "white man"

kuapmo tepm namejak, kuapmo from *kuap*: shoulder, *mo*: my, *tepm*: hot, pain, fast, *namejak*: it gives me, "my shoulder gives me pain"

kumbu amɨn, kumbu from *koñ* and *mbɨt, koñ*: "ghost," *mbu* = *mbɨt*: belly, thoughts, feelings, name of a tree through which the "ghosts" talk to the "medium," *amɨn*: man, a person receptive to powerful dreams, kind of "medium"

kunagat amɨn, kunagat: pandanus, *amɨn*: man, the "pandanus-man"

kwin wok ndima ki, kwin: above, *wok*: to go up, *ndɨma*: not, *ki*: to go, "you shall not go higher up!"

kwindañ, from *kwin*: above, *dañ*: to be, hence to be in a "hot," "above" state, "being angry"

Lepmonkwagilin from *lep = alip*: bare ass, the Yupno name for the formerly naked neighboring group, the Wantoat, *mon*: small hill, *kwa*: marking, e.g. an *umban* plant serving as a border marker, *gilin*: to be present. Meaning: a small fenced-in garden plot, a place where a Wantoat once had a garden, "garden of a bare ass"

Makumbaga, from *makum*: name of a tree, *baga*: hill, mountain, "hill of the makum tree"

Mambap from *mam = maam*: ginger, *bap*: big, "[people from the] big ginger plant"

Mambapbaga from *mam = maam*: ginger, *bap*: big, *baga*: hill, mountain, the "hill near the big ginger"

Mambapgowañ, from *mam = maam*: ginger, *bap*: big, *gowañ*: below, "below the big ginger plant"

mami from *ma = man*: name, *mi*: nonexistent, hence (for Ego) "without a name"

mandak nañ mandañamok, *mandak*: knife, *nañ*: him, *mandañamok*: has cut him, "the knife has cut him"

manimi from *mani = man*: name, *mi*: nonexistent, "without name"

manjit tepm namejak, *manjit*: back, *tepm*: hot, pain, fast, *namejak*: he gives me, "the back gives me pain"

manjit tepm tok, *manjit*: back, *tepm*: hot, pain, fast, *tok*: to exist, "backache"

mañot: red earth pigment, red soil

marasin yut, *marasin* from Tok Pisin 'marasin,' "medicine," *yut*: house, "house of medicine," term for the Teptep Health Centre

mawom: no translation, 'sangguma,' kind of sorcery, an especially evil illness causing "technique"

mawom amin, *mawom*: no translation, 'sangguma,' kind of sorcery, *amin*: man, "sorcerer"

mawom tauak, *mawom*: no translation, 'sangguma,' kind of sorcery," *tauak*: "sign," "sign of a *mawom* act"

mawom yut, *mawom*: no translation, 'sangguma,' kind of sorcery, *yut*: house, "*mawom* house"

mbaak: ice cold

mbalgerk: dried bast-like strips of the ribs of banana leaves

mbasok tauak, *mbasok*: term for the kin group of the woman, *tauak*: "sign," "sign of the kin group of the woman"

mbawo tauak, *mbawo*: term for patri- and matri-lateral persons of the second ascending generation and above, also ancestor, *tauak*: "sign," "sign of the ancestor" *mbema* from *mbe*: name of a tree which was traditionally of religious importance, and *ma*: fenced-in section around a center, hence "fenced-in section around the *mbe*-tree." *Mbema* also means men's house; it used to always stand inside the fenced-in section near the *mbe*-tree

mbema yut; mbema see above, *yut*: house, "men's house"

mbɨdok from *mbɨ= mbɨt*: belly, thoughts, emotions, feeling, *dok*: to come out, "letting out emotions"

mbɨrap: bean

mbisoñ epmdaldak, mbisoñ: head, *epmdaldak*: to scratch, "to scratch his head"

mbisoñ kɨrat, mbisoñ: head, *kɨrat*: bones, "the "skull"

mbisoñ nda, mbisoñ: head, *nda*: small, made without much effort, name for a dancing decoration

mbisoñ ndañgwan pilakndak, mbisoñ: head, *ndañgwan*: hair, *pilakndak*: to pull, "to pull the hair"

mbisoñ tepm from *mbisoñ*: head, *tepm*: hot, pain, fast, "headache"

mbɨt: belly, also the thoughts, emotions and feelings of a person (in the belly)

mbɨt kaloñ, from *mbɨt*: belly, thoughts, emotions, feeling, *kaloñ*: term for the number one, "to be one belly," 'wanbel'

mbɨt kandap, mbɨt: belly, thoughts, emotions, feeling, *kandap*: tree, wood, fire, "the belly burns," "having hot feelings," "burning thoughts," "inner fire"

mbɨt kandap kot, mbɨt: belly, thoughts, emotions, feeling, *kandap*: tree, wood, fire, *kot*: garden, but also work, "a workaholic"

mbɨt kuak, mbɨt: belly, thoughts, feelings, *kuak*: white, "cold," "the belly is cold," "the feelings are cold"

mbɨt madeptok, mbɨt: belly, *madep*: big, *tok*: to be, "swollen, inflated belly"

mbɨt njap, mbɨt: belly, thoughts, emotions, feelings, *njap*: fight, "anger," "being upset"

mbɨt opmbal, from *mbɨt*: belly, thoughts, emotions, feelings, *opmbal*: wrong, see *opmbilap*, "the thoughts are all upside down"

mbɨt pasɨl, from *mbɨt*: belly, thoughts, emotions, feelings, *pasɨl*: to frighten, to be scared, "being afraid"

mbɨt peak, mbɨt: belly, thoughts, emotions, feelings, *peak*: ripe, "increasing suspicion"

mbɨt tevan, mbɨt: belly, thoughts, feelings, *tevan*: firm, strong, "different," powerful, "to have strong thoughts"

mbɨt yawuro from *mbɨt*: belly, thoughts, feelings, emotions, *yawuro*: cool, "harmonious, cool feelings"

Mbɨvɨka, from *mbɨvɨ*: (in) two pieces (broken ground), *ka*: many, the "place of the broken-up ground"

mbobok, whereby *mbo* from *mbɨt*: belly, *bok*: no translation, meaning: "belly swells"

mbook: "sniffles (with runny nose)"

mbowañ: bark-cloth belt

mbrombak, from *mbro* and *mbɨro*: belly and breast, i.e. the front side, *mbak*: onomatopoetical, the noise made by the lizard living only in trees when moving forward, hence "breast-beater," a kind of lizard

mbumbumayut, from *mbumbuma*: on top and on top (referring to the wall with several layers of pandanus leaves, plaited 'tiktik' and split bamboo), *yut*: house, "wrapper house"

mbut mɨndak amɨn, *mbut*: pig, *mɨndak*: to cut, to chase away, also to disembowel, *amɨn*: man, "pig cutter"

mbut nduat: *mbut*: pig, *nduat*: half, rest, leftover, the remain, "a piece of pork"

meñ: mother

meñ kalap mbɨsap, *meñ*: mother, also origin, *kalap*: flesh, *mbɨsap*: knot, time, " time of the origin of the flesh"

meñ tauak, *meñ*: mother, *tauak*: mark, "mark of the mother"

meñgak: kind of frog

meñi kong from *meñi* = *meñ*: mother, *kong*: to see, special brideprice arrangement, "for the eyes of the mother"

meññan from *meñ*: mother, *nan*: father, "parents"

meññan tauak, *meñ*: mother, *nan*: father, *tauak*: "sign," "signs of mother and father"

mevɨlɨ toñ, *mevɨlɨ*: cause, origin, stem, reason, *toñ*: to exist, "a cause exists"

minam: bird

mɨndak mɨndak amɨn, from *mɨndak*: to cut, to disembowel (e.g. a pig), to chase away, to remove, *amɨn*: man, "abortion specialist"

miyaga from *mi*: nonexistent, *yaga*: to watch out, hence "not having watched out," an act to be ashamed of, "shame"

molɨt: "the people from down there"

moñan: breathe, wind, steam, breeze; it causes a human being to see, hear, smell, walk around, having his/her own personality, "breath spirit"

moñan da añakndak, *moñan*: breath, here: gust of wind, *da*: suffixed particle, *añakndak*: to make, "to catch a gust of wind," "draught"

moñan milgañ, *moñan*: "breath," "breath spirit," *milgañ*: to heat, also to prepare, "to heat the breath spirit"

monji: small

monji kuaap, *monji*: child, *kuaap*: egg, "embryo"

monji naknak altañ, monji: child, *naknak*: down, fluff (also the fine little hairs on certain kinds of grass), *altañ*: to originate, to come, "arrival of the downy child," "birth"

monji naknak yut, monji naknak: see above, *yut*: house, "a downy child in the house"

monjiyok bakok, monjiyok from *monji*: child, *yok*: container, string bag, term for the uterus, also used for the embryo in the uterus, *bakok*: to remove, "to throw out," "throw the embryo out"

morak mane kawam kuak tami, morak mane: a name of the bush-spirit *sindok, kawam*: a bird taken to be the personification of the *sindok, kuak*: white, i.e. "cold" and correspondingly to be unable to act, *tami*: leaf, meaning here: leaf with thorns, sharp edges, meaning "it will cut you," "*sindok*, you are now completely out in the cold!"

Morap from *morap*: too much, in abundance

Mpagmbewoñok from *mpagmbe*: water, *woñok*: hollow, place where water collects when it rains, "place of the emerging lake"

Mpagmbekagowañ, from *mpagmbe*: water, *ka*: many, *gowañ*: below, "below the many sources"

mum darok, mum: bosom, also milk, *darok*: dry, "no more milk"

mum ndakndak, mum: bosom, also milk, *ndakndak:* to beat, to pulse, to hurt, "breast pain"

Mundogon from *mun*: to fall down, *dogon*: to stay on the ground, "falling rocks"

murum: cool, cold. *Murum* also means the (in the Yupno region always cool) wind, cold weather

murum gen, murum: wind, cold, *gen*: language, "something that has been said, hence an utterance spread by the wind," "rumors"

nak ngakdakon nduara pasat, from *nak*: I, *ngakdakon* from *ngak*: you, *dakon*: possessive pronoun, hence your, *nduara* from *nduat*: half, rest, leftover, the remain, *pasat*: I carry, "I carry your remainder [of the misdemeanor]"

nalok: banana

nan: father, food, specifically: strengthening food. The term is based on the idea that the father feeds the baby before its birth with his semen

nandak nandak amɨn, nandak from *nandi.ak, nandi*: listen, feel, think, hear, *ak*: nominalizer, *nandak nandak*: knowledge (one has listened well, heard a lot and kept it in the memory), also thinking, *amɨn*: man, a "man with lots of knowledge"

nandak nandak opmbal, from *nandak*: see above, *opmbal*: wrong, "wrong knowledge"

nandak nandak yuki, nandak: see above, *yuki*: bad, evil, "evil thinking" *nanjok* from *nan*: father, *jok*: little, "little father"

nap mbɨsap amɨn, *nap*: string, *mbɨsap*: knot, time, *amɨn*: man, "knottier"

ndagal: kind of bird

ndak: blood

ndak wuda, *ndak*: blood, *wuda*: generic name for "wounds," "cuts," "bleeding wound"

ndak yuki, *ndak*: blood, *yuki*: bad, "bad blood"

ndakda noknda, from *ndak*: blood, *da*: suffixed particle, *nokndak*: to beat, "the blood beats, stings me"

ndakkok, from *ndak*: blood, *kok*: excrements, "bloody diarrhoea"

ndavɨl wuda, *ndavɨl*: eye, *wuda*: generic name for "wounds," "cuts," wound at the eye"

ndavɨlɨ dɨriñ, *ndavɨlɨ*: eye, *dɨriñ*: to look up, "to be cross-eyed"

ndavɨlɨ goman, *ndavɨlɨ*: eye, *goman*: red, "red eyes," "inflamed eye"

ndavɨlɨ mi, *ndavɨlɨ*: eye, *mi*: not existent, "blind"

ndavɨlɨ mpagmbe, *ndavɨlɨ*: eye, *mpagmbe*: water, "watering eye"

ndavɨlɨ pɨlɨnda, *ndavɨlɨ*: eye, *pɨlɨnda*: black, dark, dusk, "bad eyesight"

ndel yamak, *ndel*: a piece of bamboo, *yamak*: to shoot, "bamboo splinter"

ndol tepm, from *ndol*: teeth, mouth, *tepm*: hot, pain, "toothache"

ndol uroknok, *ndol*: mouth, teeth, *uroknok*: to close, "closing the mouth"

ndolɨ mi, *ndolɨ*: teeth, mouth, *mi*: nonexistent, "toothless"

nduara from *nduat*: half, rest, leftover, the remains, meaning: misdemeanor from which something remains, "guilt"

nduara abedak, *nduara* see above, *abedak*: to get, "he has gotten a remainder [of the misdemeanor]"

Ngandum from *ngan*: pandanus, *dum* = *ndom*: little mountain, "[people from the] hill of the pandanus trees"

Ngangalbuk (no splitting): those who come from far away

ngaok: betel nut

ngapma: pit, deep hole, "partner clan"

ngapma tauak, *ngapma*: partner clan, *tauak*: "sign," "sign of the partner clan"

ngesam amɨn, from *ngesam*: to soothe, *amɨn*: man, "soother"

ngɨgngekno tepm namejak, *ngɨgngek*: ribs, *no*: my, *tepm*: hot, pain, fast, *namejak*: he gives to me "my ribs give me pain"

ngɨlarɨ: from *ngɨlak.si*, *ngɨlak*: to like, to be fond of, *si*: very good, very much, "to be good"

ngodɨm: body

ngodɨm jusok, *ngodɨm*: body, *jusok*: to cook, to roast, "hot body"

ngodɨm mok, *ngodɨm*: body, *mok*: no translation, meaning: "to be only skin and bones" *ngodɨm ndapndap,* from *ngodɨm*: body, *ndapndap*: to hit, to pulse, "pain"

ngodɨm tepm from *ngodɨm*: body, *tepm*: hot, pain, "fever"

ngodɨm tepm tisok: *ngodɨm*: body, *tepm*: hot, pain, fast, *tisok*: to cook, to heat, "hot, painful body"

ngodɨm tepmtok from *ngodɨm*: body, *tepm*: pain, fast, hot, *tok*: to be, to exist, hence "the body is hot," "the body hurts," "fever"

ngom sɨt, ngom: mosquito, *sɨt*: generic noun for illness, "mosquito-illness"

Ngopmbaka from *ngopm = ngop*: covering, skin, here: shelter (under big boulders), *ba*: no translation, *ka*: many "place of many shelters"

ngopmo from *ngop*: skin, covering, *mo = no*: my, "my covering," a kind of payment

nɨmantok yut, nɨman: open, clear, not hidden, to bring into the light, *tok*: to be present, *yut*: house, name for the Teptep Health Centre

nɨmantusok, from *nɨman*: open, clear, not hidden, to bring into the light, to stand there freely, to get settled, *tusok*: to be

ninimoktak: term for trembling, shivering

njaapndak, from *njaap*: food, *ndak*: to be closed, finished, "rubbish," "leftovers"

njaapndak awedak, njaapndak see above, *awedak*: to receive, to get, "he received leftovers"

Njapnjapilin from *njapnjap*: vine for plaited ribbons, *ɨlɨn*: descending, slope, scarp, "slope of the many *njapnjap* plants"

njibu amɨn, njibu according to the Yupno a Kâte name for swollen veins where the blood is blocked in one place, *amɨn*: man, "masseur"

njɨgɨ: heavy, in the physical sense—a stone is *njɨgɨ*—as well as in a symbolic sense, "oppressing problems," 'hevi'

njɨgɨ abani wosak, njɨgɨ: "oppressing problem," *abani*: to make, to be there, to do something, *wosak*: to go up, "his 'oppressing problem' is [still] busy going up"

njɨgɨ kale pisak, njɨgɨ: "oppressing problem," *kale*: to go, *pisak*: to go down; "his 'oppressing problem' goes down"

njɨgɨ kale yawurondak, njɨgɨ: "oppressing problem," *kale*: to go, *yawurondak* from *yawuro*: "cool," *ndak*: term for something completed, finished, "his 'oppressing problem' has become [almost] cool"

njɨgɨ ni wosak, njɨgɨ: "oppressing problem," *ni*: to be, *wosak*: to go up; "his 'oppressing problem' goes up"

njɨgɨ tusokgen, njɨgɨ: "oppressing problem," *tusok*: to be there, to exist, *gen*: no translation, his 'oppressing problem' is still there"

njul: little sticks used for the brideprice

nok: cooking, also food

noñgum: black earth

nsaguo: name of a bird, Vulturine Parrot (psittrichas fulgidus) and term for the traditional wheel of feathers

nsaguo mbɨsap, nsaguo: see above, name for the wheel of feathers, the traditional dance decoration, *mbɨsap*: knot, time, "time of the *nsaguo*-wheel of feathers"

ñuak madep tok, ñuak: knee, *madep*: big, *tok*: to exist, "swollen knees"

nut: term of reference for people of the same clan (male Ego)

nut tauak, nut: term for the people of one's own clan, *tauak*: "sign," "sign of one's own clan"

obip san, from *obip*: a specific tree, *san*: a particle, hence a piece of the *obip* tree, meaning: a bullroarer

ondeñ: sweet potato

ondeñ nduat, ondeñ: sweet potato, *nduat*: half, rest, leftover, the remain, "a small piece of sweet-potato"

opmbal: wrong

opmbilap: to approach something totally wrong, to make a mistake

oskoron from *os = us*: above, up, *koron*: bush, "people from the upper bush"

pañan kalap amɨn, pañan: dog, *kalap*: meat, also generic noun for all the marsupials, *amɨn*: man, "hunting-dog man"

pat: trap, to block somebody's way

pat amɨn, from *pat*: trap, *amɨn*: man, "trap-man"

pat kɨrat, pat: trap, *kɨrat*: bone, "trap bone"

pek: to fill up, term for ego's matriline. This term is based on the concept that Ego is filled with the blood of his mother or her kinship group

pek tauak, pek: term for the kin group of the mother, *tauak*: "sign," "sign of the kin group of the mother"

pekno tauak from *pek*: name of the maternal kinship group, *no*: my, *tauak*: "sign," "sign of a maternal kinship group"

pelok: are you capable of it?, can you do it?

pieñ amɨn, from *pieñ*: name of a certain small piece of bark cloth that is burned, and with its stinking smoke chases the bush-spirit away, *amɨn*: man, "fumigator"

pɨrap: to shoot, to prick, "blood-letting"

pɨsit niroñ, pɨsit: liquid which somebody or something excretes, *niroñ*: to trickle, "semen"

pɨsit pɨsit jok, pɨsit: liquid which somebody or something excretes, here: urine, *jok*: to make, "urinate in excess"

sak: woman, grass skirt

sak amdi, sak: woman, grass skirt, *amdi* shortened from *aminti*, whereby *amin*: man, *ti*: very, true, good, "real woman"

sak amin pilañ, sak: grass skirt, woman, *amin*: man, *pilañ*: from *pi* or *pe*: big, and *ilañ*: to descend, slope, "old woman"

sak kamam, sak: woman, grass skirt, *kamam*: raw, also new, "new woman," term for newlywed woman

sak monji, sak: woman, grass skirt, *monji*: child, "little woman"

sak ngok, sak: woman, grass skirt, *ngok*: star, something small, shiny, "star woman"

sak tauak, sak: woman, grass skirt, *tauak*: "sign," "women's sign"

sak yut, sak: woman, grass skirt, *yut*: house, "women's house"

Salimbaga, from *sal*: kind of tree, *mbaga* = *baga*: hill, mountain, the "hill where the *sal* tree grows"

Sindalin from *sinda*: look here!, *lin* from *ilin*: descending, slope, scarp, "place with a view"

sindok kirat, sindok: name of the bush-spirit, *kirat*: bone, "bone of bush-spirit *sindok*"

sindok kokop, sindok: name of the bush-spirit, *kokop*: place, settlement, "place of the bush-spirit"

sindok tauak, sindok: name of the bush-spirit, *tauak*: "sign," "sign of the bush-spirit *sindok*"

sindoksak: *sindok*: name of the bush-spirit, *sak*: woman, grass skirt, "*sindok*-woman"

sindokwuli, sindok: name of the bush-spirit, *wuli*: man, used in contrast to woman, "*sindok*-man"

siñgeñ: a bird of prey

Siñgoronbaga from *siñgoron*: name for cemetery in the Kâte language, the lingua franca of the Neuendettelsau Mission on the Huon Peninsula, *baga*: hill, mountain, "cemetery hill"

sit: I burn, heat, cook," generic noun for "illness," and especially for 'poisin,' "leavings sorcery"

sit amin, sit: I burn, heat cook, generic noun of illness, *amin*: man, "burner"

sit asat, sit: I burn, heat, cook, generic noun of illness, *asat*: I make, "I am ill"

sit njigi, sit: I burn, heat, cook, generic noun of illness, *njigi*: heavy, "I am seriously ill"

sit tauak, sit: generic noun of illness, here: a special "technique," the worst cause of illness, "leavings sorcery," 'poisin,' *tauak*: "sign," "sign of leavings sorcery" *sɨt tevan, sɨt*: generic noun for illness, *tevan*: strong, firm, see *tevantok*, "serious illness"

sɨt yɨt namejak, sɨt: I burn, heat, cook, generic noun for illness, *yɨt*: grain of seed, *namejak*: he gives, "he gives seeds of illness"

sɨt yut, sɨt: generic noun for illness, here: a special "technique," the worst cause of illness, "leavings sorcery," 'poisin,' *yut*: house, "house for the leavings sorcery"

sitnɨ mɨ, sɨt: I burn, heat, cook, generic noun for illness, *ni*: no translation, *mi*: nonexistent, it does not exist, "I am not ill"

siwan: kind of rat

sulek: special stones used for rituals and by "leavings sorcery"

sut yut, sut: from Tok Pisin 'sut,' "shot," *yut*: house, "house of shoots," name for the Teptep Health Centre

talbok: "runny nose"

Talon, from *ta*: a kind of tree, lon from *ɨlɨn*: descending, slope, gradient, "[group that lives at] the slope of the *ta* tree"

tapmɨ mo mi, tapmɨm: to have strength, to be strong, *mi*: nonexistent, "weak, feeble"

tauak: "a sign, an image which appears like this"

teak kaloñ, teak: neck, also gorge, throat, thoughts, *kaloñ*: term for number one, "to be one neck," "to be one throat"

teak kandap, teak: neck, also thoughts, *kandap*: tree, wood, fire, "the throat is ablaze," "being angry"

teak ndapndap, teak: neck, also thoughts, *ndapndap* from *ndap*: to beat, hence to beat again and again, meaning: to hurt, to stir up, to incite, "repeatedly beaten, hurt thoughts"

teak opmbal, teak: neck, throat, *opmbal*: wrong, "the throat is wrong"

teak tevan, from *teak*: neck, also gorge, throat, thoughts, *tevan*: firm, strong, "different," powerful, see *tevantok*, "vital energy," "different thoughts," "being angry," "anger, jealousy"

teak tevan amɨn, teak tevan: see above, *amɨn*: man, "a man who is often looking for a fight," "a quarrelsome person"

teak tevan nda añakdak, teak tevan: see above, *nda*: her, *añakdak*: to beat, "tormenting jealousy"

tedetedetyut from *tedet*: to surround, to construct in the round, *yut*: house, "house in circles"

Teetmevilgowañ, from *teet*: kind of bamboo, *mevil*: origin, cause, *gowañ*: below, "below the *teet* bamboo grove"

tekop erap, from *tekop*: fire-saw, *erap*: bowl, meaning: to poke the embers, to light the fire anew, also: "dispute" *tepm*: hot, fast, pain

tevantok from *tevan*: to be strong, to have strength, *tok*: to exist, to be there, to be ready, "vital energy"

tilagi from *tilak*: mark, *gi*: to be, "to make a mark," (therefore) "to be different," "taboo," "forbidden"

tilagi gen: *tilagi* from *tilak*: mark, *gi*: to be, "to make a mark," (therefore) "to be different," "taboo," "forbidden," *gen*: talk, "curse"

tilagi yut, *tilagi*: to be different, *yut*: house, "exceptional, special house"

timni gorok, *timni*: nose, *gorok*: no translation, "blocked up nose"

timni njagaldak, *timni*: nose, *njagaldak*: to pull, "to pull at the nostrils"

tinyikabi from *ti*: good, *nyi*: 3rd person plural, they, *kabi*: a few, a group, "some good [people]"

tip kuakuaga, *tip*: stone, *kuakuaga* from *kuak*: white, "white stone"

tip pilin, *tip*: stone, *pilin*: black, "black stones" used for "leavings sorcery"

tira amin, *tira*: rat, *amin*: man, the "rat man"

tira goman, *tira*: rat, *goman*: red, "red rat"

tira pat, *tira*: rat, *pat*: trap, "rat trap"

tira suson, *tira*: rat, *suson*: to cook, to burn, "cooking the rats"

tira tauak penyi patogo, from *tira*: rat, *tauak*: "sign," *penyi* from *pe*: brother, *nyi*: 3.pers.pl, they, *patogo*: elder brother, "rat sign of the elder and younger brothers"

ton amin: snake

tsabom: flesh, muscles

Tsetset from *tset*: to break, to split off. When, at the dawn of history, the Yupno River flooded everything, the original lake turned into two rivers: one flows into the Nankina valley, the other, Tsetset, into the Yupno valley

tumot: navel

Tuwal, *tuwal*: keel, spit of land, "[people from] the keel"

Umban: name for different kinds of Cordyline sp., "Cordyline plant [people]"

Uskokop from *us*: above, up, *kokop*: place, "upper place"

wam suok, *wam*: stomach, *suok*: to pierce, to shoot, "piercing pain in the stomach," "stomach cramps"

wam tepmtok, *wam*: stomach, *tepm*: hot, pain, fast, *tok*: to exist, "stomach pains"

wanditit: to vomit

wau: one with the same name, a "namesake"

waunomi from *waunomeñ*, *wau*: male member of my patriline, also the one with the same name, *no*: my, *meñ*: mother, "mother of my [potential] *wau*" *waunyi* from *wau*: see above, *nyi*: 3.Pers.Pl., they, kinship term for male members of one's own patriline in the first ascending generation

wopm: image, shadow, "shadow soul"

wuda: generic name for "wounds," "cuts"

wuda bap, wuda: generic name for "wounds," "cuts," *bap*: large, "big wound"

wuda goman, wuda: generic name for "wounds," "cuts," *goman*: red, "(smaller) open, bleeding wounds

wudawuda, wuda: generic name for "wounds," "cuts," "many small wounds," "rash"

wulawula: mad, out of one's mind

yagngap mbɨsap, yagngap: moon, *mbɨsap*: knot, time, "time of the moon," "menstruation"

yawɨ nyɨvɨlɨ bapdak, yawɨ: scrotum, *nyɨvɨlɨ*: penis, *bapdak* from *bap*: big, *dak*: to be, "swollen scrotum and penis"

yawuro: cool, well tempered, the ideal state of a socially integrated, balanced person

yawuro yawuro amɨn, from *yawuro*: see above, *amɨn*: man, somebody who cools (the "heated up" patient) down to the right, "cool" condition, the generic term for various herbalists, a "cooler"

yɨmakon, from *yɨma*, whereby *yɨ*: core of something, to be inside something (see *yɨrɨ*), *ma*: fenced-in area around a center (see *mbema*: fenced-in area around the *mbe* tree), *kon*: locative, *yɨmakon* means the fenced-in space between the fence and the house, that which is inside the fence

yɨmat: traditional shell-money

yɨrɨ: seed of a plant

yut bap from *yut*: house, *bap*: big, "big house," men's house

yut kɨrat, yut: house, *kɨrat*: bones, "house posts"

Notes

Chapter 1

1 A. Young, in his contribution *The Anthropologies of Illness and Sickness* (1982), gives a concise survey of the most important trends in medical anthropology up to the beginning of the 1980s. These different methodological and theoretical approaches cover a wide spectrum; see, for example, such well-known works as Landy (1977); Wellin (1977); Foster and Anderson (1978); Kleinman (1978, 1980); McElroy and Townsend (1979); Romanucci-Ross, Moerman and Tancredi (1983); Helman (1984); Lindenbaum and Lock (1993); Good (1994); Sargent and Johnson (1996); and Brown (1998).

2 The rather demanding aim of cognitive anthropology is based on the assumption that

• whatever is relevant in a culture must be able to be communicated between the members of this culture and can therefore be investigated via the language or the respective linguistic categories respectively, and that

• culture is commonly shared knowledge and hence a mental phenomenon, since, as Goodenough expresses it in his famous definition of culture:

A society's culture consists of whatever it is one has to know or believe in order to operate in a manner acceptable to its members, and to do so in any role that they accept for anyone of themselves....it is the forms of things that people have in mind, their models for perceiving, relating, and otherwise interpreting them...culture does not exist of things, people, behavior or emotions, but in the forms or organizations of these things in the mind of people (Goodenough 1957: 167–68).

3 Frake could be criticized for unfolding in detail only a small section of the classification of disease (the skin diseases) by the Subanun, for completely disregarding therapies and only marginally treating the importance of the classificatory system of skin diseases within the Subanun culture. However, he succeeded in reaching a goal of the cognitive anthropology of the time, namely, to describe one cultural domain (the classification of skin diseases) that was linguistically well structured in terms of emic categories. While Frake's study was praised as methodologically elegant and, in 1979, assessed by McElroy and Townsend (1979: 59) as "a classical study exemplifying ethnoscientific methodology," A. Young not long afterwards (1982: 262) was already consigning it to the "prehistory of medical anthropology," which provides a further indication of how rapidly "medical anthropology" was developing.

4 See, for example, Roy D'Andrade's study *A Propositional Analysis of U.S. American Beliefs about Illness* (1976). His work was praised within cognitive anthropology as a methodologically very valuable contribution to the discovery of systems of belief since, unlike others before him, he did not compare the elements (belief statements) but put them into a causal relationship. However, medical anthropologists hardly acknowledged the study. D'Andrade himself did not deny the very complicated and demanding method of his approach.

5 The distinction between disease and illness was, according to Colson and Selby (1974: 246), initially employed by Fabrega (1971), and further elaborated by Eisenberg (1977).

6 See Fabrega (1971: 213); Lieban (1973: 1043); McElroy and Townsend (1979: 49).

7 For example, see Brown and Inhorn (1990: 189); Rhodes (1990: 165); Chrisman and Johnson (1990: 109); but also see Shweder (1988: 492), who based his criticism of Kleinman (1986) exactly on these two terms; he clearly states: "And what I think makes me confused and nervous is that shaggy distinction between illness and disease."

8 To Singer (1990: 181), for example, the "medicalization of medical anthropology [is]...reflected...in the treatment of non-Western ethnomedicine as a component of culture but biomedicine as an example of science; the assignments of afflictions not identified by biomedicine to the category of culture-bound syndromes; the development of cultural or psychological interpretations of successful healing in non-Western medicine but organic explanations for biomedicine; and efforts to test empirically the efficacy of folk healing systems but not biomedical treatment."

9 See the essays in Lock and Gordon (1988).

10 See Sinclair (1987/88) for a historical review of the development of medical anthropological writings in Papua New Guinea since the 1960s. There are also some detailed medical anthropological writings on ethnic groups in Papua New Guinea: Nelson (1971); Johannes (1976); Jones (1980); Welsch (1982).

Chapter 2

1 In the older literature, in Schmitz (1958) and in the missionary and Patrol Reports, the inhabitants are called Jupna or Yupna; the people of the valley, however, call both the river and their language *yupno* or *yupnogen* (*gen* meaning "speech," "talk," "language").

2 There are different myths about the origins, but common to many of them is the notion of the emergence of the first people from a bamboo.

3 These two differing types of landscape are only briefly described; for more detailed geological and botanical information, plus an encompassing account of economic activities, see Kocher Schmid (1991).

4 The village of Tapen, where formerly the mission station was installed, lies in the border area of the Yupno region. For administrative purposes, this village no longer belongs to the Yupno subdistrict but can be included on both cultural and linguistic grounds.

5 These estimates were made with the aid of the census book of 1985 for the Teptep subdistrict, which does not include Tapen. The numbers for the villages are: Kwembun 197, Windiluk 121, Wandaboñ 330, Bonkiman 181, and Kwaup 123.

6 In a sequence from the lowest village on the left side (the upper Yupno) across the river to the right side, the populations of the villages are: Nokopo 394, Nian 371, Kangulut 222, Taeñ (including Teptep station) 332, Uskokop 331, Gua 416, Devil and Meñan (combined in the census) 436, Tapmañge 391, Kewieñ 630, Urop 342, Isan 567, Mek 590, and Nolum 257. The figures were drawn from the census taken by the officer at Teptep. The total population (upper and lower Yupno) thus exceeds 6000 people.

7 It was written after a three weeks' stay in the Yupno region. For more recent studies, see Wassmann (1992, 1993a, 1993b, 1993c, 1994, 1997, 1998); Wassmann and Dasen (1994a, 1994b); Kocher-Schmid (1992, 1993); Keck (1992, 1993a, 1993b, 1994, 1999).

8 Several informants, after some discussion, agreed that Gua may well be a shortened version of *guammbema*.

9 In 1928, the first mission stations of the Neuendettelsau Lutheran Mission were erected at Kewieñ and Isan. The fusion of the villages and the

missionary work started there about 25 years before the village of Gua was founded.

10 The mission also had two 'komiti' elected per village as church representatives; very often the same man now holds the office of a governmental as well as a church 'komiti' at the same time. There were attempts by the administration to replace the 'luluai' with the institution of a "local government council" and its representative, the "village councillor" (which is customary in other parts of Papua New Guinea, and which for the population means being subject to taxes), but these failed because Yupno Valley people earned too little money to be able to pay them (Sailoia 1976/77: 6).

11 'Komyuniti de' is the Tok Pisin name introduced by the administration for the one day per week when all adult villagers must work for the government station or on communal tasks (like the maintenance of footpaths, building of bridges, erecting houses for administrators, installing a sports field, repairs on the school building, and so on).

12 The padlock serves less to prevent a possible burglary (the key is most often missing, anyway) than as something of a status symbol.

13 Onions, potatoes and cabbage were introduced by the missionaries or evangelists a few decades ago. The Yupno names for the latter two betray their origin: potatoes are called *kalabili* or *katopel* (from German "Kartoffel"), and cabbage is called by older people *kiraut* (from Southern German "Kraut").

14 On the classification of food, see Wassmann (1993c).

15 On Yupno immigration, see Wassmann (1992).

16 The Roman numerals added in brackets refer to the kinship diagram and are cited as a "symbol" for kinship groups (and in the case study of little Nstasiñge in Chapter 4). Not all the kinship dispositions could be included in the diagram.

17 The use of the term *nut* depends on Ego's spatial position: if he is in a foreign place (e.g. in Madang), the people of the lower Yupno Valley become *nut*, whereas he would no longer call them *nut* if he lived in the village.

18 In contrast, a female Ego calls her brother *olap* and his wife *sak* or *maniok*, her elder sister *patogo*, her younger sister *pe* and their husbands *mbasok*. Her husband's group she collectively calls *wusak*, her husband *e*, his brothers *usak*, their wives (HuBrWi) *sak* and her husband's sister *maniok*. Her husband's parents (HuFa, HuMo) are called *namda*.

19 Schmitz (1960b: 72–72) also considers these marriage rules for the Wantoat.

20 In former times, this *kasok* consisted of advantageously arranged strings of shell money (*yimat*), but today these take the modern form of two-Kina-bills strung between two sticks.

21 At least I could not discern any definite marriage relations between the villages. It needs to be remembered that Yupno villages are relatively recent formations, and there are surely certain marriage preferences among the individual partner clans (*ngapma ngapma*).

22 As will be described in detail later, the first signs of pregnancy in a newlywed woman are therefore watched with great attention by the clan and partner clan members of the husband, and at as early a date as possible are publicly proclaimed in order to discourage a woman from a possible abortion.

23 For example, a brideprice deemed to be "good" comprised: 22 pigs, 40 pieces of cloth, 22 different arrangements of bought (Western) foods, 40 grass skirts, 20 net bags, 330 Kina in cash plus separate gifts to the bride's mother (2 pigs, cash and bought presents to the value of approximately 400 Kina), which represents a total value of over 2000 Kina.

24 If the mother only has one daughter and if she is opposed to the future husband, she often resists. In one case, a mother became enraged when her daughter was taken away at night, so she brandished a knife and wounded several people who got too close to her, in a fight that escalated. The conflict was later resolved when the daughter was married off and the mother was obliged to pay a pig to those she had wounded.

25 This problem did not exist when everybody traditionally lived in the *mbema*, the "fenced-in area," since there the young unmarried men lived together in their bachelor house (*mbema yut*). People today often take advantage of the absence of young men in town to conduct a wedding.

26 It very often happens that this group is late because of bad weather or differing notions about the date arranged (up to three days later); the pork is by then often half-rotten and already smells.

27 It is questionable whether this dribbling of milk from a coconut is a traditional element or is better understood as a borrowing from the Christian ceremony of the holy water.

28 The exchange of bowls is said to still be done at times, but I was never able to see it.

29 This *ngopmo* is connected with the *amɨn ngop*, the payment to the relatives of the mother (*pek*) of the dead, see Chapter 3.3.

30 Kâte, a Papuan language originally spoken north of Finschhafen, was taken over by the Lutherans as a mission language and thus became the lingua franca of the Huon Peninsula.

31 This work under contract was welcomed by many administrators, who believed that the "backwardness" (Sailoia 1976/77: 4) of the population could thereby be reduced. "In my opinion, large recruiting potential will be found at such villages as KEWIENG and ISAN. Although many points, such as health, must be considered, I believe that a term of work for most of the young men would contribute greatly toward their progress" (Hanrahan 1955/56: 5).

32 In 1986, I met a young man who had shortly before come back from two years' work in Buka under contract with the trade company, Burns Philp, and who in the meantime had married in Kewieñ. He remained full of anger about the contract labor, and told me he had received only 21 Kina per fortnight for his strenuous work. Even though there are few opportunities to earn money in the Yupno area, no young person could nowadays be contracted for this kind of wage and this kind of work.

Chapter 3

1 As already mentioned, the Yupno villages are more recent settlements that in form are non-traditional, and it seems that some of the clans had "taken over" the *kokop kɨrat*, which originally belonged to only one clan and its partner clan, and had turned them into "village *kokop kɨrat*."

2 There is an extensive literature on ideas about human spirits or souls in Melanesia; Dalton (2002: 136, note 3) lists many ethnographic examples. See also Strathern (1994) and Stewart and Strathern (2001) for a discussion of the indigenous Hagen notions of *noman* and *min* and comparable terms found in neighboring groups, such as the Maring (studied by Rappaport and LiPuma) and the Ku Waru (Merlan and Rumsey) and, more generally for the concept of the person, Stewart and Strathern (2000). For an older overview, see Fischer (1965). In my German (and earlier English writings), I referred to *moñan* as "Körperseele" (body soul) and to *wopm* as "Freiseele" (free soul).

3 Schmitz (1960a: 204, footnote) also mentions this *koñgap*, which he describes as an "interrupted 'ajaja - ajaja.'" "This is interspersed in true mountain-dweller fashion by cheers and yodels." However, I cannot support his interpretation that the singing of this koñgap is meant to chase the ghost (*koñ*) away (Schmitz 1960a: 204). It is also possible to give a *koñgap* to highly valued animals (a man to his hunting dog, a woman to her favorite pig).

4 For these figures, I am indebted to the study by Don Niles, IPNGS, Port Moresby, who during an ethnomusicological field study in Gua

in 1987, taped hundreds of *koñgap* melodies and checked them with different informants; see also Niles (1992), and for a shorter description, Wassmann (1998).

5 This can be explained by the fact that the Yupno ascribe all the sexual attempts, that is, the active part, to the men only, seeing the women more as the "victims" of these activities. In many stories, men "cajole," "trick," "dupe," or "rape" women, but I never heard of the opposite case.

6 Not only humans are in one of these states but also animals, plants, stones, and landscapes.

7 There are "hot," "cool" (the majority) and "cold" objects. Even the "normal," "cool" objects can, with much effort, be "heated up," "charged" or "cooled down." Here, however, we are interested only in the "hot" or "cold" prototypes per se (see Wassmann and Dasen 1994b).

8 According to one informant, the *wopm* ("shadow soul") of the baby is "blown" into the mother's womb by Morap, the Yupno creator god. Today, Anutu, the Kâte name for "God," is held to be responsible for a child's *wopm*. Nothing more detailed could be learned.

9 The Melpa have a similar concept, and for them also a small child does not yet possess a *noman* ("social consciousness" or..."intention" and "will"). "*Noman* is...not the same as animation (*min*, spirit), which is in the child from birth...[note 5] having *noman* thus represents a capacity for social interaction" (M. Strathern 1968: 554–55).

10 Apart from one man who was thought to be "ancient," half-blind, almost deaf and unable to walk anymore, and whom one could have called demented or senile, all the other old people I met were mentally alert.

11 Old people who feel themselves badly treated by their children often threaten to come back after their death as "ghosts" and make life for the children and grandchildren very difficult.

12 A. Strathern notes a similar concept among the Wiru. The patrilateral relatives in the event of a death make a "death-payment" to the matrilateral relatives of the deceased. "All these payments [the death-payment and preceding payments] are said to 'buy the skin' of the person in question, first to ensure his health while alive and second to discharge the debt of 'mothering' after he is dead" (A. Strathern 1968: 550).

Chapter 4

1 The concept "therapy managing group" was introduced by Janzen (1978: 4).

2 *Plaua*, actually a Tok Pisin term for "flour"; to Yupno, who are not very well versed in Tok Pisin, a kind of sweet roll made from dough, similar to scones, which is very popular and sometimes is sold at Teptep market. Mayu wants to point out that she offered her child the very best tidbits, which a "healthy" Yupno child certainly would not refuse.

3 'Dokta' or 'doktaboy' refers to a biomedically-trained orderly, here one of the employees of the Teptep Health Centre.

4 "Normal" here means a course of illness, held by the Yupno to be appropriate according to the kind of "disorder" in terms of the intensity of pain or the duration. For example, a fractured arm from previous experience needs more time to mend than a sprain; a case of diarrhoea only becomes "extraordinary" if the patient in question feels weak or (as is rapidly the case with small children) visibly loses weight; a large cut hurts more than a small scratch, and so on.

5 An APO is a 'doktaboy' who runs a small aid post at village level.

6 As a reminder: the numbers in square brackets stand for the suspected causes of illness; see Figure 2.

7 'Kollekta' from German "Kollekte," denotes an act introduced by the Lutheran Mission that is supposed to symbolize the unanimity of all participants and the settlement of social tensions. It may also (as in the course of a Church service) indicate the end of a meeting. This ritual, new to the Yupno, consists of a collection which is paid into the account of the congregation, the church district. It is similar to the traditional action pattern according to which everybody whose misdemeanor leads to a *njɨgɨ* ("oppressing problem") gives compensation (most often a pig) to his opponent or the latter's group to "mollify" or "cool down" the latter's "hot" rage. With this payment, the "guilt" (*nduara*) is lifted.

8 All these cursorily described concepts in the context of "oppressing problems" are analyzed in detail in Chapter 5.2.

9 The various signs and their interpretations are stated in detail in Chapter 5.2.d.

10 This issue, which Mayu hints at while shouting at her husband, will be explained in greater detail in the Part d of this chapter, "Debate among the more Distant Relatives"; the essence of the reproach is Tanowe's wrong conduct at the payback for Mayu's brideprice (*pelok*).

11 This concept of "ghosts" influencing fertility is also shared by the Melpa. A. Strathern (1986: 24) gives as an example: "Thus a father may say (to his daughter): 'When I die you will have no more children.'"

12 In the currency of Papua New Guinea 100 toea equals one Kina.

13 *Sɨt* and *mawom* will be described in detail in Chapter 5.4.

14 Sandra Staub and I would here like to extend our thanks to Dr Watt, pediatrician at Modilon Hospital in Madang for granting us access to the file.

15 Haiveta (1990: 443) remarks: "The term glasman may have something to do with the examination through a microscope of blood samples on glass slides observed by local people in hospitals." These 'glasman,' also called 'wasman' ("wachman") are "culture-overlapping" in the sense that they find out several causes of sickness common to many ethnic groups in Papua New Guinea—like 'poisin,' 'sangguma,' or 'hevis'—and treat them in the same way, regardless of the causative agent or the age and sex of the patient. For the urban population, they are the specialists of the 'sik long ples,' illnesses caused mainly by social conflicts and for which biomedicine offers no treatment therapies.

16 The first aid post at Teptep has for many years been run by Dopenu, a man from Bambu (Nankina). Some years before the establishment of this aid post at Teptep, one was built at Kewieñ, probably financed initially from Kabwum, later from Saidor (Simmins 1962/63: 15). For the general development of the health system in Papua New Guinea, see Bell (1973); for its history, see Denoon (1989), Frankel and Lewis (1989b: 6-8), and Davies (2002) for the German colonial period.

17 The foods are divided into three groups: 1. "These foods give you strength, power" ('kaikai i strongim yu,' also 'kaikai bilong wok'), contain starch ('stas') and are tubers (like sweet potatoes, taro, bananas, also rice and biscuits); 2. "Foods that make the body grow" ('kaikai i kamapim body') comprise protein-rich ('protin') foods like spinach, beans, meat, fish, milk, eggs; 3. "'Food that watches over you" ('kaikai i was long yu') means food rich in vitamins ('vaitamin') and minerals, such as vegetables, papaya, and pumpkin. Posters with a similar content can be found in almost all health centers in Papua New Guinea.

18 Adequate meaning: contrary to many other health centers in Papua New Guinea, whose staff complain about chronic lack of money, the Teptep Health Centre has adequate financial means.

19 Regarding the staff hierarchy, the H.E.O., head of the health center, was trained for three years, and the nurses and the A.P.O.s for two years. The nurses are held to be slightly higher qualified than the A.P.O.s; they are trained as midwives and are allowed to assist at births.

20 The field of preventive medicine is subdivided into three groups: 1. primary prevention (i.e. exclusion of factors harmful to health, hence activities undertaken prior to the onset of disease-inducing factors, like water purification, improvement of hygiene or prevention of obesity); 2. secondary prevention (i.e. early diagnosis and treatment; for exam-

ple, the diagnosis of a still minor tumor by preventive examination with
the chance of total recovery); and 3. tertiary prevention (i.e. the limita-
tion of already present consequences of disease as undertaken, for instance, in coronary or apoplexy patients). In "developing countries," secondary and tertiary prevention usually does not take place, because it is
very expensive, limited in its effect and, in general, linked with a tech-
nically "highly-developed" (with regard to personnel) and very specialized medical system. The preventive activities at the health center thus
more precisely belong in the field of primary prevention.

21 Like the patrols, baby clinics were held far less frequently. The baby-
cards indicate that they were held every six months at most (e.g. little
Nstasiñge had not been vaccinated against anything in either Gua or
Teptep).

22 This institution of VVHWs was instigated by the WHO. Regarding its
ambiguity, see Garner (1989).

23 "Can" means that, although the technical equipment and personnel
training allowed such examinations, in fact, such examinations (contrary to the information provided by the staff) are not always performed.

24 The titles of these publications are: "Standard Treatment for Common
Illnesses of Adults in Papua New Guinea: a Manual for Health Workers
in Health Centres and Hospital Outpatient departments"; "Standard
Treatment for Common Illnesses of Children in Papua New Guinea: a
Manual for Nurses, Health Extension Officers and Doctors."

25 The patient report comprises 45 pages: eight pages are the drug sheet on
which every day the drugs administered by the 'doktaboy' on duty or the
nurse are confirmed by his or her signature; five pages consist of the
temperature chart and the fever and weight scales; three pages list the
outcome of the pathology, that is, the results of the blood, spinal fluid
and saliva analyses; and 19 pages contain the remarks of the nurses.

26 Chloramphenicol is not effective against tubercular bacteria (and hence
would be without effect in the case of tubercular meningitis); its indication
is limited to bacterial meningitis (personal communication, Dr M. Keck).

27 On some days, in the notes of the temperature, the remark "N.I.B." ("not
in bed") can be found, but it remains unclear where the child and his
mother were staying at that time.

28 According to Dr M. Keck, a treatment with Prednisolon is the usual
therapy for a recent tuberculous meningitis, whereas in Europe 30 mg
per day over a period of 4 weeks would be prescribed in most cases.

29 "Backup medication" generally means an antimicrobically-effective medication (hence aimed at bacteria) that is given if the usual therapy fails;

such a case would, for example, be the treatment of certain forms of venereal disease that do not respond to the usual therapies; such medications also exist in the therapy and prophylaxis of malaria.

30　The transfer of biomedicine to the "developing countries" does not mean that Western biomedicine is taken over as it is, but in a modified way (depending on factors such as the qualification of its representatives, technical possibilities, finances and so on.) This is but one of many reasons why it would be unsurprising to find a disease being treated in a different way in a hospital in Papua New Guinea than in Switzerland or Germany.

Chapter 5

1　Today, there are exceptions, such as the new concepts of illness, *ngom sɨt* and *sɨt tevan*, for which a new Yupno name was created (see below).

2　The treatment of the individual symptoms is described in detail in Chapter 5.1.a. and 5.1.b.

3　For these kinds of disorders, one can also visit certain people especially versed in massage techniques, the *njibu amɨn*, a kind of "masseur." Yet they are not thought of as "specialists" like the "coolers" (see below), but as "craftsmen" with better skills, who massage the body-parts in question.

4　In line with Glick's (1967: 37) division into positive and negative mobilizations of power, these treatments can be seen as positively directed, since they are primarily aimed at strengthening the afflicted person and improving his or her power of resistance, and not at fighting the illness-causing agent (for negative direction, see Johannes (1976: 172); Welsch (1982: 334)).

5　The following description is based on an ablution that Quantasañne performed on Megau (a man of the Ngandum clan) in my presence on 20.10.1987. Megau was suffering from a headache, fever and shivering fits.

6　All the plant names are translated and their botanical classifications are listed in alphabetical order in the appendices.

7　*Ndamba ɨsip* is also used against skin diseases (*wudawuda*, Tok Pisin: 'grile', fungus infection, ringworm); the leaves are crushed and rubbed onto the skin.

8　Ndondoro is the name of a mythologically relevant lake at the source of the Yupno River, Panjewik is the name of a culture hero (of the Talon clan) who brought the bullroarer, a "strength-holder of the settlement" (*kokop kɨrat*).

9 The text of this speech is not rigidly fixed and therefore is rendered here mutatis mutandis.

10 The same applies for the Lusi in New Britain, who do not have a cover term in their language to "include all the conditions that are minor, localized or superficial and that stand in opposition to the statement, *na-grivali* 'I am sick'" (Counts and Counts 1989: 281).

11 Regarding this order: mb = b, nd = d, ng = g, ñ = ng (= g), even though it is also a very Western one, it seemed to me to be the best "auxiliary solution." Exceptions: *ndak wuda* (see *wuda*), *kogɨlɨt* (see *ndakkok*), *awɨda saññamok* (see *kandapda saññamok*).

12 The biomedical terms, which are furnished by the physician Sandra Staub, were discussed with Prof. N. Gyr and also critically checked by him. The statement "not assignable" in the central column signifies that although the bodily disorder could be listed descriptively, more differentiated evaluations would be needed for a diagnosis. For example, *kwapmo tep namejak* ("my shoulder gives me pain") could be defined as "shoulder problems," but this statement is in medical terms totally unsatisfactory since, for a diagnosis and a therapy, more detailed information (as, for example, shoulder pains caused by bone problems); i.e. a differential diagnosis (DD) is necessary.

13 The plant therapy as practiced by the Yupno for these disorders has many parallels in other ethnic groups in Papua New Guinea. Just a few examples may suffice: the use of stinging nettles as a counter-irritant is mentioned in almost all the medical-ethnological studies, such as Johannes (1976: 181–84); Welsch (1987: 206); Lewis (1975: 143); Frankel (1986: 89).

14 *Ngom sɨt* and *sɨt tevan* (see below) are both new terms, which explains the use of the word *sɨt* (see also note 1).

15 The medical, manifold application of ginger against vomiting or for wounds are also widely spread in Papua New Guinea; see the examples given by Johannes (1976: 188–91); Lewis (1975: 182); Frankel (1986: 89); see also Holdsworth (1977, 1984); Woodley (1991); and the studies cited by Hill (1984) in a bibliography of traditional medical plants in Papua New Guinea.

16 An earlier discussion in Papua New Guinea regarding the acceptance of biomedicine was, for example, held in Popondetta in 1984 at a WHO workshop, under the title: "Traditional Medicine and Primary Health Care in Papua New Guinea" (see Jilek 1984) and is taken up in several articles in *The Papua New Guinea Medical Journal* (see Welsch 1986). Central to these discussions are the role of the "traditional practitioner"

(Jenkins 1984) and the relationship between traditional medicine and biomedicine (Pataki-Schweizer 1985). Earlier contributions discussed these topics predominantly from a biomedical or public health politics point of view, and rarely from the perspective of the Papua New Guineans who make use of both medical systems. More recent studies have made the emic dimension their focus (see Lepowsky 1990); various contributions in the reader edited by Frankel and Lewis (1989a) address the question of medical pluralism, of how various ethnic groups with their own medical traditions respond to theories of causation of illness new to them and to new methods of treatment, a topic Strathern and Stewart (1999: 93–114) also discuss for the Huli, Melpa and Wiru.

17 According to the study by Andreas Allemann (1989; see also Allemann, Bauerfeind and Gyr 1994), who investigated the incidence of hookworm among the Yupno, "In the area under study, there is a high rate of infection (58%) with hookworm (Necator Americanus)....In 94% of the cases, the infections are slight and cause hardly any symptoms....The hookworm infections among the Yupna [sic] (contrary to other regions of New Guinea) pose no medically relevant problem" (Allemann 1989: 3–4). As it happens, hookworm can only be detected under the microscope.

18 The physician Sandra Staub, who examined children of between 12 and 60 months of age in Gua village, obtained the following result: 45% of the children of this age-group are malnourished. The parameters on which her study is based are explained in Staub (1993).

19 See Heywood (1982) who, in the introduction to his article, comments on the necessity and futility of the American malnutrition standards (the Harvard Standard); see also Obrist van Eeuwijk (1992) for an critical anthropological study of (mal)nutrition among the Kwanga children in Papua New Guinea.

20 As studies show (see Wassmann 1992; Wassmann and Dasen 1994b), the Yupno traditionally possess a very well devised system of classification of food, according to which they compose their nutrition "correctly from the nutritional science point of view"; in many areas, it coincides with the "ideal nutrition" presented in Chapter 4, note 17.

21 This 'doktaboy bilong tit' visits Teptep once or twice a year to extract teeth and get orders for the 'giaman tit' (artificial dentures) popular among the older people. For 'giaman tit,' all a person's teeth have to be extracted.

22 No autopsies are conducted at the Teptep Health Centre.

23 Younger people call these hernias, which have been diagnosed in some women at Teptep, *mbobok* ("the belly swells").

24   There are many examples of ethnic groups classifying a common illness
      as normal; for example, Lieban (1973: 1044) mentions a skin disease
      among the Indians of the northern Amazon River, and a worm infec-
      tion among the Thonga in Africa and the Yap Islanders in Micronesia
      that both peoples believe is necessary for digestion.

25   The examinations were conducted in Gua village in a specially-prepared
      house with two rooms. It had been explained to the people that the two
      doctors were going to examine them in order to detect possible diseases,
      which they could then have treated at the Teptep Health Centre. No
      medical intervention was made, except for dressing the wounds and
      handing out medicine against worms in the relevant cases, since the two
      physicians were present only for a short time and did not want the peo-
      ple to get accustomed to a level of biomedical care in the village that
      could not have been sustained after their departure. A second reason
      was in order not to provide an alternative to the well-equipped Teptep
      Health Centre.
      All the conversations were conducted in Tok Pisin, in part with the help
      of male and female translators.
      The population had been informed in advance about this examination
      and they cooperated fully. This high acceptance of the examination is
      based on different factors: the two physicians were certainly a novelty (the
      anthropologist, in contrast, had already spent ten months in the village
      and was therefore no longer deemed very entertaining). In addition, white
      people are thought to have more medical skills (than the Papua New
      Guinean staff at the health center); however, they are thought to be com-
      pletely incompetent as far as illness-causing techniques (such as *sit*) are
      concerned, though harmless. Furthermore, the examination took place
      in the village, which meant that older, somewhat immobile people could
      also participate. Our initial apprehension that older Yupno men would
      not let themselves be examined by a European woman doctor or older
      women by a European male doctor (considerations also for the combi-
      nation of the medical team) were unfounded; on the contrary, one older
      man wanted to be examined by the female doctor three times in a row.

26   A more recent set of annual statistics was not at hand in 1987.

27   Of these 179 patients, 45 had pneumonia, 18 bronchitis, 12 fractures, 7
      arthritis, 6 diarrhoea, 6 anemia, 5 were treated for malnutrition, 4 had
      urinary tract infections, 3 malaria, 3 gonorrhoea, 2 tuberculosis, 2 lep-
      rosy, 2 inflammation of the middle ear, 44 had other, less frequent dis-
      eases; there were 20 births at the Teptep Health Centre.

28 The diseases: 3 pneumonia, 2 newborn-infection, 1 conjunctivitis, 1 urinary tract infection and gonorrhoea, 1 stomach ulcer (ulcus ventriculi), 1 malaria, 1 skin disease, 1 accident.

29 In detail: 2 malaria, 2 hernia, 1 urinary tract infection, 1 bone disease, 1 abscess, 1 malnutrition, 1 anemia, 1 newborn-infection, 1 infected ulcer, 2 births.

30 This is a statement of the staff which is rendered without further questioning. Since nobody on the staff speaks fluently Kâte either, knowledge of Kâte among the Yupno would not lessen the communication problems.

31 Barker (1989: 80) describes very similar problems with the role of APOs in Maisin society.

32 Regarding the employees, the H.E.O. is from Finschhafen and the A.P.O. are from Madang, Saidor, Popondetta and Kabwum.

33 All the same, this fear of misuse can be allayed if it is explained why these tests are necessary. When the Swiss physician A. Allemann was conducting a series of examinations that, among other things, necessitated the taking of blood and feces samples, the people were highly cooperative. This willingness may be accounted for by fact that they do not believe that white people have any knowledge of illness-causing acts like *sɨt*.

34 Physicians who base their studies more on statistical, quantitative data than through observation and qualitative methods that do not fulfil statistical requirements (but are most often better suited for statements about the actual behavior) derive from their questionnaires highly flattering statements and evidence for the acceptance of Western medicine. I learnt in conversations with some physicians, that they criticize anthropological statements based on observation as "unsound," "not empirically verifiable," "statistically insufficient" and so on. Problems that accompany the introduction of biomedicine into traditional societies are thereby glossed over rather than possibly solved.

35 As a rule, this widely known genealogy encompasses five generations, two generations above (father, grandfather), one's own, and two generations below (children and grandchildren).

36 This idea seems to be widespread in Melanesia, for example, the Melpa also know this concept: "a person who dies from his frustration [*popokl*, author's comment] may return as an angry ghost to take vengeance on those who caused him the grievance" (M. Strathern 1968: 533).

37 Since Koki's condition deteriorated nevertheless, he was carried to the Teptep Health Centre. The introductory examination revealed: fever

(39.7°C), swelling of left foot, pulse 124/min (weak), rattling noises in both lobes of the lungs. Diagnosis: pneumonia on both sides. He was treated with antibiotics and antimalarial drugs and discharged after four weeks.

38 However, Njano's condition became increasingly alarming, after even worse causes of illness like the bush-spirit *sindok* or a *sɨt* act had been excluded, so she was taken to the Teptep Health Centre. The diagnosis there was meningitis or cerebral malaria.

39 Keesing (1985) also cautions against over-interpreting the metaphors customary in a culture. "In our project of cultural translation, are we prone to attribute deeper salience to other people's way of talk than they in fact imply?" (Keesing 1985: 201).

40 Regarding the discussion of etiological concepts, see also Feinberg (1990: 322), who compares his data collected on Nukumanu to the illness-causation theories of the Huli, Gimi, and other ethnic group.

41 In this context, only the "signs" that are meaningful in connection with illness are listed. There are many more "signs" in other contexts, which are interpreted, for example, as a warning or as heralding an event.

42 Kolandi (1983: 96) very briefly touches upon the topic of the public debate on misdemeanor and its "correction" in his contribution concerning the Kiripia region; Romanucci-Ross (1978: 129), too, mentions it for the Sori (Manus).

43 The SIL bible-translators who work in the Yupno region also chose the term "Senduk" for the concept of "satan," as, for example, in the St. Mark gospel (Mareko) 1.12.

44 For a further interpretation of "explosive reactions," see Burton-Bradley (1989) and Newman (1964). Goddard (1998), presenting an elaborate case study, discusses the social construction of madness among the people of the Upper Kaugel, Western Highlands.

45 The term "technique" is not to be understood in a pejorative sense. Neither should the instrumental character of these acts be over-emphasized. "Technique" here means traditional religious knowledge on the basis of which acts solely of a logical kind can be performed. "Technique" in this sense means also the celebration of a Catholic mass.

46 The mental disturbance of a young man living in Gua was attributed to the fact that, as a boy, he had hurt himself during a *sɨt* act. Beforehand, he was said to have been a capable, bright boy (see Keck 1999: 272–73).

47 At the time of my stay, there were two such men's houses (in Kangulut and Gua), each of which was reserved for one man. Even though an informant from Kangulut openly explained everything about *sɨt* to me, a

visit to his men's house remained impossible despite various approaches made to seek permission.

48   This technique to heat or burn exuviae of the victim is widespread in Papua New Guinea; see the description by Bowden (1987: 187) for the Kwoma; by Schmitz (1959: 39–40) for the Komba. Lindenbaum's (1979: 60–67) description of *imusa* and *kuru* sorcery also emphasizes the stealing of particle intimately associated with the victim, the preparing of bundles with different leaves and so on, and the spells. In the *imusa* method, the bundle is burnt in a tree base; in the *kuru* method, the bundle is placed in the muddy ground, and as it rots, so analogously does the health of the victim deteriorate.

49   The terms "to bind" or "to tie" are found in many descriptions of this "technique"; see Schmitz (1959: 42); Knauft (1985: 96).

50   This *koñ mindak* is a variation of the ritual "chasing away of a ghost" (see Chapter 5.2.e).

51   This version was demonstrated to me explicitly by D. from K. during the night of 5 May 1987, after long preparations, with utmost secrecy and for a fee of 25 Kina. The preparation, hence the "getting into a different state" of the young men, the construction of a special house and the actual burning of the parcels (for reasons of safety empty, i.e. not filled with a *njaapndak* left-overs of a person) as well as all the acts after the performed *sɨt* act (the "cooling-down" of the boys, the "chasing away of the ghosts") were missing.

52   Indeed, Jowage's mishaps are "legend" in Gua. During my stay, he twice fell from a tree when trying to pick passion fruit. The villagers commented on these events with some derision.

53   This "technique" in various, slightly different forms is widespread in Papua New Guinea; for example, Knauft (1985: 104–6) describes it for the Gebusi; Lawrence for the Garia (1987: 26–29); Bowden (1987: 188–89) for the Kwoma; Schmitz (1959: 49) for the Wantoat; Lehner (1935: 34–35) for the Azera and Wampar; Strathern and Stewart (1999: 105–6) for the Wiru; Lewis (1975: 181) for the Gnau; Burridge (1960: 59–71) for the Tangu.

54   Pamela Stewart and Andrew Strathern (personal communication) remark: "it is curious that sangguma is invariably seen by Highlands populations as emanating from Lowland areas" (see Stewart and Strathern 1999), an observation that applies for the Yupno too. According to the inhabitants of Gua, there are specialists who know *mawom* in the villages of Nokopo, Isan and the more distant settlements of Kwembun, Wandaboñ and Windiluk, but it was very difficult to get information on

this subject as I did not have close contact with the people of those villages. After many fruitless attempts and long preparatory talks, Y., the not highly respected but all the more anxious "burner" from Gua, succeeded in winning over his friend D. from Kwembun for a long talk. The following information on the *mawom* technique is mainly based on D.'s statements.

55 This does not apply to the lower Yupno Valley where *mawom* is widespread. There, *mawom* may be performed within a village or within a clan.

56 Only in rare instances is *mawom* also performed by married men, e.g. to show it to the young men, but since they are already somewhat "cooled down" because of their sexual relations the effect decreases.

57 Each clan owns a *sindok kɨrat*, which the men of this *jalap* watch closely. It is never lent to a friendly clan since, in the event that someone falls out with this clan, it may turn against that person's own clan and cause illness (see Chapter 5.3.).

58 The way in which the *mawom* men prepare their body may vary. Some fix leaves of the *mawom* ginger to their body and take along some pieces of bark of the *wuok*, *ngup*, and *njogal* trees, and some carry some hairs from the nose of a good hunting-dog with them so they, like the dogs, can "sniff out" something hidden (the victim).

59 The injured body was repeatedly compared to a decayed house into which rain falls.

60 By "limited" is meant that not all the techniques are subsumed under this term; an exception is the "medium" (*kumbu amɨn*, see below).

61 The principle of the traps: out of branches, bamboo or reed, a rectangular plate is made, weighted with stones and supported by a little stick on one side; this stick is connected to the bait under the plate. If the animal touches the bait, the stick falls over and the animal is squashed (see Schmitz 1960a: 108–9; Schmitz 1960b: 31).

62 Schmitz (1960b: 166) describes an almost identical version of this technique, "real 'material divination,'" for the Wantoat, but without mentioning the central point of this method: the blowing of smoke on the rat with the deceased's *moñan* ("breath spirit"), which thus unmasks the culprit.

63 The specialist prepares some *ɨlok* arrows, which are stuck into a little piece of pandanus skin with a few of the deceased's hairs. At night, they are allocated a particular significance at the cemetery or the burial ground (one "represents" the Kangulut men's house, one the Kewieñ men's house, and so on), where they are lit and shot off. The men watch

closely where they fly. If a house is hit and goes up in flames, either the owner or one of the inhabitants of this house is the culprit.

64 According to Schmitz (1960b: 163), the *tawak amine* of Wantoat Valley showed "clearly the traits of a true shaman." I could only record fragments of the *kumbu amɨn* complex since the last "true" *kumbu amɨn* died some years ago. It thus has to remain open here whether the *kumbu amɨn* among the Yupno had the same skills as the *tawak amine* of the Wantoat, whether he thus has to be assigned to the realm of shamanism as defined by Schmitz or whether—which to me appears to be more likely—he originally came to the Yupno via the Wantoat Valley and was active here in an altered, less elaborate form.

65 The Wantoat call this tree *kombu* (Schmitz 1960b: 146); it is a 'soul-tree'…where the souls of the deceased dwell."

66 Apart from the instigators (the actual culprits), the *kumbu amɨn* is also able to find out the performing specialists whom he himself does not know. I was told of a case where a man from Gua died because of the *mawom* technique, and the *kumbu amɨn* named the village of the *mawom* man, Malalamai, a place on the coast, but not his name since the *mawom* man was a stranger. The deceased's relatives thereupon went to this place on the coast, found out the *mawom* man with the help of the "trap with the red liquid" (*komup pat*, see below) and practiced *sɨt* against him.

67 In Gua, there is a female "medium" who, however, is thought to be the exception. She was married to a famous "burner" and started a big fight with him when he wanted to take a second wife. Her husband beat her and he is said to have tied her to a tree in the bush naked for one night. During this night, the villagers say, the bush-spirit *sindok* had sexual contact with her and since then she has the *kumbu amɨn* skill to interpret dreams and to know things from her own dreams that are hidden to normal people.

68 This dog consists of a bone of the dog skull and a rack of *mbalgerk* (banana bast), a *kulbɨt* leaf, the bamboo *teet* and the moss *ngodan*, which represent a dog's body (with four legs).

69 A somewhat modified method is also practiced by the Wantoat (Schmitz 1960b: 166).

Chapter 7

1 The Oti and Saunu Memorial Church is named after Oti, the first evangelist from Finschhafen, who was sent to convert the Gua people, and

Sauno, an evangelist from Kewieñ, who worked for many years in Gua and was the father of Ginson Saunu.

2 Wuli says in Tok Pisin:

Tingting bilong mi i stap olsem: kantri bilong mipela i go bagarap, na gavman bilong mipela i no save bringim gutpela gutpela sevis o development i kam insait, i no planti tumas. Na planti mipela i save painim hevi long sait bilong mani na olsem skul fee, na sindaun bilong mipela insait bilong pamili haus i no gutpela tumas. Bilong wanem? Rot bilong gavman bilong mipela i senisim kantri bilong mipela na rot bilong mani i go antap moa na mipela yet mipela i nogat save na klia long wanem samting bai mipela kisim. Rot bilong mani bai kam olsem wanem? Na sevim ol pamili o? Na bilong mipela olgeta, olsem haus sik na kiap, wok didiman, wanem kainkain wok, liklik, liklik wok, mipela i no save tumas, na mipela painim hat na nau mipela stap na sindaun bilong mipela i no gutpela na mipela wok long karim planti pikinini na bihaim bai mipela karim hevi long dispela tu. Nau mipela i stap tasol.

References

Ackerknecht, E.H. 1971. *Medicine and Ethnology: Selected Essays*. Bern, Stuttgart, Wien: Hans Huber.

Aitken, I.W. [1984]. Scientific Medicine and Traditional Healing in Papua New Guinea: Pragmatic Perspectives. In W. Jilek (ed.), *Traditional Medicine and Primary Health Care in Papua New Guinea*, pp. 44–50. Port Moresby: WHO and University of Papua New Guinea.

Alcorta, F.X. 1969/70. Upper Nankina Census Division. Saidor Patrol Report No. 10 of 1969/70. Madang District. Unpubl., National Archives, Port Moresby.

Allemann, A. 1989. Praevalenz der Anaemie, des Blutverlustes im Stuhl und des Hakenwurmbefalls bei Kindern und Erwachsenen der Yupna bevoelkerung: Gesundheits-Survey bei den Yupna im Rahmen eines Projekts zur ethnographisch-kognitiven Erforschung der Yupna in Papua New Guinea. Unpubl. Dissertation, Medical Faculty of the University of Basel.

Allemann A., Bauerfeind P., and Gyr N. (1994). Prevalence of Hookworm Infection, Anaemia and Faecal Blood Loss among the Yupno People of Papua New Guinea. *Papua New Guinea Medical Journal* 37: 15–22.

Barker, J. 1989. Western Medicine and the Continuity of Belief: The Maisin of Collingwood Bay, Oro Province. In St. Frankel and G. Lewis (eds.), *A Continuing Trial of Treatment: Medical Pluralism in Papua New Guinea*, pp. 69–93. Dordrecht, Boston, London: Kluwer Academic Publishers.

Bell, C.O. (ed.) 1973. *The Diseases and Health Services of Papua New Guinea. A Basis for National Health Planning*. Port Moresby: Department of Public Health.

Boster, J.S. 1985. "Requiem for the Omniscient Informant": There's Life in the Old Girl Yet. In J.W.D. Dougherty (ed.), *Directions in Cognitive Anthropology*, pp. 177–97. Urbana and Chicago: University of Illinois Press.

Bowden, R. 1987. Sorcery, Illness and Social Control in Kwoma Society. In M. Stephen (ed.), *Sorcerer and Witch in Melanesia*, pp. 183–208. Melbourne: Melbourne University Press.

Brandewie, E. 1973. Serious Illness and Group Therapy among the Mbowamb, Central Highlands of New Guinea. *Mankind* 9: 71–76.

Brown, P.J. (ed.) 1998. *Understanding and Applying Medical Anthropology*. Mountain View, Cal., London, Toronto: Mayfield Publishing Company.

Brown, P.J., and Inhorn, M.C. 1990. Disease, Ecology, and Human Behavior. In T.M. Johnson and C. Sargent (eds.), *Medical Anthropology: A Handbook of Theory and Method*, pp. 187–214. New York, Westport, London: Greenwood Press.

Burridge, K. 1960. *Mambu. A Melanesian Millenium*. London: Methuen and Co.

Burton-Bradley, B.G. 1989. Das Amok-Syndrom in Papua und Neu Guinea. *Curare* 12: 177–82.

Chrisman, N.J., and Johnson, T.M. 1990. Clinically Applied Anthropology. In T.M. Johnson and C. Sargent (eds.), *Medical Anthropology: A Handbook of Theory and Method*, pp. 93–111. New York, Westport, London: Greenwood Press.

Colson, A.C., and Selby, K.E. 1974. Medical Anthropology. *Annual Review of Anthropology* 3: 245–63.

Counts, D.R., and Counts, D.A. 1989. Complementarity in Medical Treatment in a West New Britain Society. In St. Frankel and G. Lewis (eds.), *A Continuing Trial of Treatment: Medical Pluralism in Papua New Guinea*, pp. 277–94. Dordrecht, Boston, London: Kluwer Academic Publishers.

D'Andrade, R.G. 1976. A Propositional Analysis of U.S. American Beliefs about Illness. In K. Basso and H. Selby (eds.), *Meaning in Anthropology*, pp. 155–80. Albuquerque: University of New Mexico Press.

Dalton, D. 2002. Spirit, Self, and Power: the Making of Colonial Experience in Papua New Guinea. In J. Mageo (ed.), *Power and the Self*, pp. 117–40. Cambridge: Cambridge University Press.

Davies, M. 2002. *Public Health and Colonialism: the Case of German New Guinea 1884–1914*. Wiesbaden: Harrassowitz.

Denoon, D. 1989. *Public Health in Papua New Guinea: Medical Possibility and Social Constraint, 1884–1984*. Cambridge: Cambridge University Press.

Dyer, K.W. 1955/56. Report of a Patrol to the Upper Nankina Census Division, Saidor Sub-District, Madang District. Saidor Patrol Report No. 6 of 1955/56, Madang District, Saidor Sub-District. Unpubl., National Archives, Port Moresby.

Eisenberg, L. 1977. Disease and Illness: Distinctions between Professional and Popular Ideas of Sickness. *Culture, Medicine and Psychiatry* 1: 9–23.

Fabrega, H. 1971. Medical Anthropology. *Biennial Review of Anthropology*, pp. 167–229.

Fajans, J. 1985. The Person in Social Context. The Social Character of Bain-ing Psychology. In G. White and J. Kirkpatrick (eds.), *Person, Self, and Experience: Exploring Pacific Ethnopsychologies*, pp. 367–400. Berkeley, Los Angeles, London: University of California Press.

— 1997. *They Make Themselves: Work and Play among the Baining of Papua New Guinea*. Chicago: University of Chicago Press.

Feinberg, R. 1990. Spiritual and Natural Etiologies on a Polynesian Outlier in Papua New Guinea. *Social Science and Medicine* 30: 311–23.

Fischer, H. 1965. *Studien über Seelenvorstellungen in Ozeanien*. München: Klaus Renner.

Foster, G.M., and Anderson, B. 1978. *Medical Anthropology*. New York, Bris-bane, Toronto: John Wiley and Sons.

Frake, C. 1961. The Diagnosis of Disease among the Subanun of Mindanao. *American Anthropologist* 63: 113–32.

— 1962. The Ethnographic Study of Cognitive Systems. In T. Gladwin and G. Sturtevant (eds.), *Anthropology and Human Behaviour*, pp. 72–85. Washington, D.C.: Anthropological Society of Washington.

Frankel, St. 1986. *The Huli Response to Illness*. Cambridge: Cambridge Uni-versity Press.

Frankel, St., and Lewis, G. (eds.) 1989a. *A Continuing Trial of Treatment: Med-ical Pluralism in Papua New Guinea*. Dordrecht, Boston, London: Kluwer Academic Publishers.

— 1989b. Patterns of Continuity and Change. In St. Frankel and G. Lewis (eds.), *A Continuing Trial of Treatment: Medical Pluralism in Papua New Guinea*, pp. 1–33. Dordrecht, Boston, London: Kluwer Academic Publishers.

Garner, P.A. 1989. Voluntary Village Health Workers in Papua New Guinea. *Papua New Guinea Medical Journal* 32: 55–60.

Gatewood, J.B. 1985. Actions Speak Louder than Words. In J.W.D. Dougherty (ed.), *Directions in Cognitive Anthropology*, pp. 199–219. Urbana and Chicago: University of Illinois Press.

Glick, L.B. 1963. Foundations of a Primitive Medical System: the Gimi of the New Guinea Highlands. Unpubl. Ph.D. Dissertation, University of Pennsylvania.

— 1967. Medicine as an Ethnographic Category. *Ethnology* 6: 31–56.

— 1973. Sorcery and Witchcraft. In J. Hogbin (ed.), *Anthropology in Papua New Guinea, Readings from the Encyclopaedia of Papua and New Guinea*, pp. 182–86. Carlton: Melbourne University Press.

Goddard, M. 1998. What Makes Hari Run? The Social Construction of Mad-ness in a Highland Papua New Guinea Society. *Critique of Anthropology* 18(1): 61–81.

Good, B.J. 1994. *Medicine, Rationality, and Experience. An Anthropological Perspective.* Cambridge: Cambridge University Press.

Goodenough, W. 1957. Cultural Anthropology and Linguistics. In P.L. Garvin (ed.), *Report of the Seventh Annual Round Table Meeting on Linguistics and Language Studies,* pp. 167–73. Washington, D.C.: Georgetown University. (Monograph Series on Language and Linguistics no. 9).

Hahn, R., and Gaines, A.D. (eds.) 1985. *Physicians of Western Medicine. Anthropological Approaches to Theory and Practice.* Dordrecht: Reidel.

Haiveta, C. 1990. Health Care Alternatives in Maindroin. In N. Lutkehaus et al. (eds.), *Sepik Heritage: Tradition and Change in Papua New Guinea,* pp. 439–46. Durham: Carolina Academic Press.

Hanrahan, K.J. 1955/56. Uruwa/Yupna Divisions. Wasu Patrol Report No. 3 of 1955/56. Morobe District. Unpubl., National Archives, Port Moresby.

Helman, C.G. 1994³. *Culture, Health and Illness: an Introduction for Health Professionals.* Oxford: Butterworth-Heinemann. (1984¹).

Heywood, P. 1982. The Functional Significance of Malnutrition. *Journal of Food and Nutrition* 39: 13–18.

Hill, L. [1984]. Prelimimary Bibliography on the Traditional Medicinal Plants of Papua New Guinea. In W. Jilek (ed.), *Traditional Medicine and Primary Health Care in Papua New Guinea,* pp. 134–44. Port Moresby: WHO and University of Papua New Guinea.

Holdsworth, D. 1977. *Medicinal Plants of Papua New Guinea.* Noumea: South Pacific Commission. (South Pacific Commission Technical Paper No. 175).

— [1984]. Plants Used in Traditional Medicine in Papua New Guinea. In W. Jilek (ed.), *Traditional Medicine and Primary Health Care in Papua New Guinea,* pp. 63–67. Port Moresby: WHO and University of Papua New Guinea.

Holland, D., and Quinn, N. 1987. Culture and Cognition. In D. Holland and N. Quinn (eds.), *Cultural Models in Language and Thought,* pp. 3–40. Cambridge: Cambridge University Press.

Hughes, C. 1968. Ethnomedicine. In D.E. Sills (ed.), *International Encyclopedia of the Social Sciences,* pp. 87–93, vol. 10. New York: The Macmillan Company and the Free Press.

Janzen, J.M. 1978. *The Quest of Therapy: Medical Pluralism in Lower Zaire.* Berkeley, Los Angeles, London: University of California Press. (Comparative Studies in Health Systems and Medical Care 1).

Jenkins, C. 1984. The Role of Traditional Medical Practice in Papua New Guinea. *Papua New Guinea Medical Journal* 27: 121–22.

Jilek, W. (ed.). [1984]. *Traditional Medicine and Primary Health Care in Papua New Guinea*. Port Moresby: WHO and University of Papua New Guinea.

Johannes, A. 1976. Illness and Medical Care in a New Guinea Highland Society. Unpubl. Ph.D. Dissertation, Northwestern University.

—1980. Many Medicines in One: Curing in the Eastern Highlands of Papua New Guinea. *Culture, Medicine and Psychiatry* 4: 43–70.

Jones, B.A. 1980. Consuming Society: Food and Illness among the Faiwol. Unpubl. Ph.D. Dissertation, University of Virginia.

Kaiser, M., and Kaiser, H. [1986]. *Daunim Sik Long Ples*. Neuendettelsau: Freimund.

Keck, V. 1992. *Falsch gehandelt—schwer erkrankt. Kranksein bei den Yupno in Papua New Guinea aus ethnologischer und biomedizinischer Sicht*. Basel: Wepf. (Basler Beitraege zur Ethnologie 35).

— 1993a. Two Ways of Explaining Reality: the Sickness of a Small Boy of Papua New Guinea from Anthropological and Biomedical Perspectives. *Oceania* 63 (4): 294–312.

— 1993b. Talks about a Changing World: Young Yupno Men in Papua New Guinea Debate Their Future. *Canberra Anthropology* 16 (2):67–96.

— 1994. "Belastende Probleme" und "heisse Gefühle": ein ethno-logisches Erklärungsmodell der Yupno zu Kranksein. *Ethnologica Helvetica* 17/18: 359–79.

— 1999. Colder than Cool: Disability and Personhood Among the Yupno in Papua New Guinea. *Anthropology and Medicine* 6(2): 261–83.

Keesing, R.M. 1985. Conventional Metaphors and Anthropological Metaphysics: the Problematic of Cultural Translation. *Journal of Anthropological Research* 41: 201–17.

— 1989. Anthropology in Oceania: Problems and Prospects. *Oceania* 60: 55–59.

Kleinman, A. 1978. Concepts and a Model for the Comparison of Medical Systems as Cultural Systems. *Social Science and Medicine* 12:85–93.

— 1980. *Patients and Healers in the Context of Culture: an Exploration of the Borderland between Anthropology, Medicine and Psychiatry*. Berkeley, Los Angeles, London: California University Press.

— 1986. *Social Origins of Distress and Disease*. New Haven and London: Yale University Press.

Klemm, H.D. 1957. Tapen Annual Report 1957. Unpubl., Archives of the Evangelical-Lutheran Church in Bavaria, Neuendettelsau.

Knauft, B.M. 1985. *Good Company and Violence: Sorcery and Social Action in a Lowland New Guinea Society*. Berkeley, Los Angeles, London: University of California Press. (Studies in Melanesian Anthropology).

Kocher Schmid, Ch. 1991. *Of People and Plants. A Botanical Ethnography of Nokopo Village, Madang and Morobe Provinces, Papua New Guinea*. Basel: Wepf. (Basler Beitraege zur Ethnologie 33).

— 1993. Cultural Identity as a Coping Strategy towards Modern Political Structures: the Nayudos Case, Papua New Guinea. *Bijdragen tot de Taal-, Land- en Volkenkunde* 149: 781–801.

Kolandi, M. 1983. The Traditional Treatment of Illness in the Kiripia Area. In N.C. Habel (ed.), *Powers, Plumes and Piglets: Phenomena of Melanesian Religion*, pp. 91–96. Bedford Park: Australian Association for the Study of Religions. (1979[1]).

Landy, D. 1977. Introduction. Learning and Teaching Medical Anthropology. In D. Landy (ed.), *Culture, Disease and Healing: Studies in Medical Anthropology*, pp. 1–9. New York, London: Collier MacMillan.

Lawrence, P. 1987. De Rerum Natura: the Garia View of Sorcery. In M. Stephen (ed.), *Sorcerer and Witch in Melanesia*, pp. 17–40. Melbourne: Melbourne University Press.

Lehner, S. 1935. Die Vorstellung vom Todeszauber (Opa, Ofang, Silam, Selam oder Bumbum) unter den Eingeborenen Neu-Guineas. *Mitteilungsblatt der Deutschen Gesellschaft fuer Voelkerkunde* 6: 32–43.

Lepowsky, M. 1990. Sorcery and Penicillin: Treating Illness on a Papua New Guinea Island. *Social Science and Medicine* 30: 1049–63.

Leslie, C. 1976. The Ambiguities of Medical Revivalism in Modern India. In C. Leslie (ed.), *Asian Medical Systems*, pp. 356–67. Berkeley, Los Angeles, London: University of California Press.

— 1980. Medical Pluralism in World Perspective. *Social Science and Medicine* (Special Issue 14 B), pp. 191–95.

Lewis, G. 1975. *Knowledge of Illness in a Sepik Society. A Study of the Gnau, New Guinea*. London: Athlone Press. (London School of Economics, Monographs on Social Anthropology 52).

— 2000. *A Failure of Treatment*. Oxford: Oxford University Press.

Lieban, R.W. 1973. Medical Anthropology. In J.J. Honigmann (ed.), *Handbook of Social and Cultural Anthropology*, pp. 1031–72. Chicago: Rand McNally.

Lindenbaum, S. 1979. *Kuru Sorcery: Disease and Danger in the New Guinea Highlands*. Palo Alto: Mayfield.

Lindenbaum, S., and Lock, M. (eds.) 1993. *Knowledge, Power, and Practice. The Anthropology of Medicine and Everyday Life*. Berkeley, Los Angeles, London: University of California Press.

Linnekin, J., and Poyer, L. (eds.) 1990. *Cultural Identity and Ethnicity in the Pacific*. Honolulu: University of Hawai'i Press.

LiPuma, E. 1989. Modernity and Medicine among the Maring. In St. Frankel and G. Lewis (eds.), *A Continuing Trial of Treatment: Medical Pluralism in Papua New Guinea*, pp. 295–310. Dordrecht, Boston, London: Kluwer Academic Publishers.

Lock, M., and Gordon, D. 1988. *Biomedicine Examined*. Dordrecht, Boston, London: Kluwer Academic Publishers.

Mannheim, K. 1982. *Structures of Thinking*. London: Routledge.

McElroy, A., and Townsend, P.K. 1979. *Medical Anthropology in Ecological Perspective*. North Scituate: Duxberry Press.

Morris, B. 1994. *Anthropology of the Self. The Individual in Cultural Perspective*. London, Boulder, Colorado: Pluto Press.

Morrison, R.P. 1969/70. Yupna Census Division. Wasu Patrol Report No. 5 of 1969/70. Morobe District, Kabwum Sub-District, Wasu Patrol Post. Unpubl., National Archives, Port Moresby.

Munsel, K. 1952. Tapen Annual Report 1952. Unpubl., Archives of the Evangelical-Lutheran Church in Bavaria, Neuendettelsau.

Muskens, W.H. 1959. Report of a Patrol to the Upper Nankina Tax District, Saidor Sub-District, Madang District. Saidor Patrol Report No. 7 of 1958/59, Saidor Sub-District, Madang District. Unpubl., National Archives, Port Moresby.

Neal, M.V. 1954/55. Upper Nankina Census Sub-Division. Saidor Patrol Report No. 6 of 1954/55, Madang District, Saidor Sub-District. Unpubl., National Archives, Port Moresby.

Nelson, H.E. 1971. The Ecological, Epistomological and Ethnographic Context of Medicine in a New Guinea Highlands Culture. Unpubl. Ph.D. Dissertation, University of Washington.

Newman, P.L. 1964. "Wild Man" Behaviour in a New Guinea Highlands Community. *American Anthropologist* 66: 1–19.

Nichter, M. 1991. Ethnomedicine: Diverse Trends, Common Linkages. Commentary. *Medical Anthropology* (Special Issue: Recent Trends in Ethnomedicine) 13: 137–71.

Niles, D. 1987. Tupela boda ples i no vot. *Wantok*, namba 979, 2 Julai - 9 Julai, 1987.

— 1992. Konggap, Kap and Tambaran: Music of the Yupno/Nankina Area in Relation to Neighbouring Groups. In J. Wassmann (ed.), *Abschied von der Vergangenheit: Ethnologische Berichte aus dem Finisterre-Gebirge, Papua New Guinea*, pp. 149–83. Berlin: Reimer.

Nixon, T.R. 1965/66. Upper Nankina Census Division. Saidor Patrol Report No. 3 of 1965/66. District of Saidor-Madang. Unpubl., National Archives, Port Moresby.

Obrist van Eeuwijk, B. 1992. *Small but Strong: Cultural Contexts of (Mal-) nutrition among the Northern Kwanga (East Sepik Province, Papua New Guinea)*. Basel: Wepf. (Basler Beitraege zur Ethnologie 34).

Panoff, F. 1970. Maenge Remedies and Conception of Disease. *Ethnology* 9: 68–84.

Pataki-Schweizer, K.J. 1985. Traditional Medicine: Institutional Perceptions and Cultural Realities. *Papua New Guinea Medical Journal* 23: 211–16.

Patterson, M. 1974/75. Sorcery and Witchcraft in Melanesia. *Oceania* 45: 132–60, 212–34.

Rhodes, L.A. 1990. Studying Biomedicine as Cultural System. In T.M. Johnson and C. Sargent, *Medical Anthropology: A Handbook of Theory and Method*, pp. 159–73. New York, Westport, London: Greenwood Press.

Rivers, W.H.R. 1924. *Medicine, Magic and Religion*. London: Kegan Paul.

Robins, B.G. 1961/62. Upper Nankina Census Division. Saidor Patrol Report No. 2 of 1961/62, Madang District, Saidor Sub-District. Unpubl., National Archives, Port Moresby.

Romanucci-Ross, L. 1978. Melanesian Medicine: Beyond Culture to Method. In P. Morley and R. Wallis (eds.), *Culture and Curing: Anthropological Perspectives on Traditional Medical Beliefs and Practices*, pp. 115–38. London: Peter Owen.

Romanucci-Ross, L., Moerman, D.E., and Tancredi, L.R. (eds.) 1983. *The Anthropology of Medicine: from Culture toward Method*. New York: Praeger.

Romanucci Schwartz, L. 1969. The Hierarchy of Resort in Curative Practices: The Admirality Islands, Melanesia. *Journal of Health and Social Behavior* 10(3): 201–9.

Rosch, E., and Mervis, C.B. 1975. Family Resemblances: Studies in the Internal Structure of Categories. *Cognitive Psychology* 7: 573–605.

Rubel, A.J., and Hass, M.R. 1990. Ethnomedicine. In T.M. Johnson and C. Sargent (eds.), *Medical Anthropology: A Handbook of Theory and Method*, pp. 115–31. New York, Westport, London: Greenwood Press.

Rylands, M.W.S. 1945. Patrol Report: Uruwa and Huon Portion of Yupna Areas. Sub District Office ANGAU, Finschhafen, 7. May 1945. Unpubl., National Archives, Port Moresby.

Sailoia, P.S. 1976/77. Yupna. Patrol Report No. 3 of 1976/77. Madang District, Saidor Sub-District, Teptep Station. Unpubl., Rai Coast District 1976–1978 Volume, Department for Provincial Affairs, Madang.

Sargent, C.F., and Johnson, T. (eds.) 1996. *Medical Anthropology: Contemporary Theory and Method*. Westport, Connecticut: Praeger.

Scaletta, N.M. 1985. Death by Sorcery: the Social Dynamics of Dying in Bariai, West New Britain. In D.A. Counts and D.R. Counts (eds.),

Aging and Its Transformations. Moving Towards Death in Pacific Societies, pp. 223–47. Pittsburgh and London: University of Pittsburgh Press.

Scarlett, G. 1967/68. Uruwa, Yupna and West Sio Census Divisions. Saidor Patrol Report No. 3–4 of 1967/68. Morobe District. Unpubl., National Archives, Port Moresby.

Scheper-Hughes, N., and Lock, M. 1987. The Mindful Body: a Prolegomenon to Future Work in Medical Anthropology. *Medical Anthropology Quarterly* (New Series) 1: 6–41.

Schieffelin, E.L. 1985. Anger, Grief and Shame: Toward a Kaluli Ethnopsychology. In G.M. White and J. Kirkpatrick (eds.), *Person, Self and Experience: Exploring Pacific Ethnopsychologies*, pp. 168–82. Berkeley, Los Angeles, London: University of California Press.

Schmitz, C.A. 1958. Zur Ethnographie des Jupna-Tales im Nordosten von Neuguinea. *Acta Ethnographica* 7: 337–86.

— 1959. Todeszauber in Nordost Neuguinea. *Paideuma* 7: 35–67.

— 1960a. *Historische Probleme in Nordost-Neuguinea. Huon Halbinsel.* Wiesbaden: Franz Steiner. (Studien zur Kulturkunde 16).

— 1960b. *Beitraege zur Ethnographie des Wantoat-Tales, Nordost Neuguinea.* Koeln: Koelner Universitaets-Verlag. (Koelner Ethnologische Mitteilungen 1).

Shweder, R.A. 1988. Suffering in Style. *Culture, Medicine and Psychiatry* 12: 479–97.

Shweder, R.A., and Bourne, E.J. 1984. Does the Concept of the Person Vary Cross-culturally? In R.A. Shweder and R.A. LeVine (eds.), *Cultural Theory. Essays on Mind, Self, Emotion*, pp. 158–99. Cambridge: Cambridge University Press.

Simmins, D.R. 1962/63. Warup and Upper Nankina Census Division. Saidor Patrol Report No. 1–2 of 1962/32, Madang District, Saidor Sub-District. Unpubl., National Archives, Port Moresby.

Sinclair, R. 1987/88. Anthropological Understandings of the Relationship Between Traditional and Western Medicine in Papua New Guinea. *Research in Melanesia* 11/12: 40–65.

Singer, M. 1989. The Coming of Age of Critical Medical Anthropology. *Social Science and Medicine* 28: 1193–203.

— 1990. Reinventing Medical Anthropology: Toward a Critical Realignment. *Social Science and Medicine* 30: 179–87.

Smith, M.F. 2002. *Village on the Edge. Changing Times in Papua New Guinea.* Honolulu: University of Hawai'i Press.

Somers, P.J. 1968/69. Upper Nankina Census Division. Part of Warup Census Division. Saidor Patrol Report No. 5 of 1968/69. Madang District, Saidor Sub-District. Unpubl., National Archives, Port Moresby.

Staub, S. 1993. Nutritional Survey bei Kindern von 0 bis 10 Jahren (Yupno, Papua New Guinea). Unpubl. Dissertation, Medical Faculty of the University of Basel.

Stephen, M. (eds.) 1987. *Sorcerer and Witch in Melanesia*. Melbourne: Melbourne University Press.

Steven, A.D. 1952/53a. Upper Yupna and Upper Nankina. Saidor Patrol Report No. 1 of 1952/53. Madang District, Saidor Sub-District. Unpubl., National Archives, Port Moresby.

— 1952/53b. Nankina—Warup, Warup—Yupna and Upper Nankina. Saidor Patrol Report No. 5 of 1952/53, Madang District, Saidor Sub-District. Unpubl., National Archives, Port Moresby.

— 1953/54. Upper Nankina, Warup Yupna, Upper Yupna. Saidor Patrol Report No. 3 of 1953/54, Madang District, Saidor Sub-District. Unpubl., National Archives, Port Moresby.

Stewart, P.J., and Strathern, A. 2000. Introduction: Narratives Speak. In P.J. Stewart and A. Strathern (eds.), *Identity Work: Constructing Pacific Lives*, pp. 1–26. Pittsburgh: University of Pittsburgh Press.

— 1999. Feasting on My Enemy: Images of Violence and Change in the New Guinea Highlands. *Ethnohistory* 46(4): 645–69.

— 2001. Mind Substance. In P.J. Stewart and A. Strathern, *Humors and Substances. Ideas of the Body in New Guinea*, pp. 113–37. Westport, Connecticut, and London: Bergin and Garvey.

Strathern, A.J. 1968. Sickness and Frustration: Variations in two New Guinea Highlands Societies. *Mankind* 6: 545–51.

— [1984]. Digging out Causes—Relations Between Introduced Health Care and Traditional Medicine. In W. Jilek (ed.), *Traditional Medicine and Primary Health Care in Papua New Guinea*, pp. 26–31. Port Moresby: WHO and University of Papua New Guinea.

— 1989a. Health Care and Medical Pluralism: Cases from Mount Hagen. In St. Frankel and G. Lewis (eds.), *A Continuing Trial of Treatment: Medical Pluralism in Papua New Guinea*, pp. 115–39. Dordrecht, Boston, London: Kluwer Academic Publishers.

— 1989b. Melpa Dream Interpretation and the Concept of the Hidden Truth. *Ethnology* 24: 245–60.

— 1994. Keeping the Body in Mind. *Social Anthropology* 2(1): 43–53.

— 1996. *Body Thoughts*. Ann Arbor: The University of Michigan Press.

Strathern, A., and Stewart, P.J. 1998. Seeking Personhood: Anthropological Accounts and Local Concepts in Mount Hagen, Papua New Guinea. *Oceania* 68 (3): 170–88.

— 1999. *Curing and Healing. Medical Anthropology in Global Perspective.* Durham: Carolina Academic Press.

Strathern, M. 1968. Popokl: The Question of Morality. *Mankind* 6: 553–62.

— 1988. *The Gender of the Gift. Problems with Women and Problems with Society in Melanesia.* Berkeley: University of California Press.

Taussig, M. 1980. Reification and the Consciousness of the Patient. *Social Science and Medicine* (Special Issue B) 14: 3–14.

Terrain Handbook 14. 1943. Allied Geographical Section, South West Pacific Area, Terrain Handbook 14, New Guinea, Saidor.

Vial, L.G. 1938. Extract from Report of Patrol Officer L.G. Vial, Who, Accompagnied by Six Native Police, Carried out a Patrol on the Interior of the Huon Peninsula, Morobe District, from 27th July, to 26th October, 1936. Report to the Council of the League of Nations on the Administration of the Territory of New Guinea from 1st July, 1936, to 30th June, 1937, pp. 141–46, App. B. Canberra.

Wassmann, J. 1991. *The Song to the Flying Fox. The Public and Esoteric Knowledge of the Important Men of Kandingei about Totemic Songs, Names, and Knotted Cords (Middle Sepik, Papua New Guinea).* Port Moresby: Institute of Papua New Guinea Studies. (Apwitihire 2)

— 1992. "First Contact". Begegnungen im Yupnotal. In J. Wassmann (ed.), *Abschied von der Vergangenheit. Ethnographische Berichte aus dem Finisterre-Gebirge in Papua New Guinea,* pp. 209–60. Berlin: Reimer.

— 1993a. *Das Ideal des leicht gebeugten Menschen: eine ethno-kognitive Analyse der Yupno in Papua New Guinea.* Berlin: Reimer.

— 1993b. The Yupno as Post-Newtonian Scientists. The Question of What is Natural in Spatial Descriptions. *Man* 29(3): 645–66.

— 1993c. When Actions Speak Louder than Words. The Classification of Food among the Yupno of Papua New Guinea. *The Quarterly Newsletter of the Laboratory of Comparative Human Cognition* 15(1): 30–40.

— 1994. Worlds in Mind. The Experience of an Outside World in a Community of the Finisterre Range of Papua New Guinea. *Oceania* 64(2): 117–45.

— 1997. Finding the Right Path: the Route Knowledge of the Yupno of Papua New Guinea. In G. Senft (ed.), *Referring to Space. Studies in Austronesian and Papuan Languages,* pp. 143–74. Oxford: Clarendon.

— 1998. The Music of the Yupno. In A. Kaeppler and J. Love (eds.), *Encyclopedia of World Music, Oceania,* pp. 303–4. Washington DC: Garland Publishing.

Wassmann, J. and Dasen P.R. 1994a. Yupno Number System and Counting. *International Journal of Cross-Cultural Psychology* 25(2): 78–94.

— 1994b. Hot and Cold: Classification and Sorting Among the Yupno of Papua New Guinea. *International Journal of Psychology* 29(2): 19–38.

Wellin, E. 1977. Theoretical Orientations in Medical Anthropology: Continuity and Change over the Past Half-Century. In D. Landy (ed.), *Culture, Disease and Healing: Studies in Medical Anthropology*, pp. 47–58. New York, London: Collier Macmillan.

Welsch, R.L. 1982. The Experience of Illness among the Ningerum of Papua New Guinea. Unpubl. Ph.D. Dissertation, University of Washington.

— 1983. Traditional Medicine and Western Medical Options Among the Ningerum of Papua New Guinea. In L. Romanucci-Ross, D.E. Moerman and L.R. Tancredi (eds.), *The Anthropology of Medicine: from Culture toward Method*, pp. 32–53. New York: Praeger.

— 1986. Primary Health Care and Local Self Determination: Policy Implications from Rural Papua New Guinea. *Human Organization* 45: 103–12.

— 1987. The Distribution of Therapeutic Knowledge in Ningerum: Implications for Primary Health Care and the Use of Aid Posts. *Papua New Guinea Medical Journal* 28: 205–10.

Werner, D. 1983. *Where There is no Doctor: a Village Health Care Handbook.* London and Basingstoke: MacMillan Press. (1977[1]).

White, G.M., and Kirkpatrick, J. (eds.) 1985. *Person, Self and Experience: Exploring Pacific Ethnopsychologies.* Berkeley, Los Angeles, London: University of California Press.

WHO. 1978. *Primary Health Care. A Joint Report by the Director-General of the World Health Organization and the Executive Director of the United Nations Children's Fund. International Conference on Primary Health Care, Alma-Ata, USSR, 6–12 September 1978.* Genf, New York: World Health Organization.

Woodley, E. (ed.) 1991. *Medicinal Plants of Papua New Guinea. Part 1: Morobe Province.* Weikersheim: Josef Margraf. (Wau Ecology Institute Handbook 11).

Wright, P., and Treacher, A. (eds.) 1982. *The Problem of Medical Knowledge: Examining the Social Construction of Medicine.* Edinburgh: Edinburgh University Press.

Wurm, St.A., and Hattori, S. (eds.) 1981. *Language Atlas of the Pacific Area.* Canberra: Australian Academy of Humanities. (Pacific Linguistics C 66).

Young, A. 1982. The Anthropologies of Illness and Sickness. *Annual Review of Anthropology* 11: 257–85.

— 1983. The Relevance of Traditional Medical Cultures to Modern Primary Health Care. *Social Science and Medicine* 17: 1205–11.

Young, M. 1989. Illness and Ideology: Aspects of Health Care on Goodenough Island. In St. Frankel and G. Lewis (eds.), *A Continuing Trial of Treatment: Medical Pluralism in Papua New Guinea*, pp. 115–39. Dordrecht, Boston, London: Kluwer Academic Publishers.

Index